EMOTIONS IN HISTORY

General Editors

UTE PREVERT   THOMAS DIXON

The History of Cancer and Emotions in Twentieth-Century Germany

BETTINA HITZER

Translated by

ADAM BRESNAHAN

OXFORD
UNIVERSITY PRESS

OXFORD
UNIVERSITY PRESS

Great Clarendon Street, Oxford, OX2 6DP,
United Kingdom

Oxford University Press is a department of the University of Oxford.
It furthers the University's objective of excellence in research, scholarship,
and education by publishing worldwide. Oxford is a registered trade mark of
Oxford University Press in the UK and in certain other countries

First Edition published in 2022

Impression: 1

Published in the United States of America by Oxford University Press
198 Madison Avenue, New York, NY 10016, United States of America

British Library Cataloguing in Publication Data
Data available

Library of Congress Control Number: 2022930147

ISBN 978–0–19–286807–7

Printed and bound by
CPI Group (UK) Ltd, Croydon, CR0 4YY

To Christoph, Felix, Carlotta, and Henrietta

Contents

Acknowledgements

The topic of this book was at the centre of my thinking for many years. Sometimes it confronted me with seemingly intractable problems and at other times it pushed me to my limits—yet still it would not let go of its hold on me. I am incredibly grateful that I was able to write this book, because it allowed me to grapple intensively with questions that continue to occupy me. The process of writing gave me an opportunity to understand existentially important issues and situate them in their historical context.

Many people supported me along this path. I was very lucky that others made this project their own, helped me with questions, gave me tips, assisted with things small and large, and pushed me forward with their openness to talk, despite some initial doubts as to whether this historiographical undertaking could be realized at all.

Being able to plunge the depths of this topic over the years and conduct research in countless archives would likely have been impossible at anywhere but the place where I had the great fortune to work: the Center for the History of Emotions at the Max Planck Institute for Human Development in Berlin. I owe a profound debt of gratitude to Ute Frevert, who established the research centre in 2008 and has served as its director ever since. The intellectual community that she has assembled there provided one of the most intellectually stimulating experiences of my life as a historian. I would thus like to thank everyone who worked and researched there for periods long and short. I want to give special thanks to Monique Scheer, Gian Marco Vidor, Rob Boddice, Juliane Brauer, Pascal Eitler, Fanny Hernández Brotons, Philipp Nielsen, Susanne Michl, Soňa Mikulová, Stephanie Olsen, Kerstin Maria Pahl, Joachim C. Häberlen, and Christa Hämmerle. I received generous assistance and invaluable support from Karola Rockmann, Christina Becher (†), Anja Berkes, Adam Bresnahan, Philipp von Hugo, Kerstin Singer, Ursula Flitner, Daniela Regel, and Erna Schiwietz. I received enthusiastic, resourceful help in research and many practical matters from Marie Schubenz, Franziska Naumann, Monja Schünemann, Jonas Feldt, Flavia Citrigno, Yanara Schmacks, Sophia Gröschel, and Anne Rinke.

This kind of research project ripens through engagement with the questions and perspectives of others. I am thus grateful that I had the opportunity to discuss my work at colloquia and conferences at many places, including the Institute for the History of Medicine of the Robert Bosch Foundation in Stuttgart (Martin Dinges, Robert Jütte), the Research Colloquia on Modern History at the Heinrich Heine University Düsseldorf (Christoph Nonn, Achim Landwehr), the University of Göttingen (Petra Terhoeven, Dirk Schumann), the Technische Universität

Dresden (Dagmar Ellerbrock), the Freie Universität Berlin (Paul Nolte), the colloquium on nineteenth-century European history at the Humboldt Universität zu Berlin (Birgit Aschmann), the Institute for Ethics, History, and the Humanities in Geneva (Samia Hurst), and the colloquium of the Centre for Contemporary History (ZZF) in Potsdam (Frank Bösch, Martin Sabrow). I gained important insights in discussions with Frank Biess (San Diego), Otniel E. Dror (Jerusalem), Helena Flam (Leipzig), Michael Geyer (Leipzig), Volker Hess (Berlin), Leonhard Horowski (Berlin), Gabriele Moser (Heidelberg), Piroska Nagy (Montréal), and Anne Kwaschik (Konstanz) as well as, during my habilitation, from Paul Nolte and Uwe Puschner (both in Berlin) and Andreas Wirsching (Munich).

Every work of historical research relies on archives. During my visits to archives, I often made surprising finds because the archivists lit the path to where something might be located. I thus want to thank the workers at all the archives that I visited, and, in particular, Sabrina Zinke (Heidelberg University Archives) and Susanne Roeßiger (German Hygiene Museum Dresden). I would also like to thank Roland Jacob (Berlin) and Stephan Tanneberger (†), who, in extended discussions, told me about their work as a radiologist and chemotherapist, respectively, at the Berlin Buch Hospital, and Katharina Baltrusch (Hamburg), who generously gave me access to documents from the estate of her father Hans-Joachim Baltrusch.

Barbara Wenner helped turn the manuscript into a book. She intuitively understood what I wanted to accomplish with the book and tirelessly looked for a German publisher that would be receptive to it. Thank you! I would also like to thank Thomas Dixon and Ute Frevert, the editors of the Emotions in History series at Oxford University Press, as well as the anonymous reviewers, who made it possible for this book to be published in English.

During my research and writing, a few colleagues became my intellectual companions, reading the manuscript in part or in whole and helping me with their critical comments. I would like to thank Benno Gammerl, Alexa Geisthövel, Uffa Jensen, Anja Laukötter, Margrit Pernau, Jan Plamper, and Anne Schmidt.

I was not always able to leave this project on the desk for another day and sometimes it held me in my chair (too) late. That my life nevertheless rarely descended into chaos is largely due to the tirelessness of Doris Wüstenhagen, who over the years caringly helped me while also giving me insights from her past work as a nurse. Over the course of the project, I realized how many questions and ideas had their roots in my childhood and their first sparks in discussions with my parents Anja and Otto Hitzer. They never evaded my questions and accompanied me with curiosity every step of the way. They, along with my sister, Stephanie Mertins, gave me the resources I needed to complete this book.

My children Felix, Carlotta, and Henrietta grew incredibly fast during my work on this book, which often kept me away from them. I am so grateful for their patience with me and for their openness in expressing their desire for me to be more present. I never could have imagined the joy I would experience in their budding interest in my research and in sharing my discoveries, doubts, difficulties, and findings with them, which I got to do with steadily greater frequency the older they have become. None of this would have been possible without Christoph-Julius Hilpert, who never lost patience with my obsession for this topic, who always listened, read, questioned, and encouraged me to make my argument clearer and more pointed. I dedicate this book to him and our children.

Preface to the English Edition of *The History of Cancer and Emotions in Twentieth-Century Germany*

What distinguishes the history of cancer in Germany from the history of cancer in other parts of the world? The current pandemic has reminded us that diseases know no borders and that a virus uses the same microbiological mechanisms no matter where it is in the world. But, as the coronavirus pandemic has also strikingly demonstrated, many other aspects of disease are anything but universal. The differences range from the biological (men fall ill with Covid-19 more often and are more susceptible to severe cases) to the social (people belonging to underprivileged ethnic groups are also infected with greater frequency) to the political and national (access to vaccines, political measures to suppress the virus, healthcare systems). Similar differences define cancer, both in individual cases and in its general prevalence, even if cancer is, unlike Covid-19, not transmissible.

Among these differences is that, from the perspective of contemporary medicine, it makes little sense to speak of cancer as such. The molecular-biological dissimilarities between individual cases of cancer are too vast, so that even speaking of breast cancer as a single disease is misleading. Nevertheless, this book treats 'cancer' in general terms for one primary reason: it seeks to describe the historical entanglements between medicine, politics, and society and their various approaches to cancer over time. And during most of the twentieth century, few people outside the medical profession drew categorical distinctions between different types of cancer. 'Cancer' was perceived as an existential threat to an individual, as an extreme challenge for medicine and society. In this abbreviated form, it was turned into a metaphor for danger that evoked fear and disgust.

Fear and disgust, two powerful emotions, play a central role in this history. But so does hope. This book takes a perspective that, though uncommon in historiography, has proven especially fruitful for the analysis of the history of 'cancer' and has helped reveal numerous connections that had gone unseen by extant research. The present history of emotions aims to grasp how ideas about emotions and emotional practices shaped the experience of cancer in twentieth-century Germany and how medical, psychological, and social practices for dealing with cancer influenced the ways in which German society conceived of and acted upon certain emotions like hope, fear, and disgust. To be clear, this is *not* to argue that emotions somehow play a role in causing cancer. This is not my intention.

Determining the causes of cancer is a matter for medical science. I am writing as a historian, and part of that work involves documenting scientific ideas from the past.

This brings me back to my initial question, one that non-German readers in particular might be asking themselves: to what extent is this a specifically German story? The book details the history of cancer and emotions through five different political systems and underscores that political caesuras resonate in the immediate corporeality of the history of emotions. The narrative begins in the German Empire, a patriarchal, hierarchical society defined by gradually increasing efforts at political and social reform; a society in which medicine enjoyed high status. The German Empire was followed by the Weimar Republic. With a democratic system that suffered from instability on many fronts and that was constantly being challenged by political polarization, it was also perpetually afflicted by economic scarcity, which had a serious impact on medical care. Discussions on fundamentally reforming the healthcare system were often carried out in an acrimonious tone. In 1933, the Weimar Republic's democratic constitution was suspended. The National Socialists radicalized the discourse on health, illness, and society and ultimately translated their extreme ideas into crimes against humanity: the 'duty' to be healthy, the exclusion and, ultimately, murder of people whose lives were written off by racist eugenicists as 'not worth living'. After 1945, two new political systems were established that charted their own paths in healthcare; this book traces their histories in parallel. While the German Democratic Republic elevated socialist prophylaxis and optimism about the future to key values of a centrally organized healthcare system, the Federal Republic of Germany defined health maintenance as an individual responsibility and thus developed wholly different practices of campaigning for prevention, early detection, and therapy, all of which initially focused first and foremost on dispelling fear and panic.

Approaches towards cancer and emotions shifted with the (health) political and social conditions of the times. This book describes these shifts and analyses the complexities of cause and effect. Discussions and insights from the international scientific community that had come into being in the nineteenth century played a role in these developments. At the same time, forms of therapy and models of prevention were transferred across borders, and debates about how to treat cancer patients were carried out transnationally, too. Thus, the broader trends that this book outlines can be observed in many other countries of the Global North, if with a somewhat different temporality: the rise of psychosomatic theories of cancer aetiology between the early 1940s and the 1970s; in the 1960s and following decades, the waxing and, in recent times, waning dominance of the concept of 'emotional labour'; the first early detection campaigns, which, produced around 1900, wielded emotions with ever greater professional aptitude and played with recipients' fears in a number of ways; the increasing but by no means linear tendency towards more openness to speak about cancer; the shifting conditions that shaped the experience of being a cancer patient and their correlation with the succession of therapeutic regimes; the trend since the late 1960s of publicly discussing one's own experiences as a cancer patient and, much later, as a 'survivor'—these are all developments that transcend the German history of cancer and emotions.

But alongside these broader historical lines, there are significant differences. Listing all of them would go well beyond the limits of this preface. Moreover, readers of this book will find numerous remarks on how and why developments in Germany differed from those in Great Britain, the United States, France, and the Netherlands. Thus, I will limit myself here to noting a few distinct features of the German history of cancer and emotions.

The book describes how and why, over the run of the twentieth century, emotions were discussed in connection with cancer by medical and psychological research. Psychosomatic theories about cancer first gained traction in the United States in the late 1930s. Only in the mid-1950s did they begin to see interest in Germany, and then only in West Germany. In contrast to other European countries, discourse on the psychosomatic origins of cancer in Germany was politicized from the very beginning as a form of engagement with German guilt and repression, with a specifically German form of 'emotional anaesthesia'. In the 1960s, this evolved into a critique of the German bourgeois lifestyle. Since the early 1980s, criticisms of psychosomatic cancer aetiology have become more prevalent. In East Germany, though, such political interpretations were absent in medicine and psychology; indeed, psychosomatic cancer research was generally a rare item in the GDR. The West German discussion ultimately only found resonance in literature there, such as in the writings of Christa Wolf.

Early detection campaigns and their utilization of emotions are another topic of this book. At the end of the nineteenth century, Germany was a pioneer of such campaigns, which, in contrast to their counterparts in countries like Great Britain and the Netherlands, were aimed at laypeople from the start and, while certainly thematizing fear as a problem, also showed no hesitancy in using fear as a means of persuasion. Early on, moralizing took on multifarious guises in many countries' campaigns. German campaigns, though, more emphatically ascribed responsibility for illness to the individual. While American films depicted how turning away from the 'false path' could give rise to hope, campaigns of the late Weimar Republic focused on the stories of individuals who—early on in their stories—made the bad choice of avoiding consultations with a doctor. They repeated the message that it was now too late for that person to turn back and illustrated the terrible consequences that individual would have to reckon with. At the same time, campaigns emphasized that those who waited 'too long' to go to the doctor were accountable not only for their own suffering and death, but also for the suffering of their orphaned children and the damage they did to the 'people'. This type of moralizing was radicalized under National Socialism and then largely disappeared from the scene after 1945.

The book also engages with the various forms of talking and remaining silent about cancer as well as the concepts about emotions that informed the decision to discuss or suppress. In Germany, a minority of doctors had already endorsed speaking more openly about cancer around 1900. After 1933, this minority position was taken up by jurisprudence and by the National-Socialist brand of psychotherapy called Deutsche Seelenheilkunde, or 'German Psychotherapy', both of which interpreted it in line with Nazi ideas about 'morality'. Their key principle was that every 'German' person should have the capacity to grapple consciously with their own death, to retain their self-confidence in this crisis, and to shed their individualist concerns about self-preservation and act for the survival of the '*Volk*'. After 1945, in both East and West Germany, courts of law and the majority opinion returned to the past practice of avoiding talk about cancer, as was also common in other European countries and in the United States at this time.

Finally, the book details shifting therapeutic regimes and their effects on the emotional experiences of cancer patients. On this point in particular there is considerable overlap between, on the one hand, transnational entanglements in research and international scientific discourse, and, on the other, nationally defined healthcare systems and emotional regimes. An important dimension of this history for Germany concerns the feeling of disgust, the relevance of which has hardly been studied in work on the history of cancer in other countries. Disgust towards people with grave or terminal cases of cancer played a significant role in Germany in the early twentieth century. Doctors and care personnel used disgust—their own as well as that of other patients—as an argument to justify the exclusion of terminal cancer patients from care at clinics. Even if this disgust was rarely spoken about publicly, many doctors and nurses entertained few reservations about this practice. It remains to be determined the extent to which this was a specifically German historical phenomenon, which was prevalent during a time when physical and moral disgust were associated with antisemitic stereotypes.

The book treats many facets of the intertwining between local, national, and transnational history, which could only be touched upon briefly in this preface. The translation of the book, originally published in German, is another—much happier—example of this kind of intertwining. I'd thus like to give special thanks to the book's meticulous, resourceful, and engaged translator, Adam Bresnahan.

Berlin
October 2021

List of Figures

List of Films

Gesundheitsmagazin Praxis. Episode 'Ich hatte Krebs', directed by Sigrid Schenkenberger. Broadcast 13 April 1970 on ZDF. Produktionsarchiv des ZDF.

Jeder Achte (also appeared under the title *Ein Film gegen die Volkskrankheit Krebs*). Sound film, 17 minutes. Directed by Walther Ruttmann; script by Walther Ruttmann and Ernst Dahle; camera by Gerhard Müller; music by Wolfgang Zeller. Reviewed by the censor on 4 August 1941, B.55709: 'approved for young people; no plot; approved for holidays'. Produced by Otto Nay/Universal Film AG (Ufa) Deutschland 1941. Bundesfilmarchiv, rights held by the Murnau-Stiftung.

Jeder Fünfte . . . Ein Bericht über den Stand der Krebsforschung in der Bundesrepublik. Directed by Marianne von Arnim. Federal Republic of Germany, 1965. A copy of the film could not be found. The script is held by the German Federal Archives, as is a review from the *Stuttgarter Zeitung* 180 (6 August 1965) that evidences that the film was broadcast on television, but does not say on which channel. BArch B 145/4719.

Kampf dem Krebs. Directed by Helmut Bousset. 35mm, 37 minutes, black and white. Reviewed by the censor on 22 February 1936, B.41670: 'Only permitted at closed events of the Imperial Committee for Fighting Cancer'; on 29 August 1936, B.43197 (restricted for young people); on 19 October 1942, B.56962 ('Only permitted in events of the Imperial Society for Preventive Health Measures'). Produced by Kifo. Germany, 1935/6. Lost.

Kampf dem Krebs/Krebs ist heilbar. Directed by Nathan Schänker. Sound film, black and white, 1:06:36. Produced by the Schweizerische Nationalliga für Krebsbekämpfung (Swiss National League for Fighting Cancer). Switzerland, 1945; Germany, 1953. DVD in Daniel Kauz, *Vom Tabu zum Thema? 100 Jahre Krebsbekämpfung in der Schweiz 1910–2010* (Basel: Schwabe, 2010).

Kampf dem Krebs. Sound film, colour, live-action, 27 minutes. Commissioned by the Bundeszentrale für gesundheitliche Aufklärung (Federal Centre for Health Education). Produced by Leonaris-Film. Federal Republic of Germany, 1970. Bundesfilmarchiv.

Der Krebs. 35mm, black and white, 16 minutes, silent film with intertitles. Reviewed by the censor on 11 November 1930, B.27368 (permitted for young people). Commissioned and released by the German Hygiene Museum. Produced by Verlag wissenschaftlicher Filme GmbH, German Empire. Distributed by the German Hygiene Museum and the Filmstelle, Deutsches Reich. DHMD 2001/1655.

'Krebs ist heilbar wenn . . .', Episode of *Gesundheitsmagazin Praxis*. Broadcast 2 October 1964 on ZDF. Produktionsarchiv des ZDF.

Rauch, der uns nicht kaltläßt. 35mm, sound film, colour, live action, 6:00. Directed and produced by Gottfried Stejskal, Film-Kollektiv Dresden. German Democratic Republic, 1980. DHMD 2001/1665.

Rechtzeitig—eine Mahnung des Lebens. 16mm, sound film, black and white, 17:35. Directed by Erich Barthel; script by Kurt Bortfeldt; edited by Elfriede Böttrich; cartoons by Hugo Cernik; dramaturgy by Joachim Emuth; camera by Rudi Müller; scientific advising by head doctor Dr. Rieck. Produced by Kurt Schönbach, VEB DEFA-Studio für populärwissenschaftliche Filme. German Democratic Republic, 1956. DHMD 2001/1656.

Der Siebente. Sound film, colour, cartoon film, 35mm, 13 minutes. Directed by Walter Eckhold; scenes by Walter Eckhold, Klaus Eberhardt, and Hannelore Holz; animation by Walter Eckhold and Andre Schmidt; dramaturgy by Hans Grümmer; sound by Wolfgang Mammitzsch; edited by Renate Richter; music by Karl-Ernst Sasse; narrated by Wolfgang Jacob; concept by Heinz Becker; commissioned by the German Hygiene Museum Dresden; executive producer: Sigrid Weidhaas. Produced by VEB DEFA-Studio für Trickfilme. German Democratic Republic, 1985/6. DHMD 2001/1669.

Der Tod gibt eine Party. Sound film, colour. Directed by Fr. Herbert Engler; script by F. E. Gericke; scientific advising by Dr. Christel Schultze-Rhonhof and Dr. Hans J. Goetz. Produced by the Zentralinstitut für Gesundheitserziehung (Central Institute for Health Education) and the Deutsches Gesundheits-Museum e.V. (German Health Museum). Commissioned by the Federal Ministry of Health. Federal Republic of Germany, 1967. Bundesfilmarchiv.

Wissen heißt Leben. 35mm, sound film, colour, live-action, 16:25. Directed by Wolfgang Heyer and Ingrid Hinz; camera by Klaus Mühle; edited by Hanna Kubin; music by Karl-Ernst Sasse; scientific advising by Dr. Ahlendorf and Dr. Gibel. Produced by VEB DEFA-Studio für Kurzfilme. German Democratic Republic, 1970. DHMD 2011/1658.

List of Abbreviations

ACS	American Cancer Society
AMG	Arzneimittelgesetz (German Pharmaceutical Drug Code)
Arge	Arbeitsgemeinschaft für Krebsbekämpfung der Träger der gesetzlichen Kranken- und Rentenversicherung im Lande Nordrhein-Westfalen (Working Group for Fighting Cancer of the Statutory Health and Retirement Insurance Administrations of the State of North Rhine-Westphalia)
BArch	Bundesarchiv (German Federal Archives)
BGB	Bürgerliches Gesetzbuch (German Civil Code)
BGH	Bundesgerichtshof (German Federal Court of Justice)
CCNSC	Cancer Chemotherapy National Service Center
Dapo	Deutsche Arbeitsgemeinschaft für Psychosoziale Onkologie e. V. (German Working Group for Psycho-oncology)
DEFA	Deutsche Film AG
DHMD	Deutsches Hygiene-Museum Dresden (German Hygiene Museum)
DKFZ	Deutsches Krebsforschungszentrum (German Cancer Research Centre)
DZA	Deutscher Zentralausschuss für Krebsbekämpfung (German Central Committee for Fighting Cancer)
EBM	Evidence-based Medicine
EZA	Evangelisches Zentralarchiv in Berlin (Central Archive of the Protestant Church, Berlin)
FDGB	Freier Deutscher Gewerkschaftsbund (Free German Trade Union Federation)
GStA	Geheimes Staatsarchiv Preußischer Kulturbesitz (Secret State Archives, Prussian Cultural Heritage Foundation)
HPLC	High Performance Liquid Chromatography
HSTAD	Hauptstaatsarchiv Dresden (Saxonian Central State Archive Dresden)
HU Archiv	Universitätsarchiv Humboldt-Universität zu Berlin (Humboldt University Archive)
IKK	Innungskrankenkassen (Trade Guild Health Insurances)
LAB	Landesarchiv Berlin (Archives of the Land Berlin)
MeV	Megaelectronvolt
MPI	Maudsley Personality Inventory
NBI	Neue Berliner Illustrierte
NURSE	Naming, Understanding, Respecting, Supporting, Exploring
OLG	Oberlandesgericht (Higher Regional Court)
ORSD	Office of Scientific Research and Development
Pg.	Parteigenosse (Party Comrade)
PSA	Prostate-Specific Antigen
SARS	Severe Acute Respiratory Syndrome

SED	Sozialistische Einheitspartei Deutschlands (Socialist Unity Party of Germany)
SPIKES	Setting, Perception, Invitation, Knowledge, Empathy, Strategy, and Summary
SWR	Südwestrundfunk (Southwest German Radio)
taz	die tageszeitung
TNF	Tumor necrosis factor
TNM	Tumor Size and Grade; Nodus (= Lymph node involvement); Metastases
TPN	Total Parenteral Nutrition
VA	Department of Veterans Affairs
ZDF	Zweites Deutsches Fernsehen (Second Channel of German Television Broadcasting)

1
Writing the History of Emotions

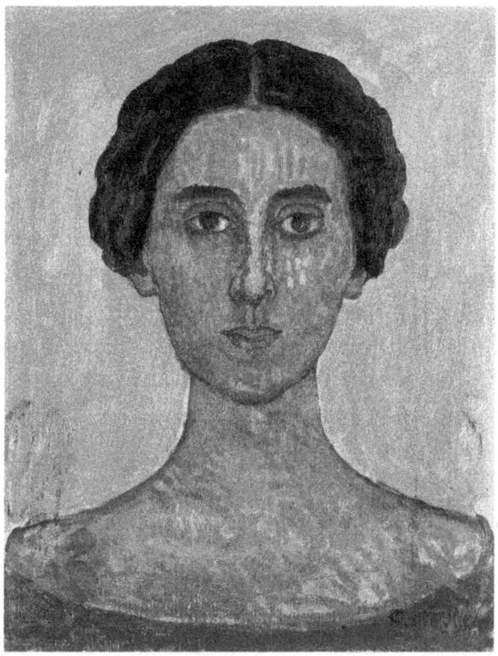

Fig. 1 Ferdinand Hodler, *Portrait of Valentine Godé-Darel*, *c.*1910.

More than one hundred years separate us from the gaze of Valentine Godé-Darel. When Swiss Symbolist and Art Deco artist Ferdinand Hodler painted her portrait in 1910 (Fig. 1), Godé-Darel, then 37 years old, had no premonition that she would get ovarian cancer, which at that time was almost always fatal. Two years after sitting for the portrait, she would suffer the disease's first symptoms and soon thereafter learn the name of her illness: cancer. Hodler, an artist who had often dealt with death in his work, captured in images Godé-Darel's illness up until the day she finally succumbed to it, 25 January 1915. More than fifty paintings and one hundred drawings document Hodler's relationship with his beloved, the deterioration of her body, and her gradual retreat into herself, as she ceased looking at the viewer.

This visual archive of a woman's life with cancer is unique, not only for the early twentieth century, but in the history of cancer more generally. A century stands between Godé-Darel and the viewer touched by her decline, the inevitability of her death, the destruction wrought by her sickness, her human capacity to suffer, the viewer's own capacity to feel sympathy, and the (im)possibility of intimacy during her final moments. In short, the images are timeless. Yet they narrate an individual experience of illness and death that was situated in a specific place and time and felt in a specific way by the painter and the cancer patient.

Towards our end of the century, acclaimed German author Wolfgang Herrndorf learned, at the age of 44, that he had an inoperable brain tumour, a glioblastoma. Over the course of three years, he blogged about his life, his thoughts, and his feelings. He wrote about operations, radiation therapy, chemotherapy, and the detrimental effect that it all had on his body, mind, and willpower. Six days before he ended his own life on 26 August 2013, he published one final blog entry. His friends later published the entirety of his blog in print form as *Arbeit und Struktur* (*Work and Structure*).[1] But despite opening up about his illness on the internet on his own initiative, Herrndorf refused readers' attempts to meet with him in person. Like Godé-Darel, he allowed people from the outside to look in, but rejected direct contact with those witnessing his decay.

In one of his last poems, he meditated on distance and closeness and the constitutive impossibility of sharing and comprehending others' feelings and their experience of life and death:

> I don't let anyone get close to me
> Up to the moment of my death.
> And at that moment, too, nobody will come.
> Nothing will come, and it is in my hands.[2]

Does Everybody Feel the Same Feelings?

These two stories touch upon two of this book's key assumptions, and they offer answers to two diametrically opposed questions. First, aren't emotions something totally personal and internal, something that can never adequately be communicated to others, especially when it comes to suffering and death, the touchstones of existential loneliness? How can a historian claim to write a history of these feelings that can be captured neither in language nor in general concepts? Second, haven't all people of all times and places been afraid of serious illnesses like the plague,

[1] Wolfgang Herrndorf, 'Arbeit und Struktur', http://www.wolfgang-herrndorf.de/; and Wolfgang Herrndorf, *Arbeit und Struktur* (Berlin: Suhrkamp, 2013).
[2] Herrndorf, 'Arbeit und Struktur', 15 July 2013, 23:12.

tuberculosis, and cancer? Don't people diagnosed with terminal illness always experience the same feelings of despair, sadness, and anxiety, resignation, hope, and rage? After all, it would seem that being terminally ill confronts every person with the same challenge: to live in the face of death. Thus, when we talk about deadly illnesses like cancer, is it not just the outer guise of emotions that changes, while their essential content remains the same?

We all want to find meaning in life and we all want to have physical and emotional contact with others. We read and view records of the past like the images of Godé-Darel as if we can understand them—or at least translate them into our own terms—with no further explanation, as if all human beings throughout history have shared a kind of basic emotional vocabulary: love, fear, despair, sadness. This view is not naïve or trivial; from an ontological perspective, it is justified. But from a historical perspective, it is questionable, because the idea that emotions remain essentially the same over time relies on a plethora of assumptions about history, feelings, and human life more generally.

Until recently, cognitive psychology and the neurosciences had made the universality of emotions into an axiom of their research, an idea most explicitly expressed in the search for a set of six or seven basic emotions.[3] But nowadays, some neuroscientists are themselves criticizing and relativizing this undertaking.[4]

A Different Perspective: Emotions and History

Historians of emotions generally reject attempts to find a universally valid definition of emotions. Broadly speaking, they opt for an approach that defines emotions on the basis of how people in particular eras, places, and cultures have described and experienced them.[5] All emotions have a corporeal dimension

[3] The concept of basic emotions comes from American psychologist Paul Ekman, who, influenced by Charles Darwin's *The Expressions of the Emotions*, spoke of six basic emotions (anger, happiness, disgust, fear, sadness, and surprise). On Ekman's own shifting positions, see Paul Ekman, E. Richard Sorenson, and Wallace V. Friesen, 'Pan-Cultural Elements in Facial Displays of Emotion', *Science* 164, no. 3875 (1969): 86–8; for an overview, see Paul Ekman, ed., *Darwin and Facial Expression: A Century of Research in Review* (Los Altos: Malor, 2006). On historical assessments of the concept, see Ruth Leys, 'The Turn to Affect: A Critique', *Critical Inquiry* 37, no. 3 (2011): 434–72, 437–40, https://doi.org/10.1086/659353; Ruth Leys, *From Guilt to Shame: Auschwitz and After* (Princeton: Princeton University Press, 2007), 133–50; and Jan Plamper, *The History of Emotions: An Introduction* (Oxford: Oxford University Press, 2015), 147–63.

[4] Chaona Chen, Oliver G. B. Garrod, Philippe G. Schyns, and Rachael E. Jack, 'The Face Is the Mirror of the Cultural Mind', *Journal of Vision* 15, no. 12 (2015): 928, https://doi.org/10.1167/15.12.928; Rachael E. Jack, Oliver G. B. Garrod, Hui Yu, Roberto Caldara, and Philippe G. Schyns, 'Facial Expressions of Emotion Are Not Culturally Universal', *Proceedings of the National Academy of Sciences of the United States of America* 109, no. 19 (2012): 7241–4, https://doi.org/10.1073/pnas.1200155109; Plamper, *History of Emotions*, 243–50.

[5] For an introduction to the history of the emotions, see Rob Boddice, *The History of Emotions* (Manchester: Manchester University Press, 2018); Barbara Rosenwein and Riccardo Cristiani, *What Is*

rooted in nervous reactions, synapses, and biochemical processes. Pain research has established that the relevance and significance of pain cannot be reduced to bodily stimuli; analogously, emotions cannot be reduced to corporeal processes either.[6] Phantom pain, chronic pain without an identifiable cause, the intangible pain of soldiers on the battlefield, and the mental regulation of pain are all phenomena that have pushed scientists to expand their view of what pain is and how it is experienced. They have long been grappling with the conundrum that, though two people's physical maladies might be the same, their experience of the associated pain can be totally different.

Just as the social sciences don't treat class as a static analytic category, so too do historians embrace the plasticity of the concept of emotions. But this requires that they define their object of research in some other way. One alternative might be to engage in historical semantics and look at the various meanings and uses of various words related to emotions. Then one could rest with a generally applicable definition of emotions as that which people have experienced and described as such. The different significations of emotion and emotions gleaned from an analysis of source material might then enable us to detect expressions of feeling even if they are not explicit. This would also make it easier to trace shifts in the meanings of emotion words.

But this approach runs into difficulties when certain concepts suddenly fall out of use or the key word 'emotion' doesn't appear in the sources. Are we still talking about the history of emotions when discussing sentiments and passions and not emotions per se? Sure, these concepts are both historically and semantically related to the younger concept of emotion, but is the gap between their respective meanings too large to justifiably argue that there is continuity here? Recent attempts to translate historical descriptions of emotions represent an ambitious, methodologically promising undertaking.[7] But it doesn't quite fit the aim of this book, which is not so concerned with writing the history of a certain emotion as it is with an analysis of the complex relation between emotions on the one hand and cancer on the other.

the History of Emotions? (Cambridge: Cambridge University Press, 2018); Ute Frevert, 'The History of Emotions', in *Handbook of Emotions*, ed. Lisa Feldman Barrett, Michael Lewis, and Jeanette M. Haviland-Jones (New York: Guilford, 2016), 49–65; Nicole Eustace, Eugenia Lean, Julie Livingston, Jan Plamper, William M. Reddy, and Barbara H. Rosenwein, 'AHR Conversation: The Historical Study of Emotions', *American Historical Review* 117, no. 5 (2012): 1487–1531; and Plamper, *History of Emotions*.

6 Rob Boddice, 'Introduction: Hurt Feelings', in *Pain and Emotion in Modern History*, ed. Rob Boddice (Basingstoke: Palgrave Macmillan, 2014), 1–15; Joanna Bourke, *The Story of Pain: From Prayer to Painkillers* (Oxford: Oxford University Press, 2014); Javier Moscoso, *Pain: A Cultural History* (Basingstoke: Palgrave Macmillan, 2012); Esther Cohen, Leona Toker, Manuela Consonni, and Otniel E. Dror, eds, *Knowledge and Pain* (Amsterdam: Rodopi, 2012); David Biro, *The Language of Pain: Finding Words, Compassion, and Relief* (New York: W. W. Norton, 2000).

7 Margrit Pernau and Imke Rajamani, 'Emotional Translations: Conceptual History beyond Language', *History and Theory* 55, no. 1 (2016): 46–65, https://doi.org/10.1111/hith.10787.

At the end of the day, this history of emotions does not seek to bring another neglected concept back onto the stage of history. The history of emotions is important because it conducts research on an object that is, at least in some respects, unique and significant in its own right. Here is where I'd like to lay out my own historically informed, if still cautiously abstract, definition of emotions, which I think can lay claim to at least some form of universal validity.

I define emotions as sensations felt by human beings that are situated on the historically variable border between the body and the non-bodily. Emotions are bound to the senses, but they're more than a mere index of a bodily state or reaction. Similarly, emotions are not just a matter of thought. What exactly the distinguishing feature of emotions consists of is not part of my elementary definition; this can only be determined by analysing different historically and culturally varying conceptions of emotions. The capacity to feel emotions is a fundamental aspect of humans' embodied, social existence. Just as humans' ability to use language is innate, though we still have to learn how to speak, so too do we (have to) learn how to feel. We learn what emotions are and how they can be good (or bad); we learn which emotions there are; we learn how they feel and how to describe them; we learn how to articulate our emotions in a manner appropriate for a given social setting; and we learn how to deal with our own feelings and those of others.

In these processes of learning, we don't just come to know the rules on how to express ourselves. These learning processes shape our emotions themselves, making real emotions out of our inborn capacity to feel. This position puts into question the distinction—dominant in Western modernity, but probably older—between inner, 'authentic' emotions and external emotional expressions guided by emotion rules,[8] because even when I perceive, name, and describe an emotion in my internal dialogue with myself, I do so with words that I learned, words that are bound up in a web of meanings, norms, rules, linguistic conventions, and bodily forms of expression. This process of navigating feelings, to borrow a term from American historian William M. Reddy, blurs the hard separation between internal and external emotions.[9] Another implication of this perspective is that the name applied to an emotion never wholly captures what a person feels. Indeed, that emotions have fuzzy borders seems to be one of their defining characteristics. Thus, the navigation of feelings often remains unfinished, picks up again at a different point, and leads to a different result than its previous

[8] Monique Scheer, 'Topographies of Emotion', in *Emotional Lexicons: Continuity and Change in the Vocabulary of Feeling 1700–2000*, ed. Ute Frevert, Monique Scheer, Anne Schmidt, Pascal Eitler, Bettina Hitzer, Nina Verheyen, Benno Gammerl, Christian Bailey, and Margrit Pernau (Oxford: Oxford University Press, 2014), 32–61; Charles Taylor, *Sources of the Self: The Making of the Modern Identity* (Cambridge, MA: Harvard University Press, 1989), 111.

[9] William Reddy, *The Navigation of Feeling* (New York: Cambridge University Press, 2001).

iteration. These repeated, ever new attempts to grasp a feeling contribute to the transformation of how certain emotions are conceived and evaluated.[10]

Emotions are thus universal (humans have an innate capacity to feel), individual (a person's to some extent unique navigation of feelings), and historical (the result of these processes of navigating feelings as communicated with others in society). This belies the notion that the fear of cancer or the fear experienced by cancer patients has always been the same. How this fear was felt changed over time, because cancer patients lived in, were housed in, and were cared for in different spaces over the run of the twentieth century, because they underwent different types of treatment, because their chances of being cured or entering into remission differed, and because doctors and nurses talked to them and approached them in different ways. And it changed because conceptions about the nature, meaning, and rationality of fear shifted. If I think that fear is an expression of cowardice, then I might detest myself for feeling it and seek out isolation to try and be rid of it or hide it. If I think that fear is undignified, then my striving to regain dignity can lend me inner fortitude—but it can also drive me into despair. If I think that fear is harmful, then my fear might cause me to fear my fear and wrestle with feelings of guilt, which might in some circumstances lead me to seek help in order to overcome it and turn it into hope.

Fear, just like any other emotion, can feel very differently depending on the person and the situation. Even if my fear is always my own, a large part of how I experience it is a factor of history. In short, fear is neither historically contingent nor is its content totally determined in advance. This book explores shifts in the ways in which emotions related to cancer were experienced, portrayed, discussed, and evaluated over the course of the twentieth century.

The History of Emotions

During the twentieth century, discussions about the significance of emotions took on an extraordinary relevance for how people thought about cancer. They defined debates about the nature of the self, the body, and death, and cancer became a common metaphor in political movements and political culture. At the turn of the twentieth century, cancer staked its claim as the paradigmatic illness of Western

[10] One might call this process the practice of trying emotions, see Benno Gammerl and Bettina Hitzer, 'Wohin mit den Gefühlen? Vergangenheit und Zukunft des Emotional Turn in den Geschichtswissenschaften', *Berliner Debatte Initial* 24, no. 3 (2013): 31–40, 37–8. On the theories and methods of the history of emotions, see also Monique Scheer, 'Are Emotions a Kind of Practice (and Is That What Makes Them Have a History)? A Bourdieuan Approach to Understanding Emotion', *History and Theory* 51, no. 2 (2012): 193–220; Benno Gammerl, 'Emotional Styles: Concepts and Challenges', *Rethinking History* 16, no. 2 (2012): 161–75, https://doi.org/10.1080/13642529.2012.681189.

Europe and the United States.[11] Certainly, cancer has existed since antiquity, and sources show that it was one of the most dreaded illnesses in the Middle Ages because it could rarely be cured and caused enormous pain.[12] Nevertheless, what medieval and early modern doctors called cancer was a relatively uncommon affliction. They normally diagnosed a person with cancer only when they had visible tumours, which is to say mostly only in cases of skin, mouth, or breast cancer. Cancer inside the body was not altogether unknown, but it was seldom diagnosed as such.

This all changed during the nineteenth century, when the discovery of etherization as well as antiseptic, and later, aseptic methods, enabled doctors to perform internal surgeries. At the same time, ideas about old age changed so that by the end of the century, it stopped being considered a pathological state in and of itself. As a consequence, many authorities no longer permitted 'old age' to be listed as the cause of death on death certificates.[13] Instead, medical examiners increasingly looked for the 'fatal' cause of death in a more restricted sense, which brought with it an uptick in the number of autopsies performed. This, in turn, led to cancer being identified as a cause of death more frequently in cases where only a few years earlier old age would have been accepted as a sufficient explanation. In an era when statistics were being collected on everything, the statistics on causes of death became more refined and discerning. The year 1905 marked the first time that statistics on cancer as a distinct cause of death were collected in the German Empire.[14] After a few years, it became clear that more people were dying of cancer than previously assumed. This elevated cancer to a highly discussed topic in both the newspapers and in internal administrative communications.

Public opinion generally agreed that the number of cancer patients and cancer deaths were on the rise. Doctors, health policymakers, and journalists termed cancer a lifestyle disease and sought to trace this development back to what they admitted were as yet poorly understood changes in the lives of people in

[11] Werner F. Kümmell, 'Krebs—die "Leitkrankheit" unserer Zeit im Licht der Geschichte', *Acta Historica Leopoldina* 39 (2004): 41–58, 41–2 and 47–56; and Wolfgang U. Eckart, 'Tumorvirologie—Linien der Forschungsgeschichte', in *100 Years of Organized Cancer Research. 100 Jahre organisierte Krebsforschung*, ed. Wolfgang U. Eckart (Stuttgart: Georg Thieme, 2000), 101–6.

[12] Patrick J. Fitzgerald, *From Demons and Evil Spirits to Cancer Genes* (Washington, DC: American Registry of Pathology, 2000), 3–22; Margaret Olszewski, 'Concepts of Cancer from Antiquity to the Nineteenth-Century', *University of Toronto Medical Journal* 87, no. 3 (2010): 181–6; Jacques Rouessé, *Une histoire du cancer du sein en Occident: enseignements et réflexions* (Paris: Springer, 2011); Siddharta Mukherjee, *The Emperor of All Maladies: A Biography of Cancer* (New York: Scribner, 2010).

[13] Stefan Schmorrte, 'Alter und Medizin. Die Anfänge der Geriatrie in Deutschland', *Archiv für Sozialgeschichte* 30 (1990): 19–21; Heiko Stoff, *Ewige Jugend. Konzepte der Verjüngung vom späten 19. Jahrhundert bis ins Dritte Reich* (Cologne: Böhlau, 2004), 210–11.

[14] Jeannette Madarász, 'Die Pflicht zur Gesundheit: Chronische Krankheiten des Herzkreislaufsystems zwischen Wissenschaft, Populärwissenschaft und Öffentlichkeit', in *Das präventive Selbst. Eine Kulturgeschichte moderner Gesundheitspolitik*, ed. Martin Lengwiler and Jeannette Madarász (Bielefeld: transcript, 2010), 137–67, 142.

industrialized countries.[15] To get a better grasp of the issue, doctors and policymakers in countries around the world established institutes to conduct research on cancer, including in the German Empire (1900), Great Britain and Spain (1902), Hungary (1903), Portugal (1904), Austria, Denmark, and Sweden (1905), France and the United States (1906), Japan (1907), and Switzerland (1910).[16]

Rudolf Virchow's revolutionary discovery of cellular pathology played a key role in thought about cancer, because it enabled cancer to be identified on the level of the cell. The same period also witnessed the finding that cancerous cells are similar to healthy cells, even if they differ in things like their rapid reproduction rate. This insight resulted in a redefinition of cancer as a 'deformation' of once healthy cells that sets in locally and then spreads. On the other hand, the methods of cellular pathology offered a seemingly deciding criterion for distinguishing cancerous tumours from other tumours that came to be defined as benevolent: the uniqueness of their cellular growth and metabolism.[17] Certainly, doctors making diagnoses on the basis of sight and touch had long differentiated between life-threatening and mostly harmless tumours. But identification in a laboratory promised much greater certainty.

Thus, while cancer had been the domain of surgeons throughout the nineteenth century, their efforts at diagnosing the disease were now bolstered by the work of pathologists.[18] And in 1900, their efforts to treat the disease got a boost by the

[15] Jacob Wolff, *Die Lehre von der Krebskrankheit. Von den ältesten Zeiten bis zur Gegenwart*, vol. 3 (Jena, 1913).

[16] Isabel Atzl and Ronald Helms, *Die Geschichte der Deutschen Krebsgesellschaft* (Germering: Zuckschwerdt, 2012), 36–7, which contains information on when many cancer institutes were founded; Joan Austoker, *A History of the Imperial Cancer Research Fund, 1902–1986* (Oxford: Oxford University Press, 1988); Patrice Pinell, *Naissance d'un fléau. Histoire de la lutte contre le cancer en France (1890–1940)* (Paris: Métailié, 2002); Daniel Kauz, *Vom Tabu zum Thema? 100 Jahre Krebsbekämpfung in der Schweiz 1910–2010* (Bern: Schwabe, 2010); James T. Patterson, *The Dread Disease: Cancer and Modern American Culture* (Cambridge, MA: Harvard University Press, 1987).

[17] Rudolf Virchow, *Die Cellularpathologie in ihrer Begründung auf physiologische und pathologische Gewebelehre*, 4th edn (Berlin, 1871), 408.

[18] The history of cancer surgery plays a significant role in a lot of historiographical works on the illness, many of which study the relation between public health campaigns and cancer treatment in the twentieth century: Patterson, *Dread Disease*; Barron H. Lerner, *The Breast Cancer Wars: Hope, Fear, and the Pursuit of a Cure in Twentieth-Century America* (Oxford: Oxford University Press, 2001); Pinell, *Naissance d'un fléau*; Kirsten E. Gardner, *Early Detection: Women, Cancer, and Awareness Campaigns in the Twentieth-Century United States* (Chapel Hill, NC: University of North Carolina Press, 2006); Robert A. Aronowitz, *Unnatural History: Breast Cancer and American Society* (Cambridge: Cambridge University Press, 2007); Ilana Löwy, *Preventive Strikes: Women, Precancer, and Prophylactic Surgery* (Baltimore: Johns Hopkins University Press, 2010); Ilana Löwy, *A Woman's Disease: The History of Cervical Cancer* (Oxford: Oxford University Press, 2011); David Cantor, ed., *Cancer in the Twentieth Century* (Baltimore: Johns Hopkins University Press, 2008); Carsten Timmermann and Elizabeth Toon, *Cancer Patients, Cancer Pathways: Historical and Sociological Perspectives* (New York: Palgrave Macmillan, 2012); Ornella Moscucci, *Gender and Cancer in England, 1860–1948* (London: Palgrave Macmillan, 2016); Carsten Timmermann, *A History of Lung Cancer: The Recalcitrant Disease* (Basingstoke: Palgrave Macmillan, 2014); Emm Barnes Johnstone and Joanna Baines, *The Changing Faces of Childhood Cancer: Clinical and Cultural Vision since 1940* (Houndmills: Palgrave Macmillan, 2014); Agnes Arnold-Forster, *The Cancer Problem: Malignancy in*

establishment of radiology as an alternative to surgery, first in the form of x-rays, and later in the form of radiotherapy. These new medical disciplines exerted an influence on how cancer was diagnosed and treated. And in a more extended sense over a longer stretch of time, they made their mark on ideas about the body and society, health and sickness, the domination and destruction of nature, what it means to fight, and what constitutes a threat.

Cancer remains one of the most talked-about diseases in the Western world. Many people are directly affected by it, either as patients themselves or as their friends or loved ones. Surveys regularly report it as one of the most feared illnesses. Medical research on oncogenes—genes that predispose a person to cancer—tends to focus on the unique characteristics of the individual. It has ignited debates about what it says about human nature that we may carry within ourselves the seeds of our own bodies' destruction. This forces us to confront the discomforting notion that cancer represents a 'distorted version of our normal selves' that we might never completely be able to 'slay' without also extinguishing our own life.[19] Our contemporary understanding of risk factors and preventative measures compels us to think about the risks we take in our lives and the risks inscribed into our very own bodies and to consider the price that we are willing to pay for a greater degree of relative security. The complexity of cancer gives urgency to questions about the therapeutic, human, ethical, and economic limits of contemporary medicine.

Since the early 1990s, 'emerging diseases' have captured the popular imagination as an equally threatening, yet wholly different medical problem.[20] These highly contagious viruses about which little or nothing is known can be transferred to humans by animals, unleashing a pandemic that doctors are incapable of harnessing. The current Covid-19 pandemic sheds a harsh light on this danger, but there have been other examples before, the most notorious being the 2003/4 outbreak of SARS, which was quickly brought under control, as well as the 2014 and 2018 Ebola epidemic. But the late 1980s also represented a different kind of turning point for perceptions of cancer.

Nineteenth-Century Britain (Oxford: Oxford University Press, 2021). On Germany there currently exists Proctor's study on cancer during National Socialism: Robert N. Proctor, *The Nazi War on Cancer* (Princeton: Princeton University Press, 2000).

[19] These were Harold E. Varmus's words in his Nobel Prize acceptance speech, awarded to him and J. Michael Bishop for their research on retroviral oncogenes. Playing on the Anglo-Saxon epic *Beowulf*, Varmus said: 'We have not slain our enemy, the cancer cell, or figuratively torn the limbs from his body. In our adventures, we have only seen our monster more clearly and described his scales and fangs in new ways—ways that reveal a cancer cell to be, like Grendel, a distorted version of our normal selves.' See Harold E. Varmus, Banquet Speech, nobelprize.org, http://www.nobelprize.org/nobel_prizes/medicine/laureates/1989/varmus-speech.html.

[20] The concept 'emerging diseases' was coined during a conference in the United States in 1989: Joshua Lederberg, Robert E. Shope, and Stanley C. Oaks, Jr, eds, *Emerging Infections: Microbial Threats to Health in the United States* (Washington, DC: National Academies Press, 1992).

In the 1970s, chemotherapy became established as a standard method of treating cancer. Its successes with Hodgkin lymphoma as well as with leukaemia, which until then had been considered uncurable, seemed to hold great promise. Around the same time, doctors began to embrace integrative oncology, which calls together all the specialists treating a person to collaborate in the development of a treatment plan. This new approach in treatment also instigated a paradigm shift in how doctors viewed cancer, as it implied that cancer was a disease of the 'whole' person. As a consequence, adjuvant therapy, which aims to strengthen the body and improve the patient's well-being during treatment, became more common. Beyond eliminating the disease, doctors came to be concerned with bettering the 'quality of life' of people 'living with cancer'—two new key terms of oncology—while psycho-oncology developed into a discipline to study and treat the relation between cancer and its psychological impact. New types of tumour centres did justice to these trends by assisting with recovery and rehabilitation and connecting patients with social services. The first West German oncological institute at the University Clinic of Essen-Duisburg, which was established in 1967, followed the model set by American Comprehensive Cancer Centres, but only in the late 1970s did others in Germany follow in its footsteps. The goals of these institutions seemed incompatible with the old practice of concealing from patients their diagnosis and thus capped off a process that had been long in the making.

Two other developments made cancer into a topic of public concern and interest: the hospice movement, which, in Germany, consisted of a multitude of local associations, and the organization of self-help groups in the 1980s. These groups have sought to imbue with greater visibility the interests, problems, demands, and feelings of cancer patients. They have enabled people to share their experiences and support one another both during and after treatment.

Only since the beginning of the 1980s has there been a significant uptick in the cure rates of many, but certainly not all types of cancer. Progressively more oncologists consider cancer a chronic illness, because many cases of cancer can be treated in such a way that the patient can either be totally cured or can live with a manageable tumour until they die of an unrelated cause. British historian Joanna Baines wrote a captivating account of this historical transformation by comparing her mother's and grandmother's illness with her own, not yet finished experience with cancer.[21]

Cancer might be seen as the paradigmatic illness of the twentieth century. The history of cancer contained in this book starts in the last years of the nineteenth century, a time when fear of cancer was growing rapidly, as French historian Pierre Darmon writes.[22] It concludes with the 1990s and compares the historical developments traced out in the book with today's cancer regime.

[21] Joanna Baines, 'Three Stories: Generations of Breast Cancer', in Timmermann and Toon, *Cancer Patients, Cancer Pathways*, 13–35, 27–8.

[22] Pierre Darmon, *Les cellules folles. L'homme face au cancer de l'antiquité à nos jours* (Paris: Pion, 1993), 143–305.

Uncertainty

A constitutive part of the history of cancer in the twentieth century was the uncertainty about the disease, and this in an epoch when security—defined by a desire for utmost certainty—was on the ascendant. Uncertainty permeated nearly every aspect of it. There was uncertainty about how to properly diagnosis it. Sure, cellular pathologists had developed criteria to identify cancerous cells under a microscope. But did cancerous cells in a sample mean that the person had cancer? Already in the early twentieth century, medical scientists observed that some cancers progressed so slowly that they would not become a deadly disease during the lifetime of the patient, while others grew rapidly, metastasized, and led to a quick death. How to distinguish the one from the other? Refined diagnostic techniques made it possible to differentiate 'abnormal' cells that, nevertheless, did not have all the features of truly cancerous ones. But were these cells always precursors to cancerous cells, as terms like *carcinoma in situ* and *pre-cancerous* suggested? And if so, did they always need to be treated as cancerous so that they never developed into cancer? Many doctors were aware of these diagnostic uncertainties, even if they generally remained unknown to patients, only entering into the broader public discussion later on in the century. Because the decision to, when in doubt, treat 'abnormal' cells as cancer in order to avoid placing the patient at risk was normally made without their knowledge or consent.

Therapy and prognosis were unsettled by the same uncertainty. A treatment that worked for one patient might fail for another with a seemingly identical type of cancer; a third patient might react well at first but then suffer from a deadly relapse or metastasis. For most of the twentieth century, these differences could be neither predicted nor explained. Only in the last third of the twentieth century did scientists discover molecular and genetic distinctions in what had until then appeared to be the same types of cancer. For example, the presence or absence of certain hormone receptors can affect the outcomes of breast cancer, and doctors can test women for a genetic predisposition to cancer in order to determine their risk for breast cancer or ovarian cancer and rule out certain forms of chemotherapy as ineffective from the outset. Doctors were similarly uncertain about their ability to predict how long a cancer patient might live. Their prognoses drew on clinical experience and statistics about how long a person with a given stage of cancer could survive, but their patients often died much sooner or lived surprisingly longer than they expected.

Aetiology was fraught with uncertainty, too.[23] In the laboratory and the clinic, scientists and doctors tested out the most diverse theories on what might cause cancer: could it be traced back to chemicals, exposure to radioactivity, injuries,

[23] On German oncological research, see Gabriele Moser, *Deutsche Forschungsgemeinschaft und Krebsforschung 1920–1970* (Stuttgart: Franz Steiner, 2011).

trauma, parasites, viral infections, genetic factors, bad habits like smoking and drinking, food, psychic disposition, emotions? And what were the deciding factors that led cancerous cells to become full-blown cancer? Was it always preceded by a more general physical debilitation, or did cancer always begin locally? At any rate, experimental and epidemiological evidence proved that certain substances were carcinogenic. Occupational cancers like Schneeberg lung disease helped doctors understand early on that exposure to some materials could cause cancer; the everyday experiences of radiology demonstrated that exposure to radioactivity could cause cancer; and psychological tests and the personality profiles deduced from them seemed to indicate that psychic factors could play a role, too. Nevertheless, the question remained open as to whether there was a single cause of cancer, and over the course of the twentieth century, medical scientists began to doubt that there was one.

American oncologist Bert Vogelstein, one of the first to sequence cancer genes, argues that each patient's cancer is unique because it arises out of the unique mutations of that individual's unique genetic makeup.[24] Although this insight is relatively new, researchers in the early twentieth century were already distinguishing between different types of cancer depending on the site of the tumour and the cancerous cells' tissue of origin. These distinctions were important for selecting which form of treatment might be most effective, but they were also decisive for how people perceived their own cancer and the pain, taboos, and vulnerability that they would have to contend with.

However, the emotional practices and emotional knowledge detailed in this book generally applied to all types of cancer, despite their differences. The commonalities were so significant that this history of cancer only analyses particular types of cancer for themselves when they spurred on distinctive emotional practices and knowledge.

The lack of certainty about cancer, perceived by many as a threat to the individual and society, opened a space in which emotions took on an extraordinary value. The need to act and make decisions (even the decision not to act) was felt to be pressing. In the face of uncertainty about what to do and how to do it, emotions helped people bridge the gap. They could ease the decision-making process and could be tapped to convince people to act in one way or another. Cancer always seemed to be a sign that death was not far off, even if those impacted often did not know how far. But in contrast to the twentieth century's influenza epidemics, cancer was not an existential threat that could strike at any second. This complexity is why cancer set off long processes of navigating feelings and trying to find the best way to relate to one's emotions and those of others. It is the history of these emotional practices that the book analyses.

[24] See Mukherjee, *Emperor*, 452.

The Spaces of Cancer and Their Emotional Meaning

In the twentieth century, cancer was both talked about and hushed in all sorts of places: on the street, at the bakery or the hairdresser, at the café, at film and TV studios, at the office, at home, in parliaments, at universities, at churches. But then there were spaces where cancer was front and centre all the time, spaces whose concrete dimensions and designs were veritably shaped by the experience of cancer and the attempt to confront it. Alongside these literal spaces were the metaphors of space in writings by doctors, journalists, politicians, and patients themselves. The notion that cancer submits its sufferers to its own rules and laws, forcing them into its regime, is a metaphor that was repeated in varying forms throughout the twentieth century; it found one of its earliest incarnations in Rudolf Virchow's concept of the cell state. These spatial metaphors and the actual existence of 'spaces of cancer' in the twentieth century suggest that we might be best advised to analyse the history of cancer and emotions in these spaces.[25]

This book explores four spaces of cancer in the twentieth century: the spaces of researching cancer, of detecting and raising awareness about cancer, of communicating a cancer diagnosis, and the space of cancer treatment, experiencing cancer, and dying from cancer. Out of these spaces emerged specific conceptions of what cancer was and what it meant, which in turn gave rise to certain practices and led to their alteration and, in some cases, overhaul. Emotions were a key component of these practices. One aspect of knowledge about cancer was knowledge about which emotions and emotional attitudes were salubrious, harmful, helpful, or disruptive. Knowledge about emotions contoured the relationship between patients and doctors, and it shaped the architecture and design of spaces and things created for the treatment of cancer. Assumptions about emotions and their effects were regularly discussed by specialists communicating their expertise to laypersons. And knowledge about emotions influenced how doctors, nurses, and other professionals talked with and comported themselves towards cancer patients during and after treatment and towards terminally ill patients who were seen as having no chance of survival.

Whether one entered these spaces in Germany, the United States, Spain, or the United Kingdom was in some respects of little significance, since many debates took place on a transnational level. Often minimal were the differences in how Western Europe and the United States described general problems and questions, and sometimes South America and Eastern Europe deviated little from the

[25] Margrit Pernau, 'Space and Emotion: Building to Feel', *History Compass* 12, no. 7 (2014): 541–9, https://doi.org/10.1111/hic3.12170; Andreas Reckwitz, 'Affective Spaces: A Praxeological Outlook', *Rethinking History* 16, no. 2 (2012): 241–58, https://doi.org/10.1080/13642529.2012.681193; Dagmar Hänel and Alois Unterkircher, 'Die Verräumlichung des Medikalen. Zur Einführung in den Band', in *Medikale Räume. Zur Interdependenz von Raum, Körper, Krankheit und Gesundheit*, ed. Nicholas Eschenbruch, Dagmar Hänel, and Alois Unterkircher (Bielefeld: transcript, 2010), 7–20.

apparently transnational consensus, too. But when it came to the concrete practices performed in these spaces, there were significant differences between countries and regions. Moreover, the design and technical outfitting of the spaces of cancer were significantly influenced by medical, occupational, and institutional traditions, as well as by healthcare systems and the amount of money invested in them—all factors that differ from nation to nation. This book concentrates on Germany, but it also looks at transnational exchanges and entanglements.

Because it begins with the turn of the twentieth century and ends around 1990, the book is confronted with the problem of how to set the story forth after 1945. I have decided against undertaking a systematic comparison of the history of East and West Germany. Instead, I write about the forty years between 1945/9 (the end of the Second World War and the founding of the two separate German states) and 1990 as a period of history that runs in two parallel paths; in fact, in some places, these paths come so close that they can be considered as a single history with different accents. In other spaces, though, the differences are more pronounced; here, I present developments in the two states separately.[26]

The first chapter introduces readers to the clinics and laboratories where research on cancer took place. These were spaces where, in the run of the twentieth century, various causes of cancer were investigated and a multitude of methods and medicines to fight it were tested. In the early twentieth century, researchers showed marginal interest in emotions' role in the genesis of cancer. It was only in the 1940s that medical doctors and psychologists working with the theory of 'psychosomatics' started to assay the relationship between emotions and cancer with increasing urgency.[27] Nevertheless, the lack of psychosomatic cancer research in the early twentieth century represents in itself an instructive fact for the history of the relationship between emotions and cancer, because an analysis of both this lack and the psychosomatic boom reveals much about how the body, emotions, and cancer were understood in the respective eras and how this understanding affected oncological research and treatment.

The chapter explores why oncologists initially thought it best to look beyond emotions in their research and the reasons why they ultimately decided to integrate emotions into their work. Metaphors of the state as a human body

[26] Frank Bösch, 'Geteilte Geschichte. Plädoyer für eine deutsch-deutsche Perspektive auf die jüngere Zeitgeschichte', *Zeithistorische Forschungen/Studies in Contemporary History* 12, no. 1 (2015): 98–114; Dorothee Wierling, 'Über Asymmetrien. Ein Kommentar zu Frank Bösch', *Zeithistorische Forschungen/Studies in Contemporary History* 12, no. 1 (2015): 115–23, 117–18.

[27] The history of psychosomatic research on cancer has been little studied; the few existing works include: Patricia Jasen, 'Malignant Histories: Psychosomatic Medicine and the Female Cancer Patient in the Postwar Era', *Bulletin canadien d'histoire de la médicine = Canadian Bulletin of Medical History* 20, no. 2 (2003): 265–97; Bettina Hitzer and Pilar León-Sanz, 'The Feeling Body and Its Diseases: How Cancer Went Psychosomatic in Twentieth-Century Germany', *Osiris* 31, no. 1 (2016): 67–93, https://doi.org/10.1086/687591; Bettina Hitzer, 'Krebs oder wie weit reicht die psychosomatische Medizin', in *Auf der Suche nach einer anderen Medizin. Psychosomatik im 20. Jahrhundert*, ed. Bettina Hitzer and Alexa Geisthövel (Frankfurt am Main: Suhrkamp, 2019), 258–72.

were central, because the merger of the individual's body and the body of the state was a key aspect of the history of psychosomatics, which claimed to work with a 'holistic', 'psychosocial' view of human health.

The second chapter studies the ways in which public health campaigns sought to communicate knowledge about cancer to laypeople. Their aim was to teach people about cancer, early detection check-ups, and prevention strategies. Stakeholders heatedly debated the meaning of emotions for public health campaigns from the very beginning. Some wondered whether knowledge about cancer should be presented in digestible forms to a broad audience at all, worrying that talking openly about the disease might strike people with fear and make them panic—potentially fatal emotional effects. Others wondered which emotions might help people be more aware of early symptoms and assume more responsibility for their own physical health. All of this took place in a period when conceptions of preventive care, health, well-being, and happiness were shifting and social hygiene, pseudoscientific race science, and eugenics were on the rise. Cultivating the right feelings and knowledge in exhibitions and advertising campaigns was another issue of contention. Doctors, health ministers, exhibition curators, and filmmakers all passionately debated how exhibition spaces should appear, which images and objects should be included, and which stories should be told in order to meet the task at hand. The techniques of knowledge transmission drew on the media psychology of their time, but they also took cues from ideas about emotions' significance in the lives and treatment of cancer patients. At the same time, these discussions left their trace on the actual treatment of cancer, even if just because the ever-increasing talk about cancer in public awareness campaigns made it more difficult to conceal a diagnosis from a sick patient.

In these first two spaces, knowledge about cancer was produced and communicated by and for people who were not themselves suffering from cancer. They could freely enter and exit them at their own leisure. This sets them apart from the spaces that envelop the second part of this book, because those who entered them were forced to. They were cancer patients, their friends and loved ones, nurses, and oncologists. Nurses and doctors could leave when they clocked out, but the patients and, often, their friends and family, could not.

Many patients describe learning about their illness as the moment when they went from being a 'healthy' person to being a 'cancer patient', even if they had suspected they were sick and were not surprised by the diagnosis. It leads a person into spaces that they had heretofore known little about, where their direct, embodied experience of these spaces' strange rules, atmospheres, usages, and instruments is defined by the existential danger confronting them. For many, this moment initiates a new form of existence that will be determined by the illness from here on out. But the diagnosis is not a static thing. It has its own history that involved questions like whether and how a doctor should tell their patients about their diagnosis, how stark the line between cancer and non-cancer was drawn, which knowledge patients and doctors brought to these talks in the first place, how invasive the treatment was, and how long it lasted. All of these factors influenced the ways in which the diagnosis was experienced and felt as a transition from one mode of being into another.

This chapter explores the history of cancer diagnoses as a moment after which nothing is as it was before, as a moment of shock, and as a chance to start over, which is how many patients today perceive it. But it also analyses the arguments that doctors, nurses, psychologists, theologists, and jurists employed in the conflict over whether and how patients should be told that they have cancer. The feeling of hope played a central role in these debates, as people asked what hope was and what its object could be, what hope might mean for human life and survival, and how destructive, permissible, or 'normal' despair was.

The fourth chapter follows patients into the spaces of cancer treatment: operating theatres, clinics, gynaecologists' offices, the few early hospitals specially designed for cancer patients, the sometimes foreboding radiology rooms, and the historically new oncology departments, where people were treated with chemotherapy. These spaces brought together patients and their loved ones, doctors and nurses, and therapeutic 'things'.[28] Places, objects, and other people moulded patients' time with cancer and the feelings they felt towards it. This chapter focuses not on the individual experience with cancer, but on the conditions that shaped it.

The different spaces of cancer treatment merged in at least three senses. First, treatment rooms and research facilities often remained opaque for patients, while they overlapped to the point of indistinction for doctors and scientists. The effects of radiotherapy and chemotherapy were tested out not only in labs, but also in the clinic itself. This intertwining of two theoretically non-identical spaces caused the spaces of research and treatment and their mutually influencing logics to permeate one another.[29]

Second, the walls between the spaces of treatment and the 'outside' world were porous. Patients, their loved ones, and doctors and nurses all brought preformed knowledge about cancer, emotions, the body, and pain into the clinic. And they had changed notions when they left, whether it be in the days between chemotherapy

[28] This concept of the therapeutic 'thing' latches onto discussions in historiography and sociology on how things and their specific materiality influence human action and are themselves altered by how people perceive, construct, and use them. See Simone Derix, Benno Gammerl, Christiane Reinecke, and Nina Verheyen (2016), 'Der Wert der Dinge. Zur Wirtschafts- und Sozialgeschichte der Materialitäten', *Zeithistorische Forschungen/Studies in Contemporary History* 13, no. 3 (2016): 387–403. On the epistemic/technological thing, see Hans-Jörg Rheinberger, *Toward a History of Epistemic Things: Synthesizing Proteins in the Test Tube* (Stanford: Stanford University Press, 1997).

[29] Peter Keating and Alberto Cambrosio, *Cancer on Trial: Oncology as a New Style of Practice* (Chicago: University of Chicago Press, 2012); Gerald Kutcher, 'A Case Study in Human Experimentation: The Patient as Subject, Object and Victim', in Timmermann and Toon, *Cancer Patients*, 57–77; Gerald Kutcher, *Contested Medicine: Cancer Research and the Military* (Chicago: University of Chicago Press, 2009).

treatments, as a cancer survivor or a terminally ill patient, as a relative giving support, or as a doctor heading home after the workday. This chapter thus engages with the interplay between the worlds inside and outside the spaces of cancer treatment and the ways in which the radically different expectations and influences they harboured defined the emotions of those who passed through their doors.

Third, the spaces of cancer treatment cannot be definitively demarcated from spaces of death and survival. When was treatment finished, when did post-treatment start, and when did the attempt to cure end because the process of dying had begun? Both doctors and patients often had a difficult time answering these questions. At the beginning of the century, the answer was generally more definite, while at its end, the lines between therapy and recovery as well as therapy and palliative care were progressively blurred. However unclear these transitions might have appeared, they still required doctors and patients to make decisions. Should (former) cancer patients be cared for after their curative treatment? How were dying people supposed to feel, and how did they feel in reality? The answers opened up new possibilities and closed off others. They defined understandings of dignity, quality of life, and what it meant to live a meaningful life. They created structures that guided people in their relations to themselves and others, structures that people infused with emotion.

Historical Perspectives: Thoughts on Morality and Linearity

> Barb, at this time in your life, it's so important to pull all your energies toward a peaceful, if not happy, existence. Cancer is a rotten thing to have happened and there are no answers for any of us as to why. But to live your life, whether you have one more year or 51, in anger and bitterness is such a waste.... I hope you can find some peace. You deserve it. We all do.[30]

This reaction and many others like it filled the replies to a post made by American columnist Barbara Ehrenreich on a self-help site for cancer patients. Under the subject line 'Angry', Ehrenreich described the side effects of chemotherapy and raged against the injustices of her health insurance provider, carcinogenic pollution, and the 'sappy pink ribbons' popularized by the Susan G. Komen Foundation. Ehrenreich saw in the comments to her entry an expression of norms that dictate that everyone greet cancer diagnosis happily as a chance at a new beginning. She responded with an attack on the American culture of positive thinking in her bitingly titled book *Smile or Die*.

[30] Barbara Ehrenreich, *Smile or Die: How Positive Thinking Fooled America and the World* (London: Granta, 2009), 32.

But such normative emotion regimes are nothing new. The appeal to open oneself to new feelings has often gone hand in hand with a denigration of other emotions and emotional dispositions. People might have a hard time dissecting why their society seems to validate certain emotions as 'natural' or 'authentic' as a matter of common sense, which exerts a power that makes it difficult to break outside its strictures. This book aims to graph the expanse and efficacy of emotion regimes and their different normative structures, because only by unearthing concrete knowledge about the historicity of these regimes, their effects, and their 'costs' and 'benefits' can we take a freer look at contemporary emotion regimes and expand our perspectives on what goes into the construction of emotions and the evaluation thereof.

As a consequence, this book does not tell a tale of simple progress in which stifling taboos were supplanted with a more emotionally liberated approach to cancer. At the same time, it does not contain a narrative of decline that laments the 'capture' of emotions by psychologists and therapists in the service of a neoliberal image of humanity.

Rather, the book gumshoes through the historical developments beyond mere linearity. Individual emotions play a significant role in this history: fear, sadness, hope; shame, disgust, rage. In the last few years much has been written about fear and anxiety.[31] Some historians, philosophers, and sociologists opine that fear and anxiety were the signature feeling of the twentieth century, alluding to W. H. Auden's 1947 poem 'The Age of Anxiety' or designating the Federal Republic of Germany as a 'republic of fear'.[32] But was fear truly the dominant emotion all the way through the century? Do emotions hold different weight in different historical periods, undergoing trends in which they are sometimes bullish, taking on greater significance and pick up momentum, and sometimes bearish, receding into the background? Did fear itself change, away from the concrete fear of external objects as the late nineteenth century defined it and towards a diffuse anxiety that blurred the old division between inside and outside and contributed to an individualization of society?[33] Where does the fear of cancer fit in this shift, and where does it fit in the twentieth-century history of fear traced by some historians, in which concepts like risk and security garnered increased

[31] For two examples from different disciplines, see Anne Springer, Bernhard Janta, and Karsten Münch, eds, *Angst* (Giessen: Psychosozial Verlag, 2011); and Lars Koch, ed., *Angst. Ein interdisziplinäres Handbuch* (Stuttgart: Metzler, 2013).

[32] Frank Biess, *German Angst? Fear and Democracy in the Federal Republic Germany* (Oxford: Oxford University Press, 2020); Wystan H. Auden, *The Age of Anxiety: A Baroque Eclogue* (Princeton: Princeton University Press, 2011); Heinz Bude, *Society of Fear* (Medford, MA: Polity Press, 2018); Cass Sunstein, *Laws of Fear* (Cambridge: Cambridge University Press, 2005); Frank Furedi, *Culture of Fear: Risk-Taking and the Morality of Low Expectation*, rev. edn (London: Continuum, 2003).

[33] Joanna Bourke, *Fear: A Cultural History* (London: Counterpoint, 2006).

importance?[34] Did other feelings central for the history of cancer and emotions undergo similar shifts and trends?

The book also analyzes the relation between the upvaluation of certain emotions and shifts in the assessment of emotions' significance more generally. The preponderant narrative says that emotional frigidity dominated in matters of feeling at the turn to the twentieth century. Peter Stearns describes the ascent of the Victorian 'cool emotionology' at the end of the nineteenth century, which helped defined the emotional habitus of scientists.[35] But hadn't the scientific ideal of rational objectivity already taken the place of fascination and wonder a hundred years previously, as Lorraine Daston and Peter Galison have shown?[36] What does empirical research tell us about the relation between the history of emotions and the history of science and their relation to history more generally? This question accompanies this history of cancer in the twentieth century. Because, if one follows Helmut Lethen, the emotional ice age remained a burden up into the 1920s.[37] Rationalization took primacy in this period, as did its associated ideals of planning, scientific calculation, and technological application. Its proponents explicitly targeted a certain form of emotionally guided action, but they also wanted to rationalize emotions themselves. Violence and emotion were key elements of the strategies of the extreme political movements of the 1920s and 1930s, which thus hitched onto this trend while at the same time themselves understanding emotions as irrational.[38]

[34] Eckart Conze, *Geschichte der Sicherheit: Entwicklung—Themen—Perspektiven* (Göttingen: Vandenhoeck & Ruprecht, 2018); Bettina Hitzer, 'Jim Button's Fear', in *Learning How to Feel: Children's Literature and Emotional Socialization, 1870–1970*, ed. Ute Frevert, Pascal Eitler, Stephanie Olsen, Uffa Jensen, Margrit Pernau, Daniel Brückenhaus, Magdalena Beljan, Benno Gammerl, Anja Laukötter, Bettina Hitzer, Jan Plamper, Juliane Brauer, and Joachim C. Häberlen (Oxford: Oxford University Press, 2014), 173–90; Frank Biess, 'The Concept of Panic in Postwar Germany: Military Psychiatry and Emotional Preparation for Nuclear War in the West German Army', in *Science and Emotions after 1945: A Transatlantic Perspective*, ed. Frank Biess and Daniel Gross (Chicago: University of Chicago Press), 181–208; Michael Laffan and Max Weiss, *Facing Fear: The History of an Emotion in Global Perspective* (Princeton: Princeton University Press, 2012); Frank Biess, 'Feelings in the Aftermath: Toward a History of Postwar Emotions', in *Histories of the Aftermath: The Legacies of the Second World War in Europe*, ed. Frank Biess and Robert Moeller (New York: Berghahn, 2010), 30–48; Frank Biess, 'Die Sensibilisierung des Subjekts: Angst und "neue Subjektivität" in den 1970cr Jahren', *Werkstatt Geschichte* 49 (2008): 51–72; Peter N. Stearns, *American Fear: The Causes and Consequences of High Anxiety* (New York: Routledge, 2006).

[35] Peter N. Stearns, *American Cool: Constructing a Twentieth-Century Emotional Style* (New York: New York University Press, 1994).

[36] Lorraine Daston and Katherine Park, *Wonders and the Order of Nature, 1150–1750* (New York: Zone Books, 1998); Lorraine Daston and Peter Galison, *Objectivity* (New York: Zone Books, 2007).

[37] Helmut Lethen, *Verhaltenslehren der Kälte. Lebensversuche zwischen den Kriegen* (Frankfurt am Main: Suhrkamp, 1997).

[38] Uffa Jensen and Daniel Morat, eds, *Rationalisierungen des Gefühls. Zum Verhältnis von Wissenschaft und Emotionen 1880–1930* (Munich: Wilhelm Fink, 2008); Ute Frevert, 'Rationalität und Emotionalität im Jahrhundert der Extreme', in *Das 20. Jahrhundert vermessen. Signaturen eines vergangenen Zeitalters*, ed. Martin Sabrow and Peter Ulrich Weiß (Göttingen: Vandenhoeck & Ruprecht, 2017), 115–40, 123–7; Biess, 'Feelings in the Aftermath', 32.

The identification of emotions and irrationality reached its zenith in post-war West Germany. Heavily resistant to the perversion of language, emotions, and many other aspects of everyday life enforced by the National Socialist regime, West Germany viewed emotions as inaccessible to reason and banished them to be managed privately by the individual.[39] In contrast, East German political leaders appealed to emotions in the 1950s to forge a bond between citizens and the state.[40] In the late 1960s, West German society gradually revaluated emotions, a change initially embraced by social movements and experimented with by the alternative left.[41] It is not clear if there was a similar trend in East German social movements.

At the same time, the scientificization of emotions picked up steam. Begun by the establishment of psychology as an autonomous discipline in the nineteenth century and driven forth by the advent of psychoanalysis, it also took hold in cultural studies and the social sciences.[42] In the 1970s, this trend fused with an unprecedented expansion of therapy, which increasingly blurred the line between the normal and the pathological and held high the ideal that emotions were endlessly plastic.[43] Emotional self-regulation seemed possible, and an army of experts, advice guides, and techniques of processing emotions stood by to help. It remains an unresolved question as to whether this development elevated the responsibility to regulate one's own emotions to the level of a moral imperative.[44]

This rough outline sketches the image of the twentieth century projected by extant research on the history of emotions. This is context of this book's exploration of the four spaces of cancer, spaces in which emotions were researched, acted out, and suffered, defined, communicated, and experienced.

[39] Biess, 'Feelings in the Aftermath', 31–3; Paul Erickson, Judy L. Klein, Lorraine Daston, Rebecca Lemov, Thomas Sturm, and Michael D. Gordin, *How Reason Almost Lost Its Mind: The Strange Career of Cold War Rationality* (Chicago: University of Chicago Press, 2013), 1–26; Anna M. Parkinson, *An Emotional State: The Politics of Emotion in Postwar West German Culture* (Ann Arbor: University of Michigan Press, 2015).

[40] Ute Frevert, *Vertrauensfragen. Eine Obsession der Moderne* (Munich: C.H. Beck, 2013), 190–4; Juliane Brauer, '"Mit neuem Fühlen und neuem Geist". Heimatliebe und Patriotismus in Kinder- und Jugendliedern der frühen DDR', in *Das Imaginäre des Kalten Krieges. Beiträge zu einer Kulturgeschichte des Ost-West-Konfliktes in Europa*, ed. David Eugster and Sybille Marti (Essen: Klartext, 2015), 163–86; Jan C. Behrends, 'Freundschaft zur Sowjetunion, Liebe zu Stalin. Zur Anthorpomorphisierung des Politischen im Stalinismus', in *Die Massen bewegen. Medien und Emotionen in der Moderne*, ed. Frank Bösch and Manuel Borutta (Frankfurt am Main: Campus, 2006), 172–92.

[41] Susanne Schregel, 'Konjunktur der Angst. "Politik der Subjektivität" und "neue Friedensbewegung", 1979–1983', in *Angst im Kalten Krieg*, ed. Bernd Greiner, Christian Th. Müller, and Dierk Walter (Hamburg: Hamburger Edition/HIS Verlag, 2009), 495–520; Judith Michel, '"Die Angst kann lehren, sich zu wehren"—Der Angstdiskurs der westdeutschen Friedensbewegung in den 1980er Jahren', in *Politische Leidenschaften. Zur Verknüpfung von Macht, Emotion und Vernunft in Deutschland (= Tel Aviver Jahrbuch für deutsche Geschichte* 38), ed. José Brunner (Göttingen: Vandenhoeck & Ruprecht, 2010), 246–69; Stefanie Pilzweger, *Männlichkeit zwischen Gefühl und Revolution. Eine Emotionsgeschichte der bundesdeutschen 68er Bewegung* (Bielefeld: transcript, 2015); Joachim C. Häberlen, *The Emotional Politics of the Alternative Left: West Germany, 1968–1984* (Cambridge: Cambridge University Press, 2018).

[42] Plamper, *History of Emotions*, 201–6.

[43] Maik Tändler, *Das therapeutische Jahrzehnt. Der Psychoboom in den siebziger Jahren* (Göttingen: Wallstein, 2016).

[44] Ute Frevert, 'Emotional Knowledge: Modern Developments', in Frevert et al., *Emotional Lexicons*, 260–73, 277; Pascal Eitler, Stephanie Olsen, and Uffa Jensen, 'Introduction' to Frevert et al., *Learning How to Feel*, 1–20, 17.

2
Researching Cancer

In the autumn of 1974, 29-year-old Frau S. ascended the stairs of the Heidelberg Clinic on Bergheimer Street. She stood for a moment in front of the tall historicist portal inscribed 'Frauen-Klinik' (women's clinic) in an old-fashioned font. Perhaps she thought about how many women had walked through this door, full of excitement or full of anxiety, in pain, or just in need of information like herself. She was just here to find out 'if it was harmless', as the resident gynaecologist had said after telling her about the somewhat abnormal result of a routine Pap smear done a few days before. She was here to undergo another gynaecological test and perhaps an x-ray. So, she was a bit surprised when a nurse led her into the doctor's room and the doctor greeted her by saying: 'We are going to conduct a few tests on you for scientific purposes, which are being done on all women in your age group.' What did this have to do with the suspicious test result? When she cautiously asked, the doctor promised her that he would explain after the test was concluded.

He first asked her about her private life and her personal history. She told him about how she met her husband and quickly married him in order to be able to move out of her parents' house. She talked about her conflicts with her husband, his lack of understanding for her feelings, and his obsession with his business. She recounted how he regularly cheated on her and how the marriage ended in divorce after ten years. The doctor also wanted to know more about her relationship with her parents and her younger brother. After some hesitation, she talked about her strict father, who only cared about her brother, and about her worrisome mother, who hardly gave her room to breathe.

She looked expectantly at the doctor: was the actual test going to begin now? Then the doctor pulled a piece of paper out of a folder, placed it on the desk, and explained: 'You can see all kinds of things in these inkblots; please tell me what you see, what you think it might be and what it reminds you of.' Frau S. looked at the images in confusion. They reminded her a bit of the pictures of butterflies that her son had proudly made by folding a piece of paper with ink on it. 'Can I turn the images?' she asked uncertainly. 'That's entirely up to you', the doctor replied matter-of-factly. She picked one up and was gripped for a moment by restlessness and irritation. She thought that she had come here to have a medical issue resolved. But instead she was now sitting here looking at some splats of ink. Then she lightly sighed and concentrated on the image.

Was she supposed to see a bat—or a moth? With a soft, interrogative voice, she attempted to answer. She was handed nine more images, some with vibrant colours, pretty, but a bit confusing. The doctor repeatedly cued in, insisting: 'Some people see more than one thing here—if that is true for you, then please tell me.' She felt a bit simple. Clearly, others knew more than her. When she had finally seen all ten images, the doctor placed all of them in front of her and read her responses aloud, inquiring into which part of this or that inkblot had led her to see a carpet or spider in it. It was finally over.

But the test still had not begun. Now she was supposed to answer questions, checking off whether a statement was true or false: 'I don't like to be around strangers.' Is that true? She got distracted and thought of the last teacher-parents' meeting she had attended: Yes, it is. The doctor observed her contemplatively while she ticked the box. Did she have cancer? After Frau S. had worked through 114 questions over the course of half an hour, the doctor said: 'This is the last test' and placed another stack of paper before her. She was again supposed to tick the statements that applied to her. Some of the forty-nine questions seemed odd to her. She stole a look at the doctor when she read: 'I find my sex life to be satisfying.' But he's a doctor, so you can check no. Then she read: 'For some people, death can be a release.' She suddenly felt cold. What's that supposed to mean? Does that have anything to do with . . . ? Just twenty-six questions to go, then she would be finished. She looked at the clock a bit apprehensively, but relieved. Nearly two hours had gone by since she had opened the clinic's heavy door. The doctor looked at her and smiled: 'Now you're finished. So let's start with the examination.'

What came after that consumed her fully. She soon forgot about the questions and strange inkblots. The cancer, the operation, the radiotherapy, and the many subsequent operations needed to make the effects of this therapy somewhat bearable took all her energy.

Frau S. was asked all these questions as part of a study conducted by doctoral student Michael Holm-Hadulla at the University of Heidelberg's women's clinic between September 1973 and September 1976.[1] In contrast to the majority of dissertations, Holm-Hadulla's was published in 1982 as a book appended to an issue of the journal *Zeitschrift für Psychosomatische Medizin und Psychosomatik* (*Journal for Psychosomatic Medicine and Psychosomatics*). The book featured a preface by the author's adviser, Walter Bräutigam, who in 1968 succeeded Alexander Mitscherlich as head of the Heidelberg psychosomatic clinic, the 'flagship' institution of West German psychosomatics. A 1977 issue of *Der*

[1] The reconstruction of this scene is based on the case study and on Holm-Hadulla's description of the test situation and procedures. See Michael Holm-Hadulla, *Psychologische Aspekte der Krebserkrankung* (Göttingen: Vandenhoeck & Ruprecht, 1982).

Spiegel even referenced Holm-Hadulla's study as a key text in contemporaneous debates on the question: 'Can cancer be caused by psychological anguish and social stress?'[2]

The findings of a single doctoral dissertation generally do not receive so much press, making the attention paid to Holm-Hadulla's seem in itself evidence of the extent to which both medical and psychological research as well as lay discourse of the 1970s were grappling with questions about the role emotions and mental factors play in the emergence of cancer. Frau S., who entered the clinic that year because her doctor suspected she might have cancer, was thus made into an object of oncological research before she had even been diagnosed. Whether she understood what the purpose of the study was remains unknown.

In the years leading up to 1977, attentive readers of large newspapers and magazines would have been able to find articles on research into psychosomatic factors as a cause of cancer.[3] But that emotions could influence whether a person got cancer was in no way an epiphany that just struck out of nowhere the scientists of this generation. For centuries, it was considered a matter of common sense that feelings of sadness could cause cancer, particularly when it cast its shadow on a life for a prolonged period of time. For instance, one of the first and most comprehensive German-language encyclopaedias of the early modern period, the *Krünitz*, stated: 'Most often, however, [cancer] seems to originate from black bile (atrabiliousness); at least experience shows that sorrow, worry, grief often occasion it.'[4]

The entry relies on the theory of humoral pathology developed by late antique physician Galen of Pergamon, who believed that an excess of black bile was associated with melancholy and that melancholic people were, in turn, more susceptible to cancer. Galen's doctrine of four bodily fluids—the other three being yellow bile, phlegm, and blood—dominated medieval medicine and remained influential far into the early modern period.[5] In the nineteenth century, 'depressing mental affects' were still being blamed for causing cancer, but the reasoning behind the blame shifted away from the outdated humoral theory and towards an emphasis on physical and mental exhaustion and an overtaxing of the nerves, which meshed better with contemporaneous conceptions of the body.[6] But by the end of the nineteenth century, doctors were discarding altogether the longstanding practice of drawing connections between cancer and emotions.

[2] 'Krebs durch Seelenschmerz und soziale Qual?', *Der Spiegel* 45 (1977): 102–16.

[3] See, for instance, 'Band des Schicksals', *Der Spiegel* 25 (1968): 129–31.

[4] '2. Krebs', in *Oekonomische Encyklopädie, oder allgemeines System der Staats- Stadt- Haus- und Landwirtschaft, in alphabetischer Ordnung*, ed. Johann Georg Krünitz, vol. 48 (Berlin, 1789), 355–423, 359.

[5] Noga Arikha, *Passions and Tempers: A History of the Humours* (New York: HarperCollins, 2007).

[6] 'Krebs', in *Meyers Konversations-Lexikon. Eine Encyklopädie des allgemeinen Wissens*, vol. 10: Kirschbaum–Luzy, 3rd rev. edn (Leipzig, 1877), 329–30. See also Bettina Hitzer, 'Healing Emotions', in Frevert et al., *Emotional Lexicons*, 118–50, 129–32, and, on the theory of physical exhaustion, see Anson Rabinbach, *The Human Motor: Energy, Fatigue, and the Origins of Modernity* (Berkeley: University of California Press, 1992).

Why did this tradition lose credibility in early twentieth-century medical science? Is it true that medical research stopped concerning itself with patients' emotions in favour of analysing cells under a microscope? What happened in the period between 1890 and 1950 to the assumption that emotions were the key to discerning the dark origins of cancer? And finally, why did psychosomatic interpretations of cancer come to be reappraised in post-war Germany? Which medical, physiological, psychological, social, and political factors influenced this shift?

Psychosomatic doctors' inquisitive interest in the personalities of their cancer patients altered the doctor-patient relationship. But it could also influence patients' experiences of their illness and perceptions of themselves. These changes did not remain limited to the doctor's office and treatment room, but implicated society, as the story of Frau S. highlights. This chapter probes the extent to which psychosomatic interpretations of cancer were transmuted into a mode of processing and discussing more general, non-oncological historical and social developments. One of the most controversial issues in psychosomatic discourse on cancer was the debate over whether individual and social pathologies were connected, and it defined a century of psychosomatic oncological research. Over time, various answers to this question came into and fell out of favour. As the later chapters will show, they exerted considerable impact on how people talked about cancer and how people lived with it.

What Causes Cancer? The Hypotheses of Early Oncological Research

Psychosomatic cancer research in the twentieth century worked on terrain largely delimited by experimental and clinical oncology. A brief overview of the concepts and laboratory methods sanctioned by the scientific community of the time is necessary to understand why and in what sense psychosomatic cancer research was relegated to the margins for so long. Conversely, it also helps explain why psychosomatic cancer research came to be accepted as a scientific fact—as Ludwik Fleck would put it—right at the moment when Frau S. was being examined for cervical cancer. Thus, this chapter's prelude sketches out the models, techniques, and institutional conditions that determined cancer research starting at the turn of the century.[7]

[7] Many histories of oncology do not discuss psychosomatics at all, such as David Cantor, 'Cancer', in *Companion Encyclopedia of the History of Medicine*, vol. 1, ed. W. F. Bynum and Roy Porter (New York: Taylor & Francis, 1993), 537–61. This is justified, since there were not nearly as many psychosomatic studies of cancer at any time in the twentieth century as there were on carcinogens, potential infectious causes of cancer, genetic mutations, oncogenetics, and tumour virology. Still, for a history of knowledge about cancer that seeks to explain the concrete medical, therapeutic, health policy, private, and public approaches to cancer, engaging with the history of the relation between psychosomatics and cancer is indispensable.

In 1905, the newly established journal *Medizinische Klinik* (*Medical Clinic*) conducted a survey of its readers' opinions about the causes of cancer. The first response printed was that of Vinzenz Czerny. One of the most prominent German surgeons of the time, Czerny had made a name for himself as a cancer specialist and was fundraising to found a centre for cancer research in Heidelberg. Czerny's contribution demonstrates the multifariousness of theories on the causes of cancer prevalent at the time.

Czerny had deep doubts about the 'cellular theory', which held that cancerous cells form out of embryonic cells that went unused during development. It postulated that these cells 'suddenly begin to grow and become malevolent because of chemical stimulation, mental anxiety, or trauma' (trauma theory developed into its own offshoot).[8] Czerny granted more credence to the theory that cancer had parasitic origins, which fit better with the paradigm of bacteriology ushered in by Robert Koch's research in the 1880s. Koch held that every illness is caused by a germ and that a categorical link between a germ and an illness could be established in three steps: first, the germ must be able to be detected in every instance in which a person gets a particular sickness. Second, it should be possible to isolate and reproduce the germ. Third, when the germ is transmitted to an animal, it should cause the same illness in the animal and then be able to again be found in the animal and isolated.[9]

The search for a cancer bacillus had already occasioned a number of experiments on animals that involved transferring cancerous cells from one mouse to another or injecting animals with human cancer serum. The experiments revealed that cancer could be passed from one animal to another in some cases, whereas in others it could not, with scientists stumped over what exactly the determining factors were. Clinical observations that some families experienced more cases of cancer than others remained ambiguous. Instances of *cancer à deux*, in which a couple each got cancer around the same time, seemed to support the notion that it was caused by a bacterial infection, but the majority of individual cases did not. Nevertheless, one thing was clear: the investigation of the causes of cancer was more complicated than bacteriology's classic success story, Robert Koch's discovery of the bacteria that causes tuberculosis.[10] Thus, Czerny admitted in his

[8] Vinzenz Czerny, 'Antwort auf: Umfrage über die Aetiologie des Krebses', *Medizinische Klinik* 1, no. 20 (1905): 496–8.

[9] Julius Koch, 'Baubeschreibung', *Das Heidelberger Institut für experimentelle Krebsforschung*, part 1, ed. Vinzenz Czerny (Tübingen, 1912), 14–46, 33. See Christoph Gradmann, 'Alles eine Frage der Methode. Zur Historizität der Kochschen Postulate 1840–2000', *Medizinhistorisches Journal* 43, no. 2 (2008): 121–48; Christoph Gradmann, *Krankheit im Labor. Robert Koch und die medizinische Bakteriologie* (Göttingen: Wallstein, 2005).

[10] Philipp Sarasin, Silvia Berger, Marianne Hänseler, and Myriam Spörri, eds, *Bakteriologie und Moderne. Studien zur Biopolitik des Unsichtbaren 1870–1920* (Frankfurt am Main: Suhrkamp, 2007); Silvia Berger, *Bakterien in Krieg und Frieden. Eine Geschichte der medizinischen Bakteriologie in Deutschland 1890–1933* (Göttingen: Wallstein, 2009).

response to the journal that there was no one cause of cancer, 'but a multitude that certainly all belong to the same group of cell moochers'.[11]

By juxtaposing the parasitic and cellular theories, Czerny was re-tracing the lines of debate drawn in the so-called carcinoma discussion held by the Berliner Medizinische Gesellschaft (Berlin Medical Society) in March of the same year.[12] But Czerny's decision to focus on the parasitic theory was motivated, in the end, by his gut feeling. At the end of his comparison of the two theories, he wrote: 'Additionally, the cellular theory of cancer is hopeless for the future of internal therapeutic treatment of and prophylaxis against cancer, while the parasite theory has an enormous heuristic value. This is the key reason why most doctors and many pathologists subscribe to the parasitic theory.'[13]

With astonishing openness, Czerny made the hope of therapeutic efficacy the highest principle in his recommendation on the direction research should take in a situation of great uncertainty.

The cellular theory on the one hand and the germ theory on the other represented the two poles of early twentieth-century thought on cancer. Though they were interpreted in different ways, produced a multitude of models, and were moulded to fit shifting laboratory methods, these two theories largely determined how research on the genesis of cancer was conducted in the twentieth century.[14] Certainly, the notion that there could be a cancer-causing bacteria was rejected by most scientists by the end of its first decade. Most respected oncologists also considered it improbable that parasites could transmit cancer, because generally, no parasites could be found in the blood and fluid samples taken from animals and humans suffering from it. Instead, some researchers held onto the germ theory by positing that viruses must be the trigger, even though they did not yet possess the technology to see viruses. Lacking empirical observations, the existence of viruses in the early twentieth century was at once a hypothesis and a model.[15] From the perspective of contemporary medical science, which has returned to the serious search for oncoviruses, the studies of American pathologist Peyton Rous were the most significant. Rous, who spent the year 1907 in Dresden, conducted experiments on tumours in chickens at the Rockefeller Institute for Medical Research. In 1911, he succeeded in infecting healthy chickens with a cell-

[11] Czerny, 'Antwort auf: Umfrage', 498.

[12] *Berliner Klinische Wochenschrift* 42, no. 12 (1905): 313–18 and no. 13: 373–9. Nevertheless, the debate was older. See Rudolf Virchow, 'Der Kampf der Zellen und der Bakterien', *Archiv für pathologische Anatomie und Physiologie und für klinische Medicin (Berlin)* 101 (1885): 1–13. On Virchow's text, see Eva Johach, *Krebszelle und Zellenstaat. Zur medizinischen und politischen Metaphorik in der Zellularpathologie Rudolf Virchows* (Freiburg: Rombach, 2008), 233–8.

[13] Czerny, 'Antwort auf: Umfrage', 498.

[14] Karlheinz Lüdtke, *Wissenschaftliche Kontroversen und die Entwicklung neuen Wissens in der Geschichte der Krebsforschung* (Berlin: Gesellschaft für Wissenschaftsforschung, 2007).

[15] Milton Zaitlin, 'The Discovery of the Causal Agent of the Tobacco Mosaic Disease', in *Discoveries in Plant Biology*, vol. 1, ed. Shain-Dow Kung and Shang-fa Yang (Singapore: World Scientific, 1998), 105–10.

free filtrate derived from chicken tumours in such a way that they themselves developed tumours. The virus later came to be known as the Rous sarcoma virus.[16] Rous was ultimately awarded the 1966 Nobel Prize in Medicine or Physiology for his research on oncoviruses; nevertheless, it initially received little attention within the scientific community.[17]

Alongside the germ theory and the cell theory, both of which were often combined with the trauma theory, oncology in the first half of the century was heavily influenced by the question as to whether inheritance and mutations might increase people's disposition to cancer.[18] Some interpreted the higher frequency of particular types of cancer in certain countries or populations as evidence of an inherited or 'racial' disposition to the disease. The realization that Jewish women were more seldom diagnosed with cervical cancer than non-Jewish women was considered to be a poignant example.[19]

In the late 1920s, numerous oncologists began conducting experiments on how the metabolism of 'healthy' cells differed from that of 'degenerated' cancer cells,[20] research that was heavily influenced by the work of Berlin-based biochemist Otto Warburg. The head of the newly established Kaiser Wilhelm Institute for Cell Physiology demonstrated that in contrast to other animal cells, cancer cells do not require oxygen to obtain energy, but instead prefer glycolysis—the fermentation of glucose to lactate. Accordingly, he found cancer cells to exhibit a high concentration of lactic acid. Warburg hypothesized that the genesis of cancer cells had its origins in dysfunctional mitochondria. The Nobel Committee bestowed him with the 1931 prize for medicine for his work on what would later be called the Warburg Effect.[21]

The founding of the Comité für Krebssammelforschung (Committee for General Cancer Research) in 1900, renamed Deutsches Zentralkomitee zur

[16] Peyton Rous, 'Transmission of a Malignant Growth by Means of a Cell-Free-Filtrate' (reprint of article from 1911), *JAMA: Journal of the American Medical Association* 250, no. 11 (1983): 1445–6, https://doi.org/10.1001/jama.1983.03340110059037.

[17] Wolfgang U. Eckart, 'Tumorvirologie—Linien der Forschungsgeschichte', in Eckart, *100 Years of Organized Cancer Research*, 101–6; Ton van Helvoort, 'Viren als Krebserreger: Peyton Rous, das "infektiöse Prinzip" und die Krebsforschung', in *Strategien der Kausalität. Konzepte der Krankheitsverursachung im 19. und 20. Jahrhundert*, ed. Christoph Gradmann and Thomas Schlich (Pfaffenweiler: Centaurus, 1999), 185–226.

[18] Karl Heinrich Bauer, *Mutationstheorie der Geschwulst-Entstehung. Übergang von Körperzellen in Geschwulstzellen durch Gen-Änderung* (Berlin: Springer, 1928).

[19] Contemporary cancer research interprets this observation differently: because the majority of Jewish women married Jewish, and thus circumcised men, they had fewer cases of human papilloma virus, which today is considered one of the primary causes of cervical cancer.

[20] Moser, *Deutsche Forschungsgemeinschaft*, 72–3.

[21] Petra Werner, *Otto Warburg. Von der Zellphysiologie zur Krebsforschung. Biographie* (Berlin: Verlag Neues Leben, 1988). By the end of the century, the hypothesis had been neither verified nor disproven. Only in 2006 and 2008 did American and German scientists publish the findings of their experiments on lab mice that supported the Warburg theory. See Michael A. Kiebish, X. Han, H. Cheng, J. H. Chuang, and T. N. Seyfried, 'Cardiolipin and Electron Transport Chain Abnormalities in Mouse Brain Tumor Mitochondria: Lipidomic Evidence Supporting the Warburg Theory of Cancer', *Journal of Lipid Research* 49, no. 12 (2008): 2545–56.

Erforschung und Bekämpfung der Krebskrankheit e.V. (German Central Committee for Researching and Fighting Cancer) in 1911, spurred oncologists to better coordinate their research—particularly as concerned the acquisition of funding—and increase public awareness of it.[22] In 1903, the committee started publishing its own professional journal, the *Zeitschrift für Krebsforschung* (*Journal for Cancer Research*).[23] A sizeable chunk of German cancer research before the 1930s was carried out at four oncological institutes in Berlin, Frankfurt am Main, Heidelberg, and Hamburg. Yet despite their prestige, they were poorly funded. They had to constantly plead for money from private donors and sometimes ran on the private funds of their directors.[24] Still, Germany was no exception here, as experimental medical research in this period almost always relied on private donations.[25]

The Nazis' seizure of power jolted the situation.[26] They branded existing oncological research as materialistic, mechanistic, misanthropic, and 'Jewish'.[27] The dismissal, expulsion, and persecution of many oncologists had a profoundly negative effect on research.[28] They also placed more weight on cancer as a threat to public health, even going so far as to declare it 'state enemy number one'.[29] Their

[22] The committee changed its name multiple times. Established in 1900 as the Comité für Krebssammelforschung (Committee for General Cancer Research), its name was changed in the same year to Komitee für Krebsforschung (Committee for Cancer Research). In 1906 it was changed to Zentralkomitee für Krebsforschung (Central Committee for Cancer Research), expanded in 1907 to Deutsches Zentralkomitee für Krebsforschung, and, finally, in 1911, to Deutsches Zentralkomitee zur Erforschung und Bekämpfung der Krebskrankheit e.V. (German Central Committee for Researching and Fighting Cancer, registered association). In 1933, the Deutsche Zentralkomitee dissolved itself. Its property, rights, and duties were taken over by the scientific committee of the Reichsausschuss für Krebsbekämpfung (Imperial Committee for Fighting Cancer), which was then dissolved in 1945 by a decree of the Allies. In 1951, the association was newly established as the Zentralausschuß für Krebsforschung und Krebsbekämpfung (Central Committee for Cancer Research and Fighting Cancer). In 1970, it was given the name that it still has today: Deutsche Krebsgesellschaft (German Cancer Society). On the history of the organization see Atzl and Helms, *Geschichte der Deutschen Krebsgesellschaft*.

[23] This remains the oldest continually published journal on oncology; in 1979, the name was changed to *Journal of Cancer Research and Clinical Oncology*. See Atzl and Helms, *Geschichte der Deutschen Krebsgesellschaft*, 25.

[24] See Blumenthal's report to the Ministry of Science, Art, and Education about the state of the oncology institutes, Berlin, 14 June 1920, HU Archiv, Charité-Direktion, 951, 24–5, and HU Archiv, Charité-Direktion, 949–54.

[25] Moser, *Deutsche Forschungsgemeinschaft*, 30–1.

[26] Wolfgang U. Eckart, *Medizin in der NS-Diktatur. Ideologie, Praxis, Folgen* (Vienna: Böhlau, 2012), 286–90.

[27] 'Das neue Berliner Zentral-Krebsinstitut. Zusammenziehung von Universitätskliniken im Krankenhaus Moabit', *Berliner Beobachter. Tägliches Beiblatt zum 'Völkischen Beobachter'* 44, 13 February 1935, BArch R 86/2764.

[28] Birgit Hellmann-Mersch, 'Institutionen zur Krebsforschung und Krebsbekämpfung in Deutschland. Historischer Überblick und Analyse' (PhD diss., RWTH Aachen, 1994), 148–9; Peter Voswinckel, *Erinnerungsort Krebsbaracke. Klarstellungen um das erste interdisziplinäre Krebsforschungsinstitut in Deutschland (Berlin, Charité)* (Stuttgart: Georg Thieme Verlag, 2014), 134–5.

[29] Fritz Lickint, *Die Krebsfrage im Lichte der modernen Forschung* (Berlin: F.A. Herbig, 1935), 5.

motivations were economic and racist. Accordingly, National-Socialist health policy focused on early detection and preventive care. Funding for research also shifted towards the search for simple diagnostic methods and testing on substances suspected to be carcinogenic. Particular energy was dedicated to studying chemicals that had become prevalent in processed foods and modern everyday pleasures, particularly tobacco consumption. Researching the negative effects of tobacco meshed well with Nazi ideology's castigation of 'decadence'. But they were more ambivalent about the substances in the sights of many oncologists at the time, namely hormones and vitamins, which were popularly perceived as contributing to vitality and youthfulness.[30]

The concentration on potentially carcinogenic chemicals and hormones did not mark a break with, but rather an intensified continuation of the tendencies of the 1920s. Similarly, the path that oncological research took under National Socialism was not radically different from that pursued by scientists in other European countries, the United States, and the Soviet Union.[31]

After the end of the Second World War, oncological research booked few gains,[32] as combatting infectious diseases like typhus took priority.[33] Certainly, as early as 1948, an Institut für experimentelle Krebsforschung (Institute for Experimental Cancer Research) was founded in Heidelberg. But besides that, the bulk of the little financing granted to oncological research went to the so-called Hinterzartener Kreis; founded in 1950, the group met once a year to discuss findings and methods in oncological research far away from the eyes and ears of the public.

Still, German oncology in the immediate post-war period was primarily characterized by major continuities, both in the people doing the research and in the things being researched. Both before 1945 and after, Karl Heinrich Bauer, Adolf Butenandt, and Hermann Druckrey in West Germany along with Heinrich Cramer and Arnold Graffi in East Germany remained the most influential names. All born between 1890 and 1910, they were 'men in their best years' and occupied key positions in oncology in divided Germany for lengthy periods. Though all were, to varying degrees, involved in the Nazi movement and politics,

[30] Heiko Stoff, *Wirkstoffe: Eine Wissenschaftsgeschichte der Hormone, Vitamine und Enzyme, 1920–1970* (Stuttgart: Franz Steiner, 2012).

[31] Moser, *Deutsche Forschungsgemeinschaft*, 315–16. [32] Ibid., 239–40.

[33] Melanie Arndt, *Gesundheitspolitik im geteilten Berlin 1948–1961* (Cologne: Böhlau, 2009); Udo Schagen, 'Die Gesundheitspolitik in der Sowjetischen Besatzungszone—Umsetzung sozialdemokratischer Forderungen', in *'Gesundheitsschutz für alle' und die Ausgrenzung von Minderheiten*, ed. Udo Schagen and Sabine Schleiermacher (Berlin: Institut für Geschichte der Medizin, 2006), 63–72; Dagmar Ellerbrock, *Healing Democracy. Demokratie als Heilmittel. Gesundheit, Krankheit und Politik in der amerikanischen Besatzungszone 1945–1949* (Braunschweig: Veröffentlichungen des Instituts für Sozialgeschichte, 2004).

this fact hindered their careers little in the long run.[34] Research on what caused cancer or increased one's risk to get it also stuck to the topics that had dominated before 1945: chemicals, hormones, vitamins, and, somewhat less prominently, viruses.[35]

More and more oncological research was being conducted in labs. In West Germany, the close link between research and clinical praxis, particularly championed by the pre-war iteration of the Heidelberg cancer institute as well as the Berlin Oncology Institute, largely fell to the wayside. In the German Democratic Republic (GDR), in contrast, the Akademie-Institut für Medizin und Biologie (Academy Institute for Medicine and Biology) in the Buch district of Berlin brought laboratory and clinic under a single roof. East Germany continued to set forth the pre-war tradition with the 1972 establishment of the Zentralinstitut für Krebsforschung (Central Institute for Cancer Research) and the Robert-Rössle-Klinik attached to it.[36]

The difference between the countries grew as the Federal Republic of Germany accelerated the decoupling of research and clinical practice by building the first largescale research centre exclusively dedicated to cancer. Construction on the Deutsches Krebsforschungszentrum (DKFZ—German Cancer Research Centre) in Heidelberg began in 1964 and was finished in 1972.[37]

Its creation took place in a sobering period when even American researchers, whose work on oncology was considered cutting edge, stated that the riddle of how cancer is caused had yet to be solved. Many states pumped more money into oncological research, an international exemplar being Richard Nixon's signing of the National Cancer Act in December 1971, which was intended to translate that January's declaration of war on cancer into action. The law was passed in the wake of the Apollo programme's spectacular success of rocketing a man to the moon and held an analogous promise of a breakthrough in oncological research (and assist Nixon to an electoral victory in the face of the increasingly unpopular Vietnam War).[38] The Nixon Administration granted the National Cancer Institute—which, established in 1937, provided the prototype for West

[34] Volker Wunderlich, '"Mit Papier, Bleistift und Rechenschieber." Der Krebsforscher Hermann Druckrey im Internierungslager Hammelburg (1946–1947)', *Medizinhistorisches Journal* 43, no. 3/4 (2008): 327–43; Robert N. Proctor, 'Adolf Butenandt (1903–1995). Nobelpreisträger, Nationalsozialist und MPG-Präsident. Ein erster Blick in den Nachlass', http://www.mpiwg-berlin.mpg.de/KWG/Ergebnisse/Ergebnisse2.pdf; Eike Wolgast, 'Karl Heinrich Bauer. Der erste Heidelberger Nachkriegsrektor. Weltbild und Handeln 1945–1946', in *Heidelberg 1945*, ed. Jürgen C. Heß, Hartmut Lehmann, and Volker Sellin (Stuttgart: Franz Steiner, 1996), 107–29.

[35] Moser, *Deutsche Forschungsgemeinschaft*, 278–313.

[36] Heinz Bielka, *Geschichte der Medizinisch-Biologischen Institute Berlin-Buch*, 2nd edn (Berlin: Springer, 2002), 73–4 and 99–101.

[37] Gustav Wagner and Andrea Mauerberger, *Krebsforschung in Deutschland. Vorgeschichte und Geschichte des Deutschen Krebsforschungszentrums* (Berlin: Springer, 1989), 83 and 100.

[38] Cantor, 'Cancer', 550.

Germany's DKFZ—broad financial autonomy within the National Institutes of Health and set aside 100 million dollars for cancer research.

That large oncology centres represented a pragmatic approach to research was also highlighted by new discoveries. Since the 1950s, a consensus had been developing around the belief that cancer did not have a single cause, but could be induced by a number of different factors, and that it might begin not as a local illness, but as a systemic issue.[39] The assumption that cancer resulted out of the dysfunction of cell parts amplified the multi-cause theory and made close cooperation between different research institutes more attractive. In 1973, David Comings published a widely read book on the causes of cancer that argued for a synthesis of tumour virology and oncogenetics.[40] In principle, the cell dysfunction model seemed compatible with research on carcinogens and studies on the relation between cancer and the immune system, since it was assumed that cell functions could be disturbed both by environmental factors as well as by a weakened immune system.[41] The 'discovery' of interferons and their immunological effects drew media attention to this branch of oncological research. And big pharmaceutical companies ogled at the profits to be gained from interferon therapy. They stirred up hopes that were, however, already dashed in the early 1980s by their side effects and limited therapeutic value.[42]

Investigating cellular regulatory mechanisms necessitated costly laboratory equipment. The more expensive research got, the more important the profit potential became. Thus, since the 1970s, foundations and pharmaceutical corporations have been working parallel to state-funded studies, financing cancer research and marketing the results to generate enormous revenue streams.

As oncological research was expanding rapidly and gaining in significance for health policy, private enterprise, and society more generally, clinical research developed a renewed interest in the link between psychosocial factors, emotions, and cancer. Was it a coincidence that this question underwent a renaissance at precisely this moment? Did it just pop up out of nowhere after largely going missing after the end of the nineteenth century? Answering these questions demands more than simply looking at the specific historical moment when oncologists decided to seriously consider that emotions might causatively contribute to a person getting cancer. It requires beginning in the early twentieth

[39] Ralf Bröer, 'Das Mammakarzinom als Systemkrankheit. Die Entstehung eines neuen tumorbiologischen Konzeptes und seine Beziehungen zur Therapie', in Eckart, *100 Years of Organized Cancer Research*, 107–11.

[40] David E. Comings, 'A General Theory of Carcinogenesis', *Proceedings of the National Academy of Science USA* 70, no. 12 (1973): 3324–8.

[41] Michel Morange, 'From the Regulatory Vision to the Oncogene Paradigm, 1975–1985', *Journal of the History of Biology* 30, no. 1 (1997): 1–29, 8, https://doi.org/10.1023/A:1004255309721.

[42] Toine Pieters, 'The Biography of a Wonder Drug: The Interferon', in Eckart, *100 Years of Organized Cancer Research*, 149–55.

century, a time when, at least according to common knowledge, emotions played an insignificant role in cancer research.

The Fragmentary History of the Psychosomatics of Cancer

In a 1934 article in the renowned *Praktische Karzinomblättern* (*Practical Carcinoma Journal*), Danzig-based doctor Erwin Liek polemicized with the preceding decade: 'The successful cancer doctor mobilizes—consciously or unconsciously, willingly or dismissively—mental powers against cancer. Previously, no doctor was permitted to utter or even write such a thought without being punished with exclusion from the scientific community, and all the more so in the case of cancer.'[43] As discussed in detail below, Liek was blowing the horn of the Neue Deutsche Heilkunde (New German Medicine). Its adherents lambasted mainstream medicine of the 1920s as 'mechanistic', 'rationalistic', and, with antisemitic invective, as 'Jewish'. But was Liek's assessment of cancer research necessarily incorrect? Doctor and psychoanalyst Georg Groddeck came to a similar conclusion in the same year. In one of his last writings, he reflected on the 'psychic conditions of cancer' and voiced his concern that: 'The medical world's interest in the psychophysics of healthy and sick people is constantly growing. It is all the more astonishing that there have been almost no attempts to find the psychic roots of the illness most discussed in modern times, cancer.'[44] Vinzenz Czerny likely would have only half-heartedly agreed with Groddeck. In his 1905 response to the survey by *Medizinische Klinik* on the causes of cancer quoted above, he matter-of-factly stated that psychological factors were part of the discussion by referring to an article published in that same year by gynaecologist Wilhelm Alexander Freund (1833–1917).[45] Freund's piece drew on a plethora of case studies to argue that a disposition to cancer would only develop into cancer when stimuli, and particularly 'physical or mental states of depression', trigger its growth.[46] But Groddeck was thinking about something else when he bemoaned the lack of interest in uncovering the psychic causes of cancer, because he was specifically concerned about research conducted within the framework of psychoanalytic theory.

The distinction is significant for a number of reasons. First, it underscores that doctors who embraced psychoanalysis had been discussing the extent to which the

[43] Erwin Liek, 'Stand und Zukunft der Krebsbekämpfung', *Praktische Karzinomblätter* 1 (1934): 1–7.

[44] Georg Groddeck, 'Von der psychischen Bedingtheit der Krebskrankheit', in *Psychoanalytische Schriften zur Psychosomatik*, ed. Günter Clauser (Wiesbaden: Limes, 1966), 380–5, 380.

[45] Czerny, 'Antwort auf: Umfrage', 497.

[46] Wilhelm Alexander Freund, 'Zur Naturgeschichte der Krebskrankheit nach klinischen Erfahrungen', *Zeitschrift für Krebsforschung* 3, no. 1 (1905): 1–33, 23.

psyche can make the body sick since the 1910s. But it also reveals that psychoanalysts and psychologists alike had largely forgotten older models of the interaction between mind and body. The new concept of the psyche did not overlap with the traditional concept of the mind, necessitating that thinkers reformulate their inquiry into the position of the emotions in the psyche-body relation.[47]

An important forum for discourse on these kinds of questions were conferences. One noteworthy conference took place in April 1926 in Groddeck's hometown of Baden-Baden: 419 men and women (who were, nevertheless, in the minority) travelled from all around Germany, Switzerland, Austria, and the Netherlands to the first Allgemeiner ärztlicher Kongreß für Psychotherapie (General Medical Congress for Psychotherapy), where they discussed the role of psychotherapy in various aspects of medical practice. Thus, present were not just doctors who already practiced psychotherapy. They ranged from a—perhaps to be expected—large number of neurologists and psychiatrists to internists, gynaecologists, and child therapists, and included doctors who worked in private practices, clinics, and hospitals.[48] Drawing the conference to a close, Ernst Simmel (1882–1947), cofounder of the Berliner Psychoanalytische Vereinigung (Berlin Psychoanalytic Association), euphorically predicted that the event would chime in a 'new era' of clinical medicine.[49] But Groddeck, who had also attended, hardly would have recognized the conference as the beginning of a new era, and not just because of his tense relationship with Freud, who did not attend. The reason lies in most participants' subscription to an understanding of the body, psyche, and emotions that did not go far enough for Groddeck. For instance, August Meyer (1876–1968), director of the Tübingen University women's clinic, did argue that clinicians and researchers should be on the lookout for potential mental causes of cancer, placing 'unpleasurable affects, fear, anxiety' at the top of the list. But he explicitly asserted that they could only exert an effect in cases where a 'local organic ailment' could be ruled out with certainty. He wrapped up with the categorical statement: 'Just so that I am not misunderstood, I would like to emphasize that so-called major gynaecology will not be affected by these things. In its domain, the scalpel will retain its dominance and will continue to have its healing effect.'[50]

Mayer's position lagged behind the concept of psychosomatics that Felix Deutsch (1884–1964), a pioneer of psychoanalytic psychosomatics, had already articulated in 1921. In a talk on psychoanalysis and physical sickness, Deutsch

[47] Thomas Dixon, *From Passions to Emotions: The Creation of a Secular Psychological Category* (Cambridge: Cambridge University Press, 2003).

[48] Vladimir Eliasberg, ed., *Bericht über den I. Allgemeinen ärztlichen Kongreß für Psychotherapie in Baden-Baden, 17–19 April 1926* (Halle: Marhold, 1927), 319–27.

[49] Ibid., 318.

[50] August Mayer, 'Über psychogene Entstehung gynäkologischer Symptome', in Eliasberg, *Bericht über den I. Allgemeinen ärztlichen Kongreß für Psychotherapie in Baden-Baden*, 85 and 95.

wrote 'that a not insignificant part of the symptoms of organic illnesses can be effectuated purely by the psyche'.[51] In his eyes, the psychogenesis of organ illnesses originated in a conflict that, because it was repressed, escalated into neurosis. This, he thought, led nervous stimuli to be detoured through the vegetative nervous system, bringing about an alteration of function and, ultimately, 'material damage'. Thus, a stomach ulcer could be caused by psychological factors, but the lasting organ damage could no longer be cured by psychoanalysis alone, but only through the collaboration of internist and analyst.[52] However, his account failed to mention stomach cancer, which afflicted many men at the time. This blind spot bothered Groddeck. He lamented that most German-speaking doctors interested in psychoanalytic psychosomatics ignored cancer, as if it were absurd to even think about the possibility that psychic complexes might play a role in its causation.

Groddeck was the only Germanophone psychosomatic therapist who read this silence as indicative of a research gap, and the only one spurred by it to reflect on how the psyche might contribute to the emergence of cancer.[53] Groddeck's work on the psychosomatics of cancer helps explain why most others did not attempt to study the potential connection between the psyche and cancer. Later on, his ruminations—understood as a kind of intuitive knowledge not wholly confirmed by science—influenced medical praxis and attracted great interest in the wake of the 1960s' fascination with psychology and psychotherapy.

In contrast to many other psychosomatic doctors, Groddeck worked neither in a clinic nor in private practice, and it is likely that this fact was key to him discovering cancer as a psychosomatic illness. In 1900, Groddeck had founded a small sanatorium with fifteen beds in Baden-Baden, where he primarily treated chronically and terminally ill patients. Incurable by the standards of medicine at the time, the patients received a combination of older and newer treatments. Daily massages, foot baths, and a special diet were supposed to aid the circulation of bodily fluids, while hypnosis, suggestion, and psychoanalysis were supposed to unearth repressed conflicts. This unconventional potpourri of therapeutic methods underscores that the 'wild analyst', as Groddeck called himself, conceived of body and psyche not as two separate entities, but as interwoven attributes that

[51] Felix Deutsch, 'Psychoanalyse und Organkrankheiten', *Internationale Zeitschrift für Psychoanalyse* 8, no. 3 (1922): 290–306, 294.

[52] Ibid., 290, 300, and 306.

[53] Outside Germanophone psychosomatics, too, only few examples exist of psychosomatic perspectives on cancer. One exceptional case was American Elida Evans's depth-psychological study that she published in 1926 with a short, but laudatory introduction by Carl Gustav Jung: Elida Evans, *A Psychological Study of Cancer* (New York: Dodd, Mead & Co., 1926). Wilhelm Reich (1897–1957) only studied cancer after 1933, first in exile in Scandinavia, and after 1939 in exile in the United States; this work would play a crucial role in his late work. See, for instance, Wilhelm Reich, *The Cancer Biopathy* (New York: Farrar, Straus and Giroux, 1974). See also: James E. Strick, *Wilhelm Reich, Biologist* (Cambridge, MA: Harvard University Press, 2015), 186–217.

could influence one another.[54] In his 1917 essay on 'Psychic Conditioning and the Psychoanalytic Treatment of Organic Disorders', he wrote:

> The fact that man blushes when he is ashamed, goes pale when he is alarmed, sheds tears when he is sad, breathes hard or with difficulty, that his heart beats faster or stops in passion, that the intestinal tracts move faster when he is anxious and that there is a sweat of fear is well enough known, apparently too well known for notice to be taken of it. Should it be so impossible that an organism's temperature balance, like its system of circulation and its growth, be governed by psychological influences and that fever could have psychological causes? Of course it could be so, because the unconscious does not make a distinction between body and soul; according to its own purposes it uses the body in some cases, the soul in others.[55]

Groddeck flipped the 'why' of modern medical science, which was guided by the bacteriological paradigm and its search for *the* single cause of an illness, into a 'what for'. He theorized that illness did not arise because some physical or psychological issue caused it, but because the unconscious wanted to express a repressed conflict with it. The maverick analyst interpreted cervical cancer as an escape tunnelled by women's unconscious to escape the moral dictates against female pleasure: 'To relieve the senseless torture inflicted by this hypocritical environment woman is helped by her unconscious. It gives her dizziness, fainting, heartburn, deformation of the body, unpleasant smell, white discharge, infection of the ovaries and the womb, unpredictable bleeding, and finally cancer; all this keeps temptation away and repels everything that might excite her desires.'[56]

In the 1934 text referenced above, Groddeck connected these thoughts on the unconscious 'gain from illness' with speculation about how cancer might be the id's way of 'punishing' a woman (or man) for failing to have a child.[57] The later essay opted for a different understanding of body and emotions, shedding the 1917 text's claims about the deep symbolic significance of cancer. It replaced the physiological model of blushing as an effect of shame with an endocrinological concept of physiology centred on hormones. Many cancer researchers were doing the same, though they drew totally different conclusions. The observation that tar caused cancer in mice and contained substances similar to some chemicals in female sex hormones led Groddeck to surmise that cancer must have something to do with the 'mother-child relation'.[58] He found further evidence in medical

[54] Michael Giefer, ed., *Briefwechsel Georg Groddeck—Sigmund Freud* (Frankfurt am Main: Stroemfeld/Roter Stern, 2008), 176–7.

[55] Georg Groddeck, 'Psychic Conditioning and the Psychoanalytic Treatment of Organic Disorders', in *The Meaning of Illness: Selected Psychoanalytic Writings*, trans. Gertrud Mander (New York: International Universities Press, 1977), 109–31, 120–1.

[56] Ibid., 119. [57] Groddeck, 'Von der psychischen Bedingtheit', 381. [58] Ibid., 380.

statistics, which showed that women were primarily stricken with cancer of the reproductive organs. He also riffed on the common denotation of cancer as a 'new formation' (*Neubildung*) and the perception that the embryo represented the true 'new formation' in the human body. The essay painted cancer as a 'terrible shapeshifter' that the id let grow in a woman's body in order to punish her with the pain and destitution she had done upon herself by not having a child as society demanded of her.[59] Groddeck explained men's susceptibility to cancer by analogizing that an unborn 'brainchild' could harbour pain and sadness and trigger a similar need to self-flagellate. The most common sites of cancer among men in Groddeck's time—mouth, stomach, and colon—were the body parts that 'receive, shelter, and expel' the 'brainchild'.[60]

Even though the aetiological mechanisms sketched out by Groddeck were supposed to apply to both men and women alike, the model was undoubtedly provided by women's body, sexuality, and emotions. Associating cancer with unactualized female sexuality and childlessness is an idea often repeated in the modern history of psychosomatics. It can probably be traced back to older ideas about the special intensity of women's emotions that supposedly destabilize the female body and make female sexuality a conundrum.[61] Scientific oncology did not show any interest in the assumption that cancer derives from repressed feelings and a faltering sex life until the 1950s. But there is evidence that doctors took it for granted as a sort of self-explanatory, if unproven bit of wisdom. For example, many doctors recycled the recommendation of renowned surgeon Ferdinand Sauerbruch (1875–1951) to his supervising doctors that they enter into sexual relationships with nurses in order to prevent the latter from developing cervical cancer.[62]

Thus, Groddeck's appeal to gender stereotypes could not be blamed for his model's failure to gain traction among psychosomatic doctors and oncologists of the interwar period.[63] It was clearly epistemologically suspect, inquiring not into cancer's cause, as the bacteriologists and pathologists of the time did, but into its purpose (what end does the illness serve?). Many medical scientists did accept Freud's claim that sickness might provide some kind of benefit to the patient, but this did not inhibit them from looking for its psychic and organic causes.[64]

The loaded concept of 'gain from illness' evoked scepticism outside the epistemological debate, too. The notion that sadness and guilt felt about the lack of a

[59] Ibid., 381–2. [60] Ibid., 382. [61] Jasen, 'Malignant Histories'.

[62] A reference to Sauerbruch's recommendation can be found in 'Krebs durch Seelenschmerz', *Der Spiegel*, 110.

[63] Herbert Will, *Die Geburt der Psychosomatik. Georg Groddeck, der Mensch und Wissenschaftler* (Munich: Urban & Schwarzenberg, 1984), 52–3.

[64] As early as the 1920s, however, Viktor von Weizsäcker had emphasized the central significance of a patient's biography in the interpretation of their illness, a model that is comparable to Groddeck's in its consequential turn away from trying to quantify the causes of disease.

child would occasion the id to 'give' its body cancer probably seemed ludicrous to most who saw cancer patients suffer and die during a time when being diagnosed with cancer was almost always a death sentence. Moreover, cancer often caused unbearable pain that could not be tempered by medicine. Just as well, the idea that an organism could choose to fall ill with a disease that ended in death contradicted the concept of self-preservation so important not only to evolutionary theory, but also to physiology, a discipline that served as the bedrock of psychology and psychosomatics.[65]

Two further reservations clipped the plausibility of Groddeck's theses. The first was its pessimism about the potential of therapy, as even he himself spoke not of curing, but 'only' of helping.[66] Second, Groddeck was unable to explain how sadness and guilt could cause healthy cells to 'degenerate' into cancerous cells. Of course, Groddeck did refer to the findings of medical research, but in a fairly associative fashion. Above all, the complexity of the emotions that his model was based on made it impossible to verify through experiments on humans and tissues and, perhaps most importantly for cancer research of the era, on animals.

It is thus no coincidence that fear and anxiety occupied a central position in many debates on psychosomatics in the 1920s, with Felix Deutsch asserting: 'Every disease is an anxiety disease.'[67] Whether fear and anxiety were conceived of as a drive, an affective state, or an emotion, hardly a single researcher doubted that animals could feel fear and anxiety. They could be intentionally produced in experiments like those of Russian physiologist Ivan Pavlov (1849–1936), who sought to quantify the effects of conditioned reactions by measuring the saliva that dogs produced when they heard a noise that they had learned to associate with food.[68] Early psychologists like Wilhelm Wundt (1832–1920) chose different physiological indicators to measure emotions, such as pulse rate, blood circulation, and the excretion of stomach acid. Groddeck's concept of emotions, in contrast, could not be reduced to physiological factors. Still, while Groddeck was publishing his thoughts on the relation between cancer and psychological conditions shortly before his death, Erwin Liek took another perspective on the question.

[65] Friedrich Kraus, 'Die Abhängigkeitsbeziehungen zwischen Seele und Körper in Fragen der inneren Medizin', *Ergebnisse der Inneren Medizin und Kinderheilkunde* 1 (1911): 1–46, 10. From 1921 to 1933, Kraus was the president of the Deutsche Zentralkomitee zur Erforschung und Bekämpfung der Krebskrankheit.

[66] Deutsch, 'Psychoanalyse und Organkrankheiten', 302; Groddeck, 'Von der psychischen Bedingtheit', 385.

[67] Felix Deutsch, 'Der gesunde und der kranke Körper in psychoanalytischer Betrachtung', *Internationale Zeitschrift für Psychoanalyse* 12, no. 3 (1926): 493–503, 502.

[68] On the reception of Pavlov in Germany and on further physiological experiments on human beings, see Kraus, 'Abhängigkeitsbeziehungen', 32–6; Georg Nicolai, *Erforschung der Tierpsyche* (Leipzig, 1907).

New German Medicine: A Movement Gone Awry?

Erwin Liek (1875–1935) was one of the most outspoken proponents of the movement against the mainstream medicine of his era. In 1926, the professional surgeon published the book *Der Arzt und seine Sendung* (*The Doctor and His Mission*), which revolved around his stark distinction between doctors and medical scientists.[69] He criticized scientists for labouring on the 'microscopic horizon' and staring at the mechanisms of illness and their symptoms with 'cellular shortsightedness'. Meanwhile, his idealized doctor took a holistic perspective on the mind and body of the sick patient, making him the most important part of what Liek described as human-centred medical practice.[70] No question in which camp Liek saw himself. By subtitling the book 'Thoughts of a Heretic', Liek underscored that his text was not just a critique of the medical profession in the Weimar Republic, but the manifestation of a full-fledged *Weltanschauung*.

But in truth, Liek's ideas were not so heretical. His was just one more voice in the polyphonic debate about whether the world was best to be understood through its individual parts or whether proper knowledge could only be gained by analysing how things are connected—in short, whether the whole was more than the sum of its parts. The 'search for the whole', particularly pronounced in many spheres of early twentieth-century German culture, was nourished by the feeling that the trusted beliefs and institutions that gave life meaning had been lost. Holism was a reaction to industrialization, urbanization, and secularization just as much as it was a reaction to the experiences of the First World War, the end of the German Empire, and the heatedly contested democratization of the Weimar period.[71] In Germany, the holistic movement had a strong bond with cultural pessimism, which lashed out against the 'disenchantment' that Max Weber had diagnosed as a defining feature of the modern world. This trend shored itself up on binaries like community and society, culture and civilization, soul and mind.[72]

But the yearning for holism was also the end result of feelings of disappointment that the grand expectations conjured up by the scientific discoveries of the nineteenth century had not entirely been translated into reality. Shadows had even fallen on bacteriology, because it had not been able to trace many diseases back to a single germ. The limits of bacteriology were cast in dramatic relief by its inability to identify the germ that caused the 'Spanish flu' pandemic, which claimed about 50 million lives between 1918 and 1920.[73] This summoned up serious doubts about the 'rationalist', 'mechanistic', 'reductionist', 'materialist' view of the world.

[69] Erwin Liek, *Der Arzt und seine Sendung. Gedanken eines Ketzers* (Munich: J. F. Lehmanns, 1926), 105.

[70] Ibid., 121–2; Liek, 'Stand und Zukunft', 5.

[71] Anne Harrington, *Reenchanted Science: Holism in German Culture from Wilhelm II to Hitler* (Princeton, NJ: Princeton University Press, 1996).

[72] Ibid., 17.

[73] Berger, *Bakterien*, 283–90.

Thus, the very diverse, not exclusively conservative search for wholeness was not just a hobby of disgruntled 'heretics'. Prominent professors like biologist Hans Driesch (1867–1941) and gestalt psychologist Max Wertheimer (1880–1943) were part of this loose movement, as were people at the margins of academic life like environmental biologist Jakob von Uexküll (1864–1944).[74] The movement was not confined to Germany but spread throughout the Western world.[75] Many holists found teleological questions fundamentally more important than the cause-and-effect inquiries dominant in science. The concepts of equilibrium, system, and (self-)regulation were some of the central heuristic devices of holistic thought. They signalled that the world could only be understood if one did *not* dissect it into its parts. The logical consequence was scepticism about whether the world even existed outside our perception of it, or at least about whether we could gain knowledge of it that is independent of perception. Was there a 'thing in itself', or just that which I perceive?

Even if Erwin Liek's ideas generally meshed with this intellectual trend, he subscribed to a very specific sort of organicist holism. His position was, on the one hand, defined by the political and ideological radicalization of the late 1920s, while on the other, he joined in Weimar Germany's widespread discontent with the 'crisis of medicine', which represented more than a failure of established models and explanations.[76] Hyperinflation and the Great Depression worsened the state of hospitals and meant losses for doctors. The social safety net was expanded, which many doctors criticized as an intolerable paternalistic intervention in strictly medical concerns. They clamoured even louder that social insurance created false incentives and thereby contravened the health and productivity of 'the people' by artificially lengthening the lives of the 'sick' and 'disabled'. In their eugenicist perspective, social insurance brought about a form of 'negative selection', since they thought it might give the 'unfit' advantages over the 'fit' and thus might enable them to produce large numbers of 'sick' or 'disabled' children.[77]

It was no coincidence that Liek deeply reflected on cancer,[78] because the discrepancy between impressive findings in oncological research, the development of new diagnostic tools, and radical expansions of therapy on one side and low cure rates on the other was jarring. Many doctors shared his impression that

[74] Harrington, *Reenchanted Science*, 34–71 and 103–39.

[75] Charles Rosenberg, 'Holism in Twentieth-Century Medicine', in *Greater than the Parts: Holism in Biomedicine, 1920–1950*, ed. Christopher Lawrence and George Weisz (New York: Oxford University Press, 1998), 335–55.

[76] Michael H. Kater, 'Die Medizin im nationalsozialistischen Deutschland und Erwin Liek', *Geschichte und Gesellschaft* 16, no. 4 (1990): 440–63.

[77] 'Erwin Liek, Arzt und Volksgesundheit', *Münchener Medizinische Wochenschrift* 73 (1926): 112–16, 113. On the 'crisis of medicine', see Detlef Bothe, *Neue Deutsche Heilkunde 1933–1945* (Husum: Matthiesen, 1991), 16–37.

[78] Erwin Liek, 'Gedanken über den Krebs', *Hippokrates* 3 (1929): 287–305; Erwin Liek, *Krebsverbreitung, Krebsbekämpfung, Krebsverhütung* (Munich: J. F. Lehmanns, 1932); Erwin Liek, *Der Kampf gegen den Krebs* (Munich: J. F. Lehmanns, 1924).

cancer could be beat neither with 'humans' formulaic laws' nor with ever more drastic operations and radiation treatments.[79] For their part, many of these critics belonged to the ranks of the New German Medicine movement, which received official sanction from Reich Doctors' Leader Gerhard Wagner in 1933. As Julius Streicher wrote in his antisemitic medical journal *Deutsche Volksgesundheit aus Blut und Boden* (*German People's Health from Blood and Soil*), which touted a particularly radical version of New German Medicine, the goal was to tear down the decrepit house of scientific medicine in order to open space for natural medicine, homeopathy, mesmerism (curative magnetism), and physiological medicine.

After 1933, the New German Medicine movement lashed out against established medicine. With blatant antisemitism, it denounced 'natural-scientific medicine' as a 'Jewish' attempt to infiltrate the health of the German *Volk*. Many of its proponents saw this charge confirmed in the fact that a large number of scientists at the Berliner Oncology Institute were, in the definition of the Nazis, Jewish. As Liek offensively wrote in 1934, the rejection of 'Jewish' experimental research was supposed to dethrone the 'rodent as the measure of man'.[80]

The New German Medicine sought to place human beings front and centre in the clinic and in research; in this sense, neither the movement nor Liek were in principle opposed to laboratory experiments. Rather, they shunned a certain type of laboratory practice that sought to verify isolated effects in experiments on animals. Thus, Liek rushed to announce that one of the few renowned scientists who had been allowed to remain at the Berlin Oncology Institute, cell biologist and head of the department for experimental cell research Rhoda Erdmann (1870–1935), had turned towards questions of human diet and away from animal experiments, which had been the focus of her work for years.[81] Liek conveniently ignored the fact that financial considerations and the threat of losing access to laboratory space probably influenced her decision, just as he failed to mention that she had been briefly arrested by the Gestapo in 1933 after being denounced and was stripped of her teaching licence in 1934. In ill health, she tried to save her life work. She died in 1935—the same year as Liek—but not before being subject to further harassment.[82]

Shortly before his death, Liek witnessed his vision of medicine take the day with the Nazi-sanctioned New German Medicine. At the same time, he realized how this paradigm ushered in a shift in assumptions about what causes cancer and how

[79] Diedrich Kulenkampff, 'Über die Krebskrankheit', *Hippokrates* 3 (1929): 271–86; E. Silber, 'Magenkrebs', *Deutsche Volksgesundheit aus Blut und Boden* 5 (1934): 5–7; Bernhard Fischer-Wasels, 'Die Bedeutung der besonderen Allgemeindisposition des Körpers für die Entstehung der Krebskrankheit und die Möglichkeiten ihrer Bekämpfung', *Strahlentherapie* 50 (1934): 5–78.

[80] Liek, 'Stand und Zukunft'. [81] Ibid., 6.

[82] Hans-Christian Jasch, *Rhoda Erdmann (1870–1935). Leben und Karriere einer frühen Krebsforscherin zwischen internationaler Anerkennung und nationaler Marginalisierung* (Berlin: Be.bra Wissenschaft, 2017), 24–33.

it should be treated. Certainly, oncologists did not abruptly change how they conducted experiments, as Liek seemed to suggest in his comments on Rhoda Erdmann. But the Nazis did direct more money to research projects that studied the metabolism of cancerous cells and the oncological significance of hormones and vitamins. Interest had been growing in these areas since the 1920s and they overlapped with the concerns of the New German Medicine.

But oncologists experimenting in the labs were open to psychosomatic models, too. For instance, pharmacologist Wolfgang Heubner, who was testing the pathological effects of aniline on haemoglobin, wrote in 1934: 'The often-heard opinions that the reproductive system is involved in the formation of cancer have affinities with better-supported views. Whether expressions like "nervous weakness", "disturbed mental life", "incorrect mental attitude" are seeking to articulate the same thoughts is a different matter.'[83]

Heubner fused aspects of a Groddeck-style psychoanalytic psychosomatics with the New German Medicine's attempt to revive the 'old' theory of humoral pathology by cloaking it in the language of modern endocrinology. Dr Werner Tiegel followed a similar line of thought in his response to the question 'What is sickness?' According to him, sickness was a reaction to a false way of thinking and a false way of life; it represented the organism's self-defence and its attempt to 're-establish the old balance'.[84] Part and parcel of the 'false way of thinking and false way of life' were 'false' feelings like worry and sorrow, which threw the body's equilibrium off kilter and wore down the body and nerves.[85] In essence, his answer was a syncretic combination of the old humourism—which assessed melancholy ('black bile') as the cause of cancer—and the updated version of it that worked within the nineteenth-century paradigm of nerves and nervous exhaustion.

But with its concern with equilibrium, the New German Medicine was also taking up a key concept of contemporaneous physiology. In the late nineteenth century, the concept had played a central part in French physiologist Claude Bernard's research on the 'milieu intérieur'. American physiologist Walter B. Cannon developed it further with his notion of homeostasis, defining the body as a system open to its environment that seeks to maintain physiological equilibrium through automatic self-regulation.[86] Cannon's fight-or-flight theory detailed how emotions could affect physiological equilibrium, with fear being a

[83] Report from Prof. Dr Heubner (Pharmacological Institute of the University of Berlin), Transcription of a Meeting of the Scientific Committee of the Imperial Committee for Fighting Cancer on 13 April 1934 in Berlin, BArch B 142/412, 275–96, 282.

[84] Werner Tiegel, 'Was ist Krankheit? Ein Gang durch die Jahrhunderte', *Deutsche Volksgesundheit aus Blut und Boden* 2 (1934): 12–13.

[85] Silber, 'Magenkrebs'.

[86] Walter B. Cannon, 'Organization for Physiological Homeostasis', *Physiological Reviews* 9, no. 3 (1929): 399–431. See also Steven J. Cooper, 'From Claude Bernard to Walter Cannon: Emergence of the Concept of Homeostasis', *Appetite* 51, no. 3 (2008): 419–27, https://doi.org/10.1016/j.appet.2008.06.005.

physiological mobilization to flee and anger being a mobilization to fight. Erwin Liek and other doctors of the New German Medicine latched onto these new ideas and instrumentalized them against the field of cellular pathology.[87]

At the same time, doctors interested in alternative and natural medicine were rediscovering the old notions of constitution and disposition, which helped them explain why cancer occurred with greater frequency in certain families (constitution) and why emotions could, over the long run, increase a person's disposition to cancer. In this respect, too, the alternative doctors of the 1930s were not much different from their scientifically oriented colleagues, who worked with some of the same concepts, even if they did not define them in the same way. Even a renowned pathologist like Bernhard Fischer-Wasels, long-time director of the Senckenbergisches Pathologische Institut (Senckenberg Institute of Pathology), wrote in 1934 that the emergence of cancer was dependent upon both local factors and an inherited disposition. Over months, Fischer-Wasels injected mice and rabbits with small doses of tar or arsenic to demonstrate that this could increase their general disposition to cancer. He showed that while a tumour that grew as a reaction to the local poisoning with tar could be removed locally, the animal's altered general disposition would ultimately lead to further tumour growth on other, non-contaminated parts of their body.[88]

Though Fischer-Wasels drew his conclusions on the basis of animal experiments, he agreed with Liek about their clinical meaning. He frowned on operations, surmising that they might 'open the flood gates' of a person's general disposition, and believed that diet played a key role in human cancer.[89] A similar argument was put forward by Ernst Günther Schenk, whose interest in the 'natural' diets so central to National-Socialist health policy helped him climb the Nazi Party career ladder. He was named dietary inspector of the Waffen SS in 1940; as a member of the SS Main Economic and Administrative Office, he began supervising 'dietary experiments' at the Mauthausen concentration camp in 1943. In 1944, he advanced to become surgeon general and dietary inspector of the Wehrmacht.[90] But in 1936, when he was still a senior physician in Heidelberg, he penned a text on the 'problems of cancer treatment' that asserted: 'But for us, it is totally grotesque and unacceptable when people believe that the analysis of a single state of being or process offers a way to correct complex functions that have become afflicted . . . '. This assessment led Schenck to call on doctors to have an open mind about methods like homeopathy, to acknowledge the importance of

87 Tiegel, 'Was ist Krankheit?'.

88 Fischer-Wasels, 'Die Bedeutung'.

89 Ibid., 10–12 and 65–9.

90 Gine Elsner, *Heilkräuter, 'Volksernährung', Menschenversuche. Ernst Günther Schenck (1904–1998). Eine deutsche Arztkarriere* (Hamburg: VSA, 2010).

'natural' diets, and to consider psychological factors, one among them being the patient's confidence in the effectiveness of therapy.[91]

Thus, like Groddeck's psychosomatics, proponents of alternative natural medicine also referenced physiology to argue that emotions were a matter of the body of the 'whole human'. But their concept of what constitutes an emotion diverged from his. Psychosomatics maintained that while emotions were partially physiological in nature, their meaning could only be deciphered by a doctor's interpretation of the patient's life history and the formations of their unconscious. In contrast, practitioners of alternative medicine described emotions as something immediately perceptible that had a direct, physiological effect on bodily equilibrium. As such, they understood emotions as an outgrowth of a person's lifestyle, reasoning that, just as one can choose what one eats (at least so long as food is available in sufficient quantity and quality), so too can one influence one's own feelings. This line of thought was captured succinctly in Dr Silber's 1934 contribution to Julius Streicher's antisemitic medical journal *Deutsche Volksgesundheit aus Blut und Boden*: 'We don't want to forget that staying healthy requires proper mental behaviour! "It is the spirit that makes the body!"'[92] This was a direct adaptation of the first two of Erwin Liek's ten rules for 'protecting oneself from cancer' that he formulated in 1932: '1. Do not think about cancer; instead, plan to die at 90 years of age after a long working life . . . . 2. Do not allow yourself to be too influenced by joy and suffering. Everything passes. Believe in immortality and the eternal return. Only the form is destructible, not the being.'[93] This made the question of who would get cancer into one of willpower and attitude towards life, since, after all, everybody could choose whether or not to be optimistic about the future and avoid exhausting emotional extremes. Liek unmistakably relied on an understanding of the body and emotions that was developed out of mesmerism and its theories of suggestion and autosuggestion, which, for their part, were enjoying a renaissance among early proponents of positive thinking.[94]

At the same time, these ruminations prioritized 'cancer prevention', with one reviewer bemoaning that Liek's book was a 'terrible disappointment' for people already stricken with cancer.[95] The swing towards prevention, valourized as an individual duty to the *Volk* and oneself, shifted the focus of medicine away from curing the sick and towards maintaining the healthy. This shift did not just define the New German Medicine. It defined the entirety of National Socialist health policy. After naming Leonardo Conti Reich Health Leader in 1939, and perhaps

[91] Ernst G. Schenck, 'Probleme der Krebsbehandlung', *Hippokrates* 25 (1936): 653–61, 656–7, and 659.

[92] Silber, 'Magenkrebs', 7.

[93] Liek, *Krebsverbreitung*, 230.

[94] Oscar Schellbach, *Mein Erfolgssystem: Das positive Leben in Theorie und Praxis* (Hamburg: Schellbach, 1929); Dale Carnegie, *How to Win Friends and Influence People: A Self-Help Book about Interpersonal Relations* (New York: Simon and Schuster, 1937).

[95] Alfred Neumann, 'Erwin Lieks Krebsbuch', *Praktische Karzinomblätter* 3 (1933): 42–5.

even before, Nazi medicine began turning away from the New German Medicine in favour of ever further radicalization.[96]

National-Socialist 'New German Psychotherapy'

The Nazis' seizure of power kneecapped Germanophone psychosomatics in the same way that it hurt oncological research, as psychoanalysis was tabooed as 'Jewish' and the writings of Sigmund Freud were publicly burned in 1933. In the face of these events and the first wave of antisemitic legislation, many psychosomatic therapists and psychoanalysts left Germany, and, a bit later, Austria too: Wilhelm Reich and Kurt Goldstein in 1933, Ernst Simmel and Otto Fenichel in 1934, Felix and Helene Deutsch in 1936, Sigmund Freud and his daughter Anna in 1938. Others like Franz Alexander and Karen Horney had already left before 1933.[97]

But more than a few remained, and psychosomatics was integrated into the institutions and discourses of medicine in Nazi Germany. As early as 1933, the Deutsche Allgemeine Ärztliche Gesellschaft für Psychotherapie (German General Medical Society for Psychotherapy) was established at the behest of the National-Socialist government as a parallel organization to the Deutsche Psychoanalytische Gesellschaft (German Psychoanalytical Society), which was founded in 1910 and dissolved by the Nazis in 1938. In 1936, the Berliner Psychoanalytische Institut, founded in 1920 by Karl Abraham and Max Eitingon, was absorbed into the Deutsches Institut für psychologische Forschung und Psychotherapie (German Institute for Psychological Research and Psychotherapy). Leadership of the institute was given to doctor and psychotherapist Matthias Göring almost solely because he was a relative of Reichsmarschall Hermann Göring.[98]

Göring and many others who had remained in Germany called their new brand of psychosomatics the Deutsche Seelenheilkunde (German Psychotherapy).[99] This underscored its kinship with the New German Medicine while also attacking what they lambasted as the '*Entseelung*' (de-spiritualization) instigated by scientific medicine and 'Jewish' psychoanalysis's 'soul-devouring overestimation of the drives'.[100] They pulled the plug on the study of libidinously tangled drives and

[96] Eckart, *Medizin in der NS-Diktatur*, 164–73.

[97] Michael Schröter, '"Hier läuft alles zur Zufriedenheit, abgesehen von den Verlusten..." Die Deutsche Psychoanalytische Gesellschaft 1933–1936', *Psyche* 63, no. 11 (2009): 1085–1130.

[98] Ibid., and Geoffrey Cocks, *Psychotherapy in the Third Reich: The Göring Institute*, 2nd edn (Piscataway: Routledge, 1997).

[99] Matthias H. Göring, ed., *Deutsche Seelenheilkunde: Zehn Aufsätze zu den seelenärztlichen Aufgaben unserer Zeit* (Leipzig: S. Hirzel, 1934).

[100] The words used to defame Freud's writings when they were burned in Berlin in 1933. See Christoph Jahr, 'Die nationalsozialistische Machtübernahme und ihre Folgen', in *Die Berliner Universität zwischen den Weltkriegen*, ed. Michael Grüttner (Berlin: Akademie, 2012), 295–324, 303.

shifted their efforts to an analysis of the *Seele*, or 'mind and soul', its emotions, and their visible effects on the body. As such, they embraced a concept of emotions that was nearly indistinguishable from that of Liek's holistic organicist medical theory.[101] And the New German Psychotherapy distanced itself from psychoanalysis in another respect, too, as the introspection it fostered was supposed to serve a 'greater' purpose—to liberate the patient's inner and outer powers from the grip of illness and egoism, so that every individual could put themselves at the service of the community and 'efficiently' work for the ethnically defined '*Volksganze*', the 'whole of the people', as New German psychotherapist and later founder of neo-psychoanalysis, Harald Schultz-Hencke, put it.[102]

Cancer hardly played a role in New German Psychotherapy though, as proponents doubted that psychological treatment could have any serious impact on it. This also held true for the so-called Heidelberg School of Psychosomatics and its most prominent representative, neurologist Viktor von Weizsäcker (1886–1957). Weizsäcker veered sharply away from the theory that bodily illnesses could have psychogenic origins and its concomitant focus on fear and anxiety. His conceptual ruminations and clinical practice centred neither on individual emotions nor on any one of the then prominent ideas about the body-mind dualism. Instead, he posited that psychic conflicts were an outgrowth of the subject—the ego with its complex life history—and that their gears ground behind the scenes of the 'corporeal action' and encompassed both body and mind.[103] The theory of hidden conflicts was, indeed, a sign of Freud's influence, but Weizsäcker's concept of the subject was different. He believed that the true illness was neither the bodily nor psychic affliction, but the conflict lurking behind them. Accordingly, he thought doctors should not train their energies on diagnosing and treating the illness as an objective phenomenon, but instead on teasing out the subjective meaning concealed in the symptoms. Weizsäcker's anthropological medicine depicted the doctor's job as a complex act of listening, understanding, and interpreting the

[101] This turn away from the drives as the primary force of human psychic life was also apparent in the attempt to weed out or 'spiritualize' words associated with drives and sexuality. See Mechthilde Kütemeyer, 'Die Sprache der Psychosomatik im Nationalsozialismus', in *'Gift, das du unbewußt eintrinkst...' Der Nationalsozialismus und die deutsche Sprache*, ed. Werner Bohleber and Jörg Drews (Bielefeld: Aisthesis, 1991), 61–82.

[102] See Matthias H. Göring, 'Die nationalsozialistische Idee in der Psychotherapie', in Göring, *Deutsche Seelenheilkunde*, 15 and Harald Schultz-Hencke, 'Die Tüchtigkeit als psychotherapeutisches Ziel', in Göring, *Deutsche Seelenheilkunde*, 84–97. See also Ulrich Schultz-Venrath and Ludger M. Hermanns, 'Gleichschaltung zur Ganzheit. Gab es eine Psychosomatik im Nationalsozialismus?', in *Neues Denken in der Psychosomatik*, ed. Horst Eberhard Richter and Michael Wirsching (Frankfurt am Main: Fischer, 1992), 83–103.

[103] Viktor von Weizsäcker, 'Körpergeschehen und Neurose. Analytische Studie über somatische Symptombildungen', in *Gesammelte Schriften*, Vol. 6: *Körpergeschehen und Neurose, Psychosomatische Medizin*, ed. Peter Achilles (Frankfurt am Main: Suhrkamp, 1986), 119–238.

patient's life story. And yet, while he thought that this model was generally applicable, he doubted its validity for cancer, a reservation that could not exclusively be traced back to the limitations that might have been imposed on him by his interests and everyday experiences as a head doctor of neurological clinics, first in Heidelberg and later in Breslau.[104] He clearly dedicated considerable thought to the topic and, in one of his first publications after 1945, he framed the lack of an answer as a central issue for research on the limits of anthropological medicine:

> What about the psychology of cancer? Sure, it is not all that seldom that a person who has little more to expect from life now gets cancer. One sees that often. But it seems that the cases where fatal illness grabs onto blossoming life are much more frequent.... But our question is the extent to which we can use psychology to grasp the organic process. Does doing so have limitations, and what are they?... It is very simple: we *understand* much more about organic illnesses when we view them from the perspective of natural science and leave out psychology; moreover, we can help the patient a lot when we do so. We have not yet succeeded in curing organic illnesses with psychological approaches; at least that is how it seems. And so, a *split* develops, both in body and mind and in the methods used to treat them. This is discomforting, because it destroys the unity of the human being. But might there not be other ways?...Must the psychic, the human approach break apart so early upon the granite of material processes?[105]

Weizsäcker's concerns here clearly reveal uncertainty as to whether cancer really marked the limit beyond which the 'subject' faltered and the laws of biology reigned exclusively. Theory was unable to solve the problem. Like Vinzenz Czerny forty years before him, the doctor in Weizsäcker decided that surgery was the most promising way to cure cancer.

As early as 1943, Weizsäcker confided in a letter to his former student Wilhelm Kütemeyer (1904–72) that he had, despite his best efforts, been unable to figure out 'what happens when we transition from neurosis to organic illness or even psychosis'.[106]

[104] For example, he treated a 47-year-old woman whose breast cancer was operated on in 1919 and who was sent to the neurological clinic in 1922 because doctors thought it might be metastasizing, UA Heidelberg LV Acc. 30, 01.888/22; in 1931, he treated a 59-year-old man who had undergone an operation for stomach cancer in 1930 and was transferred to Weizsäcker's clinic because doctors suspected multiple metastases, UA Heidelberg LV Acc. 30, 01.445.31. 1+2.

[105] Viktor von Weizsäcker, 'Klinische Vorstellungen I–VI', *Psyche* 1, no. 2 (1947): 258–93, 290–1 [emphasis in original].

[106] Letter from Viktor von Weizsäcker to Wilhelm Kütemeyer, 22 December 1943, Deutsches Literaturarchiv Marbach, A: Sternberger, 89.10.6952/9.

Emotional Anaesthesia and the Issue of Guilt after 1945

Kütemeyer's ideas deserve some attention, because even if most influential psychosomatic doctors after him did not adopt them, they ignited an important discussion on what constitute scientific standards in psychosomatic medicine. And they set off a debate about the interrelation between individual and social pathology, particularly in regards to cancer. These debates defined the more general West German discourse on cancer, emotions, and society, while they received little publicity in the East.

Exactly when Kütemeyer began studying cancer is difficult to tell. Up until he completed his dissertation in 1953, his work was primarily concerned with whether psychosomatic medicine had anything to say about psychosis.[107] In all likelihood, though, he probably began thinking about the psychosomatic aspects of cancer around 1945, because his writings from the period wrestled with how to demonstrate that the psychic, somatic, metaphysical, and moral dimensions of the human being are all intertwined and mutually influence every human event. Kütemeyer first articulated these concerns in a 1946 lecture that his mentor Weizsäcker enthusiastically praised.[108] Indeed, it is not implausible that Weizsäcker's thoughts on cancer quoted above were inspired by his discussions with Kütemeyer.

The year 1945 seems to represent a caesura in Kütemeyer's development for other reasons, too. As a new doctor at Heidelberg's Krehl Clinic, he probably had his first contact with cancer patients. He later recounted that he invited cancer patients to talk at a lecture he held in the winter semester of 1955/6. Around the same time, he published one of his first longer medical articles, which dealt with a case study of Hodgkin's lymphoma.[109]

But his fascination with moral philosophy and politics probably contributed just as much to his interest in the psychosomatics of cancer as did his work with cancer patients. In the 1920s, he had translated works by Søren Kierkegaard, and his writings up until the end of his life evidenced his deep engagement with the Danish philosopher's concept of despair as a sickness unto death that could only be 'cured' by confronting existential anxiety. Not doing so, Kierkegaard thought,

[107] Wilhelm Kütemeyer, *Körpergeschehen und Psychose* (Stuttgart: Ferdinand Enke, 1953).

[108] The lecture occupies a prominent place in a volume of Kütemeyer's essays published in 1951. A lack of documentation makes it impossible to determine the extent to which he revised it for the publication: Wilhelm Kütemeyer, 'Wandlungen medizinischer Anthroplogie. Ein Vortrag 1946', in *Die Krankheit Europas. Beiträge zu einer Morphologie*, ed. Wilhelm Kütemeyer (Berlin: Suhrkamp, 1951), 139–86. Hans Stoffels, 'Gelebtes und ungelebtes Leben. Zum 100. Geburtstag von Wilhelm Kütemeyer (1904–1972)', *Viktor von Weizsäcker Gesellschaft*, 24 March 2005, quotes from Weizsäcker's letter from 20 May 1946 containing the praise; it is in the private possession of Dr Mechthilde Kütemeyer.

[109] Wilhelm Kütemeyer, 'Psychosocial Aspects of Cancer' (paper, Fourth International Conference on Psychosomatic Aspects of Neoplastic Disease, 1965), 2; Wilhelm Kütemeyer, 'Anthropologische Medizin in der inneren Klinik', in *Viktor von Weizsäcker: Arzt im Irrsal der Zeit. Eine Freundesgabe zum 70. Geburtstag*, ed. Paul Vogel (Göttingen: Vandenhoeck & Ruprecht, 1956), 243–65.

would inevitably cause the self to perish and lead to a consequential failure to grasp the meaning of one's own life and human existence in general.[110]

These questions probably took on a new dimension for Kütemeyer during the Second World War. For a time, he worked at the sanatorium in Wiesloch, which was located on a site where the Nazis were carrying out their euthanasia programme.[111] Doctors employed there sent over 2,000 people to facilities where they were either murdered or left to die from malnourishment and inadequate care. The Wiesloch complex also housed a euphemistically named children's department, where children were killed with phenobarbital and other drugs so that employees could conduct pseudoscientific experiments on their brains to determine the causes and effects of childhood psychiatric illnesses.[112] Working at the Wiesloch military hospital meant that Kütemeyer probably knew that crimes were being committed at the Wiesloch sanatorium, although he did not himself have a hand in euthanasia.[113]

Even though they did not explicitly refer to his time at Wiesloch, his writings composed immediately after the war intensively grappled with issues of illness, the guilt of the individual, and 'superindividual organisms', for which he offered the crimes of the Nazi euthanasia programmes as an example. In January 1947, shortly after the beginning of the Nuremberg Doctors' Trial, he published an article in the weekly *Die Zeit* titled 'Germany: guilty or sick?'.[114] A more in-depth articulation of his thoughts was published in 1948 under the same title in Dolf

[110] Søren Kierkegaard, *The Concept of Anxiety: A Simple Psychologically Orienting Deliberation on the Dogmatic Issue of Hereditary Sin*, ed. and trans. Reidar Thomte (Princeton: Princeton University Press, 1981); Søren Kierkegaard, *The Sickness unto Death: A Christian Psychological Exposition for Upbuilding and Awakening*, ed. and trans. Howard V. Hong and Edna H. Hong (Princeton: Princeton University Press, 1983).

[111] Almost all publications lack information about where Kütemeyer worked before 1945. The only clue is in the obituary written by his student Heinrich Huebschmann: 'he first worked as a doctor for the mentally ill under the supervision of Alfred Schweninger [sic] at the asylum in Wiesloch, then a military hospital.' See Heinrich Huebschmann, 'Zum Tode Wilhelm Kütemeyers', RN 2, 20 July 1972. UAH, PA 4711. More precise dates are hard to find. However, the archives of the Deutsche Dienststelle für die Benachrichtigung der nächsten Angehörigen von Gefallenen der ehemaligen deutschen Wehrmacht (German Agency for Informing the Family Members of Fallen Members of the Wehrmacht) suggest that Kütemeyer worked between the summer of 1941 and September 1944 in Wiesloch as a member of the Heeres-Sanitäts-Staffel Heidelberg (response of the archive from 19 October 2015).

[112] Franz Peschke, 'SCHRECK's Abteilung—Die Wieslocher "Kinderfachabteilung" im Zweiten Weltkrieg', *Schriftenreihe des Arbeitskreises 'Die Heil- und Pflegeanstalt Wiesloch in der Zeit des Nationalsozialismus'* 2 (1993): 19–41. On Wiesloch more generally, see Franz Peschke, *Ökonomie, Mord und Planwirtschaft. Die Heil- und Pflegeanstalt Wiesloch im Dritten Reich* (Bochum: Projekt, 2012).

[113] Alfred Schwenninger, Kütemeyer's supervisor in the neurological clinic of the military hospital was interrogated by the Combined Intelligence Objectives Sub-Committee: he told them that he knew of the euthanasia murders and protested against them multiple times before remaining silent upon threat of being sent to a concentration camp. See the report by Leo Alexander of 19 August 1945, a copy of which can be viewed at Stuart D. Stein's Web Genocide Documentation Centre of the University of the West of England: http://www.phdn.org/archives/www.ess.uwe.ac.uk/genocide/alexrep6.htm#Alfred.

[114] Wilhelm Kütemeyer, 'Deutschland schuldig oder krank?' *Die Zeit* 4, 23 January 1947, 3.

Sternberger's monthly journal *Die Wandlung* (*The Changing*).[115] Kütemeyer drew parallels between individual and social pathology by tracing them both back to the anaesthetization of emotions and self-betrayal, a diagnosis that explicitly drew on Kierkegaard's concept of the sickness unto death. He asserted that Germany was both guilty *and* sick, a unique position in the debate started by the Allies on Germans' collective guilt for the crimes of Nazism.

He opined that Germany's illness evolved out of its unwillingness to confront its despair about its own divisions, instead repressing it by anaesthetizing the emotions of all. A case study of a male patient with an early onset of psychosis helped him illustrate his claim that this incapacity to feel not only made possible euthanasia and the other crimes of Nazi Germany, but facilitated them. According to Kütemeyer, the patient had been incapable of adequately processing his own grief and the suffering of others since he was a child. His relationship to others' pain was one of mere 'curiosity', a sort of academic distance, and so he felt nothing but 'interest' for the feelings of a group of women who he shot in order to overcome the general panic on a boat transporting refugees. The doctor's account explained that the patient tried to fill his inner emptiness by seeking out dangerous situations where he could prove his own fortitude to himself. And this, Kütemeyer argued, was the juncture where individual and superindividual pathologies reinforced one another, reasoning:

> Can there be for such people a more fortuitous situation than war? . . . But to be clear: not because of their readiness to sacrifice, but because, while they never feel totally calm in this world, they nowhere feel more relatively calm than in the kind of danger that best reflects the state of their tortured souls . . . . The unleashing of all the contradictory forces bound up in them is where they find the highest expression of their lives. Because they know nothing of what actually motivates them. They are just obscurely driven by their inner conflicts, which remain hidden from them themselves.[116]

Thus, he thought that existential angst and despair could be repressed beyond the reach of consciousness when the self turned its back on itself and lost touch with its own feelings. In turn, he offered this as an explanation of both individual and superindividual psychosis. Kütemeyer's ideas particularly occupied people calling for political, moral, and cultural reforms in Germany, among them the aforementioned Sternberger along with Werner Kraus, Alfred Weber, and Kütemeyer's close friend Werner von Trott zu Solz.[117] Margret Boveri, who would soon publish

[115] Wilhelm Kütemeyer, 'Deutschland—schuldig oder krank?' *Die Wandlung* 2 (1948): 106–19.
[116] Ibid., 116.
[117] Kütemeyer had been friends since the early 1930s with Werner von Trott zu Solz, whose brother Adam was one of the close confidantes of Claus von Stauffenberg, who tried to assassinate Hitler.

her extensive analysis of betrayal as a defining feature of life in the twentieth century, also thought highly of Kütemeyer's politically infused psychosomatic medicine. It interested her 'as a chronicler and impacted person greatly, because [Kütemeyer's case studies] deal with situations in which people have to choose between different types of betrayal'.[118]

Kütemeyer, too, ultimately concluded that his cancer patients engaged in a subliminal form of self-betrayal. Nevertheless, his notes in the only preserved medical records of one of his cancer patients say little about which clinical experiences might have led him to this conclusion. Under the heading 'personal-social matters', he wrote of the 55-year-old patient 'Fräulein K.W.': 'She was expelled from Lorraine together with her brother in 1919. She lives alone and works as a seamstress. She has a very good relationship with her neighbours. Since her brother died, she has always supported his family in Lorraine a lot. Her sister-in-law and nephew live there and they always take care of her. She earns enough to get by on.'[119] The records reveal that she only told her doctor at a very late stage about her serious symptoms, loss of appetite, weight gain, and physical weakness, which she explained: 'It came on its own, and it will go away on its own.' In an entry from 19 May 1947, Kütemeyer suggested that her denial of her own fear might have been behind her 'naïve' assessment of her situation, noting that the unchangingly 'dull' patient repeatedly said: 'So long as it's not cancer, then it's alright.'[120]

We cannot know with certainty how Kütemeyer interpreted the case from a psychosomatic perspective, because he never referred to it in his publications. But that the mentioned statements were the only two that he quoted verbatim in his report indicates that he likely judged them to be significant. It is conceivable that he viewed both statements as effects of the woman's self-deception about the reality of her health. In turn, he may have thought that her self-deception had its origin in her yearning to dispel her fear, something that also expressed itself in her relatively unremarkable, seemingly conflict-free existence, because these are attributes that Kütemeyer analysed in detail in his first published case study of a cancer patient, which was printed in 1956.[121]

In contrast to 'Fräulein K.W.', the 34-year-old Hodgkin's lymphoma patient knew of his illness. Though uncurable with the means available at the time, he talked about it in a detached way. In Kütemeyer's assessment, the young man's knowledge of his deadly illness, '*in itself* of cardinal importance for his existence', had lost '*for him* all of its affective content'.[122] His diagnosis of this cancer patient matched that of the psychosis patient discussed above: emotional anaesthetization

[118] Margret Boveri, 'Körpergeschehen und Psychose. Eine Studie aus der Landschaft des Verrats', *Merkur* 8, no. 74 (1954): 371–8, 372.

[119] Krankenakte Fräulein K.W., UAH L-I Acc. 1/96 2029/47.

[120] Ibid.

[121] Kütemeyer, 'Anthropologische Medizin', 250–1.

[122] Ibid., 251 [emphasis in original].

and emptiness had made the war seem 'like the best time of his life'.[123] Kütemeyer inferred from this the more general notion that cancer was a form of madness embedded 'in the structure of the material', i.e. the body. Thus, he thought it arose out of the same pathological complex as psychosis, with the only difference being that cancer expressed itself in the body instead of in the mind.[124] This conclusion was facilitated by Kütemeyer's conviction—derived from his clinical experience—that the metaphysical and physiological aspects of the self were united through the psyche.[125]

Kütemeyer's theory posited that emotional anaesthetization had its origins in a traumatic childhood contortion of the self, which he suggested might also be grasped as a form of self-betrayal. In the 1956 case study, he wrote that his patient had a very close relationship to his mother, while his father cheated on her and hit her. At some point, the patient ceased loving his mother and took the 'side of violence'. He began to justify his father's actions and consequently made authority and obedience into his core values; meanwhile, his emotions were 'blunted': 'This is the underbelly of the smooth conformity with the business of life and society, which followed his ruined childhood.'[126]

Under the veneer of normality was an alienated, unfeeling person whose inner conflicts and hatred remained concealed both to himself as well as to others and could only find an outlet in illness. On the one hand, Kütemeyer offered his theory as an explanation of how National Socialism was ever possible in the first place, while on the other, he wanted to avoid placing personal moral blame on his patients for the grip that their pathology had on their lives. A lecture that he held in June 1965 emphasized this motivation. Citing Primo Levi's and Jean Cayrol's descriptions of their experiences in concentration camps, he analogized that cancer patients were captured by their general inclination to obedience in the same way that liberated camp prisoners could not easily escape the psychological terror imposed on them by camp guards: 'He [the camp prisoner as well as the cancer patient] remains at his master's feet, singing his favourite melodies with a feeble voice, in order to amuse and appease him.'[127]

The comparison now seems reprehensibly irresponsible, because it posits a fundamental psychic affinity between concentration camp prisoners and people who, according to Kütemeyer's case studies, described the Nazi war of aggression as the happiest time of their lives. But at the time, nobody publicly reproached this form of historical-psychological interpretation, because it dovetailed well with psychiatric discussions about the long-term trauma suffered by concentration camp prisoners.[128] Moreover, as he noted elsewhere, he wanted the reference to

[123] Ibid., 252. [124] Ibid., 261, n. 6. [125] Ibid., 265. [126] Ibid., 264.

[127] Kütemeyer, 'Psychosocial Aspects of Cancer'.

[128] Svenja Goltermann, *Die Gesellschaft der Überlebenden. Deutsche Kriegsheimkehrer und ihre Gewalterfahrungen im Zweiten Weltkrieg* (Munich: DVA, 2009), 312–19.

Nazi Germany to help underscore the urgency of his demand that medicine undertake fundamental reforms.[129]

But Kütemeyer's psychologizing of everything somatic and his approach to the case studies so essential to his work did run up against resistance. One particularly loud critic was Alexander Mitscherlich (1908–82), who at first glance seems like he might have been destined to be a supporter. When Kütemeyer presented his observations on the deeper pathological structure underlying cancer at a conference in Turin in the summer of 1965, the Heidelberg medical faculty had already been debating the scientific value of his work for about seven years. At stake was whether he should be certified to become a professor or should at least be granted an honorary professorship. The key question was the extent to which psychosomatic medicine could be applied to somatic ailments and the scientific standards that should be used to judge experiments' findings. Mitscherlich was, like Kütemeyer, also a student of the deceased Viktor von Weizsäcker and would come to leave a lasting mark on West German psychoanalysis, psychosomatics, and the heated social discourse on how to come to terms with Germany's Nazi past.[130]

The conflict over Kütemeyer's work was amplified by the fact that psychosomatic medicine was establishing itself as a serious, socially relevant science. In 1949, the Deutsche Gesellschaft für Innere Medizin (German Society for Internal Medicine) dedicated a section of the first conference it held after the war to psychosomatics. In 1950, the first psychosomatic clinic in West Germany was founded in Heidelberg, with Mitscherlich as its first director. Mitscherlich had also advocated for psychosomatics as a more humane alternative to National-Socialist medicine in his extensive reporting on the Nuremberg Doctors' Trial, which was published in book form in 1947 and in English translation in 1949 under the title *Doctors of Infamy*. Initially, his articles were only received by an expert readership, which was generally enraged by them. But in 1960, Mitscherlich and Fred Mielke published a new edition of the book in paperback that ignited a vigorous public debate.[131] They laid exclusive responsibility for the Nazis' murderous medical experiments at the doorstep of so-called natural-scientific medicine. Because the text did not contain a single reference to psychosomatic medicine, it gave the (wrong) impression that no doctors working with psychosomatic methods had

[129] Wilhelm Kütemeyer, *Die Krankheit in ihrer Menschlichkeit* (Göttingen: Vandenhoeck & Ruprecht, 1963), 184.

[130] On his life, work, and influence, see Martin Dehli, *Leben als Konflikt. Zur Biographie Alexander Mitscherlichs* (Göttingen: Wallstein, 2007), and Tobias Freimüller, *Alexander Mitscherlich. Gesellschaftsdiagnosen und Psychoanalyse nach Hitler* (Göttingen: Wallstein, 2007).

[131] Mitscherlich and Fred Mielke published three reports on the Doctors' Trial: *Das Diktat der Menschenverachtung. Eine Dokumentation. Der Nürnberger Ärzteprozeß und seine Quellen* (Heidelberg: Lambert Schneider, 1947), published in English translation as *Doctors of Infamy: The Story of Nazi Medical Crimes* (New York: Henry Schuman, 1949); *Wissenschaft ohne Menschlichkeit. Medizinische und eugenische Irrwege unter Diktatur, Bürokratie und Krieg* (Heidelberg: Lambert Schneider, 1949); and, finally, the book *Medizin ohne Menschlichkeit. Dokumente des Nürnberger Ärzteprozesses* (Frankfurt am Main: Fischer, 1960).

embraced the Nazi view of human life or participated in forced sterilizations and euthanasia killings.[132]

The debate in Heidelberg over the validity of Kütemeyer's work thus took place at a time when many psychosomatic doctors were hoping to elevate the status of their field, both as a science and as a moral authority inside and outside the medical world. Mitscherlich's assessment was decidedly negative: asked to evaluate Kütemeyer's work by the Heidelberg University medical faculty in 1964, he faulted as 'arbitrary' Kütemeyer's tendency to place a single case study at the heart of his texts—an approach that Kütemeyer had adopted from Weizsäcker—and warned that the international community would ignore his research on account of its methodological flimsiness.[133] But the latter charge did not hold true. A contribution to Thure von Uexküll's *Lehrbuch der Psychosomatischen Medizin* (*Textbook of Psychosomatic Medicine*) highlighted Kütemeyer's findings: the author was psychologist Claus Bahne Bahnson, an internationally recognized name in the psychosomatics of cancer and a professor at Philadelphia's Jefferson Medical College; the volume, a standard work of its time, was published in 1979, a full fifteen years after Mitscherlich's dismissal of his colleague's work.[134]

Presumably, Mitscherlich was most interested in preserving his own position as an internationally acclaimed researcher. But by knocking Kütemeyer, Mitscherlich was also distancing himself from the biographical medicine of his teacher Weizsäcker and thus from his own intellectual past. Coupled with his turn towards psychoanalysis, Mitscherlich had begun this shift in the 1950s, when he maintained that a human being's psychosomatic unity could be dismantled by serious physical illness. Even though detrimental illnesses might have their origins in what Mitscherlich had conceptualized as a two-phase process of repression, he claimed that they could separate themselves off from the psyche and attain a sort of secondary autonomy.[135] His standard example was, in the 1960s and after, the carcinoma.[136] This admission allowed him to defend himself against accusations that doctors and psychotherapists in his clinic had overestimated the effectiveness of treating physical illnesses like cancer with the methods of psychosomatics,

[132] Dehli, *Leben als Konflikt*, 145–75; Schultz-Venrath and Hermanns, 'Gleichschaltung zur Ganzheit'.

[133] Letter from Alexander Mitscherlich to the Dean of the Medical Faculty, Prof. Dr Friedrich-Wilhelm Brauss, 14 January 1964; Report, UAH, PA 10389, 10, Dr Wilhelm Kütemeyer.

[134] Claus Bahne Bahnson, 'Das Krebsproblem in psychosomatischer Dimension', in *Lehrbuch der psychosomatischen Medizin*, ed. Thure von Uexküll (Munich: Urban & Schwarzenberg, 1979), 685–98, 688.

[135] Alexander Mitscherlich, 'Zur psychoanalytischen Auffassung psychosomatischer Krankheitsentstehung', *Psyche* 7, no. 10 (1954): 561–78, 571.

[136] Alexander Mitscherlich, 'Anmerkungen über die Chronifizierung psychosomatischen Geschehens', *Psyche* 15, no. 1 (1962): 1–25, 5; Alexander Mitscherlich, 'Über die Behandlung psychosomatischer Krankheiten', *Psyche* 18, no. 11 (1965): 643–63, 644–5.

denying that they were responsible for the death of patients by providing them inadequate care.[137]

Moreover, he acknowledged that his version of psychosomatics had its limits and could only function in tandem with other fields of medicine. In doing so, he discarded Weizsäcker's challenge to all doctors to take a holistic approach to their work. Kütemeyer criticized the shift in a review of Alexander and his wife Margarete von Mitscherlich's diagnosis of post-war German society as one incapable of properly mourning the loss of the '*Führer*'. He chided their book's 'resignation towards the importance of material processes in history' as if history were solely determined by 'the inhuman mechanisms of these material processes'.[138]

In the 1960s, practitioners and researchers of psychosomatics in Germany increasingly expanded psychosomatic interpretations to all bodily ailments and the conflict and emotions that define them, despite Mitscherlich's reservations about doing so. But before their work could be recognized both by the scientific community and the public more broadly, they needed to find a way to make their assumptions both verifiable and reproducible in experiments. Thus, Mitscherlich's critique of Kütemeyer's overreliance on case studies was not for nothing: the depth psychology and biographical medicine practiced by Kütemeyer (and his teacher Weizsäcker) could not be verified in laboratory experiments. Their results could only be confirmed retrospectively and could not be checked using standardized test procedures as was customary in psychological research. Indeed, Kütemeyer's insistence on the uniqueness of individual biographies was fundamentally at odds with the principle of generalizability. For him, the case study was not just a narrative form intended to illustrate the features of an illness. It was a central component of diagnosis; writing a case study was at once analysis and method.[139]

But in other parts of the world, another scientific standard was on the rise. In his evaluation of Kütemeyer's dissertation, University of Amsterdam professor of psychology Pieter Cornelius Kuiper (1919–2002) admonished 'that we must work with comprehensible concepts and must develop methods that lead to verifiable results'.[140] By verifiable, he meant first and foremost that the findings be statistically relevant, experimentally reproducible, and thus generalizable.

The relatively new, but ever more influential concept of stress offered a middle way. It opened the door to animal experiments that German psychosomatics, with its complex models of emotions and conflict, had long rejected.

[137] Freimüller, *Alexander Mitscherlich*, 209 and 221–2.

[138] Wilhelm Kütemeyer, 'Psychoanalyse der Geschichte? Zu Alexander Mitscherlichs Ideen über den Frieden', *Evangelische Kommentare* 11 (1969): 662–4, 664.

[139] Alexa Geisthövel, 'Aktenführung und Autorschaft. Ärztliches Schreiben in der Subjektmedizin Viktor von Weizsäckers (1920er bis 1950er Jahre)', *Medizinhistorisches Journal* 51, no. 3 (2016): 180–208.

[140] Copy of the report by Prof. Dr P. C. Kuiper to the dean of the Heidelberg medical faculty, Amsterdam, 8 March 1964. UAH, PA 10389, Dr Wilhelm Kütemeyer.

Dominant Mothers and Emotionless Daughters: Cancer Personalities and the Problem of Quantifying Subjectivity

A younger generation of doctors and psychologists born in the 1930s saw psychosomatics as a chance to fundamentally reform medicine. At the same time, they avoided getting caught up in antinomic debates with 'natural-scientific' medicine like their early post-war predecessors in Heidelberg had done. Their desire was to incorporate psychosomatics into mainstream everyday clinical practice.[141] Stepping outside the traditional bounds of psychosomatics and other fields of medicine provided them with fruitful alternatives.

In the United States, where psychosomatics had already achieved considerable recognition in the 1930s, psychosomatic cancer research started gaining traction in the 1940s.[142] One of the most influential early American studies on the links between psychosomatics and cancer was carried out by psychiatrist and neurologist Milton Tarlau and psychologist Irwin Smalheiser at the New York City Cancer Institute, a hospital for late-stage cancer patients. They published their findings in 1951 in *Psychosomatic Medicine*, the official journal of the American Psychosomatic Society.[143]

Their study sought to discern whether patients with a particular type of cancer had personality traits similar to one another but different from patients with other types of cancer, or if the personality structures of all cancer patients were similar to one another, but markedly divergent from the healthy control group. They interviewed eleven breast cancer patients and eleven patients with cervical cancer. The assumption that there might be important personality differences between breast cancer patients on the one hand and cervical cancer patients on the other was rooted in a guiding principle of American psychosomatics of the era, specificity theory. The principle was formulated in 1939 by Austrian émigré Franz Alexander in the first issue of *Psychosomatic Medicine* and was essentially an extension of the theory of psychophysiology developed by Friedrich Kraus in the early twentieth century.[144] It postulated that every emotion is correlated with a specific physiological reaction (fear is expressed by a racing heart, for instance). As a consequence, it held that an emotionally laden conflict situation or an emotion that persists over an extended period of time could lead to long-term changes to

[141] Mechthilde Kütemeyer, 'Neurologie und Psychosomatik. Erinnerungen an die Janz'sche Klinik', in *Die Wahrheit der Begegnung: anthropologische Perspektiven der Neurologie*, ed. Rainer M. E. Jacobi, Peter C. Claussen, and Peter Wolf (Würzburg: Königshausen und Neumann, 2001), 191–214.

[142] Bettina Hitzer and Pilar León-Sanz, 'The Feeling Body and Its Diseases: How Cancer Went Psychosomatic in Twentieth-Century Germany', *Osiris* 31, no. 1 (2016): 67–93, 83–7, https://doi.org/10.1086/687591.

[143] Milton Tarlau and Irwin Smalheiser, 'Personality Patterns in Patients with Malignant Tumors of the Breast and Cervix: An Exploratory Study', *Psychosomatic Medicine* 13, no. 2 (1951): 117–21.

[144] Franz Alexander, 'Psychological Aspects of Medicine', *Psychosomatic Medicine* 1, no. 1 (1939): 7–18.

an organ or bodily system. The core of the theory was that every illness could be traced back to a specific, repressed, and therefore 'chronic' emotion and the physiological reaction associated with it. Alexander believed that he had discovered a generally applicable pathological principle that was particularly pronounced in seven illnesses that would later come to be known as the 'holy seven' psychosomatic afflictions.[145] Thus, it was their adherence to specificity theory that occasioned Tarlau and Smalheiser to select patients with different types of cancer for their test group.

No coincidence either were the types of tumour they selected. The introduction to their article explained that these two types of cancer comprised the majority of cancer cases among American women. But the questions they asked and the tests they conducted reveal that their choice was also informed by assumptions about female emotions and sexuality that they did not explicitly articulate. This is underscored by the fact that neither Tarlau and Smalheiser nor any other American psychosomatic doctors of the period conducted any comparable studies on men with lung or stomach cancer, even though these were the most common forms of cancer among men.

Everything in Tarlau and Smalheiser's questionnaire revolved around a single topic—the women's 'psychosexual' personality development. It inquired into their relationship with their mother and father in early childhood, how old they were when one or both of their parents died, their first sexual experiences, their reaction to their first menstrual period, and their marital life. The other tests probed whether and how much the women stood in conflict with their female self, how strongly they repressed, came to terms with, or acted out negative feelings, and their ability to react to emotional stimuli. Working with the assumption that childhood experiences played a formative role in the women's relationship to their own femininity, sexuality, and emotions, the researchers hypothesized that their 'psychosexual' profile was directly responsible for the emergence of cancer in their bodies. Tarlau and Smalheiser believed that the tests confirmed their hypothesis.

They extrapolated some commonalities among the women from the test results. They concluded that all of them rejected their female role because they had had dominant mothers who did not show them affection. This, in turn, caused them to develop a negative attitude towards their own sexuality, which inhibited them from leading a 'normal' sex life. But while the breast cancer patients had marriages that, at least on the surface, appeared stable and happy, the cervical cancer patients' sexual dysfunction was decidedly more manifest.[146] The researchers

[145] They were peptic ulcers, asthma, rheumatoid arthritis, ulcerative colitis, hypertension, neurodermatitis, and Crohn's disease. See Franz Alexander, *Psychosomatic Medicine: Its Principles and Applications* (New York: W. W. Norton, 1950).

[146] Tarlau and Smalheiser, 'Personality Patterns', 121.

based this inference on their observation that the latter group had had premarital sexual relations, had married very early, and were unhappy with their husbands.

The two scientists were convinced that they had established a connection between abnormal female sexuality and cancer. The idea was not new. Both Georg Groddeck's and Elida Evans's case studies in depth psychology had put forward similar claims. Groddeck surmised that the connection developed out of women's suffering under the weight of gendered social expectations. Tarlau and Smalheiser took a different approach: they articulated their own psychosomatically informed ideal of 'healthy' female behaviour and then deduced normative expectations from it. But by painting a picture of two different types of female 'cancer personality' that, from the outside, seemed to be diametrically opposed, they revealed just how much the experiences of the war had transformed understandings of gender roles. Their analysis of the test results labelled as healthy neither the women active in premarital or extramarital sexual relationships nor the women living in a stable marriage and conforming, at least superficially, to gender norms. The authors appealed to psychoanalysis' dynamic concept of emotions in support of their assessment that the repressed, insufficiently developed emotions hiding behind the façade of conformity played a causative role in cancer.[147]

But which particular female emotions they chose to problematize also represented a sharp departure from older social discourses on femininity. The issue for the two researchers was not the emotionally wild woman who had a difficult time bringing her feelings under control; neither of the cancer personalities drawn by Tarlau and Smalheiser were characterized by passion or intense emotions. Rather, the trouble was that both types had difficulty getting in touch with their emotions and feeling 'authentically'.

In both cases, the two doctors placed the guilt squarely in the hands of the mother, thus following a trend in Anglo-American psychiatry that had begun in the 1940s and would develop into the dominant paradigm of psychology and psychiatry in the post-war United States and Western Europe. Influenced by psychoanalysis, this shift was foundational for much social discourse on how children should be raised so that they would grow up to become productive, responsible, healthy, psychologically and physically stable citizens.

While early Freudian psychoanalysis revolved around the drives, by the 1930s a new generation of analysts were homing in on how social relations and the environment shape human beings and their emotions. Still, early childhood maintained its primacy during this shift, and the person's relation to their mother continued to be seen as especially formative. This perspective was summed up pointedly in 1940 by British psychoanalyst Donald Winnicott: 'There is no such

[147] On the 'hydraulic' model of emotions, see Barbara Rosenwein, 'Worrying about Emotions in History', *American Historical Review* 107, no. 3 (2002): 821–45, 834.

thing as an infant . . . whenever one finds an infant one finds maternal care, and without maternal care there would be no infant.'[148] In the 1930s and during the Second World War, many British paediatricians and child therapists worked with children who were temporarily or permanently parentless: children brought to the countryside to protect them from German air raids, Jewish children sent to Great Britain, and war orphans. Doctors remarked how extended periods of time without their mothers could cause children to regress emotionally and mentally and become physically fragile.[149] The observation was expanded upon by psychoanalysts in the United States like Austrian émigré René Spitz, who had similar experiences in his work in orphanages.[150]

This confluence of events instigated a shift in child psychology away from the dominant paradigm of behaviourism—which defined human behaviour in line with the stimulus-response model as the sum of conditioning—and placed the blame for abnormalities on overly protective mothers. In its place stepped the psychoanalysis of early childhood and its emphasis on motherly affection as the foundation of healthy psychological development. John Bowlby's 1951 book *Maternal Care and Mental Health* catapulted the theory's political and social influence well beyond the borders of the United States and Great Britain.[151]

Known as attachment theory, this new model placed considerable pressure on mothers to be emotionally devoted and available. But the ideal of a mother who successfully crafted her child's emotional stability and capacity to forge bonds with others had a flipside: the image of a mother who literally drove her child mad.[152] In the immediate post-war era, more and more psychologists and psychiatrists agreed that mothers were responsible if their child became schizophrenic, even going so far as to coin a new concept to describe them. The schizophrenogenic mother was described in sometimes self-contradictory terms: she was overbearing, cold towards her child, and lacking 'authentic' love.[153]

Thus, in a striking parallel to developments in psychosomatic cancer research, a psychic illness that had previously been explained as the result of physical brain damage was now interpreted as the endgame of an emotionally unfulfilling, loveless mother-child relationship. This shift from a material aetiology to an

[148] Donald Woods Winnicott, 'The Theory of Parent-Infant Relationship', *International Journal of Psychoanalysis* 41, no. 6 (1960): 585–95, 587.

[149] See, for instance, Dorothy Burlingham and Anna Freud, *Young Children in War-Time in a Residential War Nursery* (London: G. Allen & Unwin, 1942).

[150] René A. Spitz, 'The Role of Ecological Factors in Emotional Development in Infancy', *Child Development* 20, no. 3 (1949): 145–55.

[151] John Bowlby, *Maternal Care and Mental Health: A Report Prepared on Behalf of the World Health Organization as a Contribution to the United Nations Programme for the Welfare of Homeless Children* (Bulletin of the World Health Organization 3) (Geneva: WHO, 1951), 355–534.

[152] Anne Harrington, 'Mother Love and Mental Illness: An Emotional History', *Osiris* 31, no. 1 (2016): 94–115, 106–9, https://doi.org/10.1086/687559.

[153] Frieda Fromm-Reichmann, 'Notes on the Development of Treatment of Schizophrenics by Psychoanalytic Theory', *Psychiatry* 11, no. 3 (1948): 263–73.

emotional aetiology took place in the context of a more general transformation in the history of emotions. Sociologists, political scientists, and economists cast a leery eye at emotions, their mistrust feeding off the perception that emotions had seized the masses and thus opened the gates for fascism and its derailing of morals and laws.[154] Many post-war sociological and political theories largely ignored the role of emotions in society and politics and developed models of decision-making procedures based on a 'rationality' devoid of emotions.[155] In contrast, doctors, psychologists, and psychiatrists researched emotions more fervently.[156] But the concept of emotions they were working with was more nuanced than the dominant tendency to write them off as irrational. They were not trying to find ways to shut off emotions or avoid feelings deemed too intense. Rather, they explored the relations between authority, obedience, and 'authentic' emotions, thus anticipating the 1960s' critique of the superficial lifestyle of 'square' post-war society.[157] At the same time, their research might be read as an alternative approach to the historical experiences of fascism and world war.

Back to Tarlau and Smalheiser's study. The experiment that they conducted with the twenty-two female cancer patients at the New York City Cancer Institute established a prototype for two decades of psychosomatic studies, including Michael Holm-Hadulla's that opened the chapter. They combined three different psychological tests and read their results against one another to obtain greater validity, a practice still standard in psychology today. The women answered the questions discussed above during a one- to two-hour dialogue and were then asked to take a Rorschach test. At the end, they had to draw three human figures: a man, a woman, and themselves.[158] The Rorschach test was the centrepiece. One of the standard psychological tests of the time, it was employed in a broad spectrum of diagnostic procedures.[159]

[154] Frank Biess and Daniel M. Gross, 'Emotional Returns', in *Science and Emotions after 1945: A Transatlantic Perspective*, ed. Frank Biess and Daniel M. Gross (Chicago: University of Chicago Press, 2014), 1–4; Biess, 'Feelings in the Aftermath', 34–5.

[155] Ute Frevert, 'Passions, Preferences, and Animal Spirits: How Does Homo Oeconomicus Cope with Emotions?', in Biess and Gross, *Science and Emotions after 1945*, 300–17; Helena Flam, 'The Transatlantic Element in the Sociology of Emotions', in Biess and Gross, *Science and Emotions after 1945*, 318–41; Erickson et al., *How Reason Almost Lost Its Mind.*

[156] American historian of emotions Peter Stearns claims that the 1950s were dominated by attempts to master feelings and dampen their intensity. Frank Biess supported this position in his work on soldiers returning home from war and West German policies on civil defence. See Stearns, *American Cool*; Frank Biess, '"Everybody Has a Chance": Civil Defense, Nuclear Angst, and the History of Emotions in Postwar Germany', *German History* 27, no. 2 (2009): 215–43, https://doi.org/10.1093/gerhis/ghp003.

[157] See the section of this chapter: 'The Risks of Diagnosing Society: The (In)ability to Mourn, Be Angry, and Feel Rage'.

[158] Eleanor Holtz-Eakin and Ida Sue Baron, 'Human Figure Drawing Tests', in *Encyclopedia of Clinical Neuropsychology*, ed. Jeffrey Kreutzer, John De Luca, and Bruce Caplan (New York: Springer, 2011), 1269–71.

[159] Joni L. Mihura and Gregory J. Meyer, 'Rorschach Inkblot Test', in *Encyclopedia of Clinical Psychology*, ed. Robert L. Cautin and Scott O. Lilienfeld (Chichester: Wiley-Blackwell, 2015), 2491–6, 2491.

Hermann Rorschach, student of Eugen Bleuler and a psychiatrist at the asylum in Herisau, Switzerland, published the test's ten inkblots in 1921 in a book titled *Psychodiagnostics*.[160] In contrast to the inkblot tests that preceded it, Rorschach's test did not aim to gather information about a person's faculties, such as their imagination. Rather, the Swiss psychiatrist wanted to determine the person's *Erlebnistypus*, or experience type,[161] a concept that was informed by a singular understanding of the self. While psychologists had generally conceived of the self as the sum of a person's abilities, Rorschach thought the key lay in how a person perceived and processed experiences, which involved a number of different cognitive and affective capacities.[162] By asking the subject about their impressions of inkblots that are in themselves meaningless, the test 'forces' them to imbue them with significance and thus generates knowledge about how they process experiences. Thus, the test relies neither on the subject's introspection nor on the psychoanalytic theory of the unconscious.

The test was used to interpret various aspects of the subject's responses (or lack thereof). During the first phase, the subject described what they saw in each image and then explained what parts of the image led them to see a spider, flower, or a chicken. What surprised many people was that *what* they perceived in the pictures played a subordinate role, a fact communicated to them neither before nor after the test. Decisive were other factors, which the psychologist sitting behind or in front of them was supposed to inconspicuously note down. Among them were whether what they saw comprised the entire image, or just a part or some details; whether what they saw was more centred on the image's form, or whether its colour or the illusion of movement held more significance. The psychologist was supposed to count how many times the subject saw a human, an animal, or a thing, whether the responses lined up with those of a majority of other test-takers, or if their associations were uncommon or unique. Whether the person saw just one or multiple things in the image also counted in the final assessment. Their reaction time was measured, too, in order to ascertain whether an image shocked them and thus led to a delayed reaction.[163]

The psychologist or psychiatrist who administered the Rorschach test entered all these parameters into a table. The guidelines that helped them judge which parameters stood for which personality attributes evolved over the course of the test's history. Rorschach himself had put forward some interpretations, which were then refined over the course of millions of applications and the construction

[160] Hermann Rorschach, *Psychodiagnostik. Methodik und Ergebnisse eines wahrnehmungs-diagnostischen Experiments (Deutenlassen von Zufallsformen)* (Bern, 1921).

[161] Hermann Rorschach, *Psychodiagnostik. Methodik und Ergebnisse eines wahrnehmungsdiagnostischen Experiments (Deutenlassen von Zufallsformen)*, ed. Walter Morgenthaler, 10th edn (Bern: Hans Huber, 1983), 113–14.

[162] Peter Galison, 'Image of Self', in *Things That Talk: Object Lessons from Art and Science*, ed. Lorraine Daston (New York: Zone Books, 2004), 257–94, 276–7.

[163] Rorschach, *Psychodiagnostik*, 19–46.

of new personality profiles that were generated through juxtaposition with other tests and diagnostic tools. The Rorschach test promised to reveal whether groups like Tarlau and Smalheiser's breast cancer and cervical cancer patients had personality traits in common with one another and whether their traits significantly deviated from those of a 'normal group'. Thus, from the perspective of its administrator, the Rorschach test offered a measure to quantify the personalities of the most diverse groups because it was supposed to have a level of objectivity that was, at the time, described as being similar to that of an x-ray.[164]

In comparison to the control group, Tarlau and Smalheiser's patients' interpretations were much more austere than those given by the control group and they predominantly derived what they saw from the whole image. From this the researchers concluded that the women's inner lives were desiccated and their critical faculties meagre. Because the women rarely saw humans in the inkblots, and almost never moving humans, Tarlau and Smalheiser characterized them as people who were unable to accept themselves and their own desires and dreams, and thus as people with immature, brittle personalities. When the patients did see a human, however, it was almost always a man, leading the researchers to conclude that the women rejected their femininity and fostered masculine emotions. Perceptions of animals were supposed to be an indicator of the women's acceptance of their sexual drives. The breast cancer patients generally saw 'weak' animals like butterflies and bats, read as a sign that their sex life was undeveloped, and their reactions to the colour inkblots differed little from their reactions to the black-and-white ones. From this the researchers inferred that they were incapable of emotionally reacting to external stimuli.[165] In contrast, the cervical cancer patients often saw inanimate objects and shadows, read as a sign of fear and anxiety. The breast cancer patients, in turn, frequently focused on the inkblots' form and thus betrayed their high level of inner control and rigidity.

It might seem surprising that a person's free associations about what they see in ten inkblots could lead researchers to draw such broad conclusions about their personality and even about the connection between their personality and their illness. In recent years, psychologists and others have begun raising doubts about the legitimacy of using Rorschach tests to make assessments so weighty for an individual's life.[166]

But when Tarlau and Smalheiser published their study in 1951, the test and the conclusions they deduced from it still seemed plausible to most of their peers.

[164] Galison, 'Image of Self', 292. The comparison to x-rays was made at the time, see Lawrence K. Frank, 'Projective Methods for the Study of Personality', *Journal of Psychology* 8, no. 2 (1939): 389–413, 397–8, https://doi.org/10.1080/00223980.1939.9917671.

[165] The assessment along with the table can be found in Tarlau and Smalheiser, 'Personality Patterns', 118–20.

[166] James M. Wood, M. Teresa Nezworski, Scott O. Lilienfeld, and Howard N. Garb, *What's Wrong with the Rorschach? Science Confronts the Controversial Inkblot Test* (San Francisco: Jossey-Bass, 2003).

Nevertheless, their study was criticized for other methodological deficits. In 1955, a review published by John Wheeler and Bettye McDonald Caldwell in the journal *Psychosomatic Medicine* listed some of the study's most severe methodological issues. First, the data for Tarlau and Smalheiser's 'normal' group was taken from a 1942 study of Rorschach tests completed by fifty soldiers ages 18 to 33 who had been sent to the psychiatric section of the Fort Dix Station Hospital for various mental disturbances.[167] Moreover, Wheeler and Caldwell raised their eyebrows at the notion that the Rorschach tests of a group of severely ill women under the influence of painkillers and anti-anxiety drugs could offer any insights into their *Erlebnistypus*. They were sceptical about inferring any conclusions about the women's personalities from the draw-a-person test that complemented the Rorschach, too. That the breast cancer patients only drew 'primitive' figures probably had more to do with the fact that they had all undergone mastectomies, Wheeler and Caldwell reproofed, because due to the operation and the lymphatic obstruction in the arms that often followed it, they could probably only draw under serious pain and duress.[168]

These faults induced Wheeler and Caldwell to repeat the study on more solid methodological ground. Alongside a group of breast cancer and cervical cancer patients, they tested a control group of women with the same average age and similar socio-economic and familial status. The control group had come to the clinic suffering from different ailments than the test group, but had never had cancer. The test group, in contrast, were all in outpatient treatment. In Wheeler and Caldwell's assessment, the differences between the three groups' Rorschach tests and draw-a-person tests were insignificant. Still, they did not close the case on whether cancer patients might have specific personality traits, concluding cautiously: 'the relationship between these group tendencies and the neoplastic transformation remains an unsettled issue.'[169] Their recommendation was to keep on researching the question.

Over the course of the following decade, studies out of the United States, Canada, and Europe followed suit. But doctors in the United States became increasingly wary of this brand of psychosomatic oncological study.[170] Another article in *Psychosomatic Medicine* accelerated the trend by highlighting the studies' methodological problems and assumptions even more penetratingly than the

[167] Captain James A. Brussel and Private Kenneth S. Hitch, 'The Rorschach Method and Its Uses in Military Psychiatry', *Psychiatric Quarterly* 16, no. 1 (1942): 3–29, https://doi.org/10.1007/BF01561244.

[168] John I. Wheeler and Bettye McDonald Caldwell, 'Psychological Evaluation of Women with Cancer of the Breast and of the Cervix', *Psychosomatic Medicine* 17, no. 4 (1955): 256–68, 258 and 262.

[169] Ibid., 267.

[170] At the same time, the psychosomatic explanation of stomach ulcers lost in significance, see Robert A. Aronowitz, 'The Rise and Fall of the Psychosomatic Hypothesis in Ulcerative Colitis', in *Making Sense of Illness: Science, Society, and Disease*, ed. Robert A. Aronowitz (Cambridge: Cambridge University Press, 1998), 39–56, 48–52.

piece by Wheeler and Caldwell.[171] Some psychosomatic oncologists tried to counter this criticism with less fallible methods, testing men and women who came to the clinic because they suspected that they might have cancer but did not yet know. This was supposed to rule out the potential influence that the knowledge of suffering from a serious illness might have on the personality profile. But others turned their attention towards the older inquiry into the experimentally provable physiological mechanisms through which emotions could play a causative role in cancer. Key to this strain of research was the yet relatively young concept of stress.[172]

Stress and Personality

Anglo-American psychosomatic cancer research really began to strike roots in Germany—East and West—in the early 1960s. With its mixture of hard science and personality psychology, it seemed to offer precisely what Alexander Mitscherlich had found so sorely missing in Wilhelm Kütemeyer's writings: evidence, statistical representativeness, a methodology recognized by natural scientists, and engagement with international research. Increasing discomfort with established cancer therapies and their middling success rates made oncologists more open to alternative approaches.

The expansion of the psychosomatics of cancer in Germany brought together two somewhat contrary developments. While psychosomatic cancer researchers in the United States and United Kingdom were facing tough criticism and appealing for international support, German doctors and psychologists wanted to up the standing of an approach that had until then received little appreciation in their home country. In 1960, the International Psychosomatic Cancer Study Group was established to provide a forum for interested doctors, psychologists, sociologists, biologists, and cultural anthropologists.

It was organized by two internationally renowned psychosomatic oncologists, David M. Kissen of the Glasgow Department of Psychological Medicine and Lawrence LeShan of the New York Institute of Applied Biology, as well as a less prominent clinical psychologist from Oldenburg, West Germany named Hans-Joachim F. Baltrusch. At first sight, it might seem surprising that a 33-year-old with little to his name would be setting up an international research group

[171] George M. Perrin and Irene R. Pierce, 'Psychosomatic Aspects of Cancer', *Psychosomatic Medicine* 21, no. 5 (1959): 397–412, 411.

[172] Roy R. Grinker, 'Psychosomatic Aspects of the Cancer Problem', *Annals of the New York Academy of Science* 125 (1966): 876–82, https://doi.org/10.1111/j.1749%966632.1966.tb45439.x.

alongside two seasoned professionals.[173] But Baltrusch's 1957 curriculum vitae fused in exemplary fashion threads that would come to define the history of German psychosomatic cancer research.[174]

Baltrusch entered medical school in Bremen in 1947, where he became increasingly steeped in philosophy and psychology as his studies went on. He took off in 1949 to spend a year at the Institut für Psychotherapie und Tiefenpsychologie (Institute for Psychotherapy and Depth Psychology) in Stuttgart. Erected in part on the initiative of Viktor von Weizsäcker, the multidisciplinary institute trained psychotherapists and special educational needs teachers, and the parental counselling centre attached to it evidenced an affinity for the child psychology of Melanie Klein, Anna Freud, and John Bowlby. After Stuttgart, Baltrusch headed to the University of Lund in Sweden, where he completed a degree in psychology in 1954. The choice of school was significant, as Lund was, in European comparison, very strongly influenced by Anglo-American personality psychology.[175]

Gudmund Smith, one of Baltrusch's professors in Lund, worked for the Swedish military during the Second World War, where he had intensively studied psychometrics and personality tests. Baltrusch headed back to Oldenburg after completing his studies in Lund and was hired as a clinical psychologist at the town's Lutheran Hospital. His boss was Helmut Bohnenkamp, who had been a professor of internal medicine at Freiburg in the 1930s and a formative figure in Wilhelm Kütemeyer's development during his time there.

Thus, the intellectual biography of this young, ambitious, reformist clinical psychologist bridged pre-war psychosomatics with the ideas of the newer psychosomatics defined by Anglo-American theories of personality and psychodynamics. Baltrusch mixed them all together in his clinical work as well as in his research projects, which probed the relations between personality structure, emotions, and illness, particularly in the lives of children with leukaemia.[176]

Leukaemia was a priority in American psychosomatic research, too, though for different reasons than breast and cervical cancer. At the time, it was one of the most feared forms of cancer, as there existed no viable therapy and the chances of

[173] In 1960, Baltrusch worked as a clinical psychologist at the Elisabeth Children's Hospital in Oldenburg. He temporarily filled a visiting doctor position, but apparently only part-time, probably alongside his yet unfinished medical studies. Employee file of Hans-Joachim Baltrusch, inventory 113, no. 83, Stadtarchiv Oldenburg.

[174] Curriculum vitae, signed Oldenburg (Oldb), 25 August 1957, Hans-Joachim F. Baltrusch. Private collection of Hans-Joachim Baltrusch, inventory 113, no. 83, Stadtarchiv Oldenburg. I would like to thank his daughter Katharina Baltrusch in Hamburg for providing me further information on his life.

[175] Ingvar Lundberg, 'Zeitgeist, Ortgeist, and Personalities in the Development of Scandinavian Psychology', *International Journal of Psychology* 36, no. 6 (2001): 356–62, https://doi.org/10.1080/00207590143000.

[176] Hans-Joachim Baltrusch, 'Leukämien und andere maligne Erkrankungen des haematopoetischen, lymphatischen und reticulo-endothelialen Systems in psycho-somatischer Hinsicht. Teil II (Schluss)', *Zeitschrift für Psycho-somatische Medizin* 8, no. 1 (1962): 12–23, 21 (n. 33b).

real recovery were slim to none. And in distinction to solid tumours, it was easier to conceive of leukaemia as a dysfunction of the body's regulatory mechanisms and thus to treat it as a systemic illness. For the psychosomatics of the 1960s, which had been shaped by object relations theory and ego psychology, leukaemia was interesting from another perspective, as both adults and children suffered from it.

The latter fact was resonant for psychosomatics in two ways. First, it deflated the importance of psychosexual development, while giving more weight to research on the child's emotional development and the decisive role played by their mother in it. The portrait that Baltrusch and others painted of children ill with leukaemia was of a child whose relation to their mother was fragile because the mother did not 'properly' love them. Their mothers spoiled them or were overprotective because they themselves had not received enough love and attention from their own mothers.[177] This concern with the historical 'heritage' of insufficient motherly love likely gave expression to two more general social-historical phenomena: the real historical experience of the loss of one's mother during the war, and the stresses placed on motherhood by war, flight, and expulsion, an issue that was hardly being discussed elsewhere. For instance, in 1947, Marburg radiologist Else Pulvermacher described flight and expulsion from Germany's former eastern territories as a 'mass experiment' that enabled scientists to witness in real-time how the 'diminishment of physical and mental strength' relates to the genesis of cancer. Her own clinical observations led her to the conclusion that refugees from the east who got cancer had worse than average outcomes and more frequently suffered from late metastases and relapses.[178]

But in the observation of psychosomatic doctors, the volatile relation between mother and child did not in itself cause cancer. Rather, it left traces on the child's personality and negatively impacted their ability to grapple with emotional stress.[179] The introduction of stress into the theoretical toolbox of psychosomatics opened a range of new courses of action. It functioned as a kind of boundary concept, because stress could affect the body in many ways, including by making the body's hormonal balance go haywire, by exhausting the nervous system, or by inhibiting the immune system.[180]

[177] Ibid., 17–18.

[178] Else Pulvermacher, 'Über Einflüsse der Umwelt auf die Entstehung und den Ablauf der Krebskrankheit', *Strahlentherapie* 76, no. 4 (1947): 556–61.

[179] Bahnson, 'Das Krebsproblem', 692–5.

[180] Ilana Löwy, 'Unscharfe Begriffe und föderative Experimentalstrategien', in *Die Experimentalisierung des Lebens. Experimentalsysteme in den biologischen Wissenschaften 1850–1950*, ed. Hans Jörg Rheinberger and Michael Hagner (Berlin: Akademie, 1993), 188–206, 189–90. See also Lea Haller, Sabine Höhle, and Heiko Stoff, 'Stress—Konjunkturen eines Konzepts', *Zeithistorische Forschungen/Studies in Contemporary History* 11, no. 3 (2014): 359–81; Mark Jackson, *The Age of Stress* (Oxford: Oxford University Press, 2013); David Cantor and Edmund Ramsden, eds, *Stress, Shock,*

Thus, the concept of stress provided an opportunity for researchers to knot together knowledge on psychosomatic cancer research from different historical eras. First, they could draw on the nineteenth-century notion of nervous exhaustion, which, as discussed above, set the paradigm for the pre-psychoanalytic period. This concept also had affinities with new experiments on animal psychology being conducted in the wake of Pavlov's work. Second, stress could absorb the endocrinological focus of psychophysiology, which had spearheaded studies on the aetiological significance of vitamins and hormones in cancer. Third, hypotheses that stress could affect the immune system were gaining in plausibility, enabling psychosomatic research on stress to benefit from cutting-edge oncological studies. Finally, psychosomatic cancer research conceived of these three bodily systems—nervous, endocrine, immune—not just as self-contained units, but as interlocking circuits. This made it into a kind of third-order cybernetics, thus putting it in contact with yet another field of knowledge, which was, as an aside, enjoying great popularity at the time.

Stress also helped psychosomatic cancer research escape the search for the one single cause of cancer. Stress could be caused by intra-psychological as well as social or natural factors. Similarly, stress need not be the exclusive cause of cancer, but could be one aggravating factor among others.[181]

The 'stress turn' thus pushed psychosomatics away from sniffing out causes towards the search for correlations.[182] This made it easier for the insights of psychosomatic research to be integrated into clinical practice, which doctors indeed capitalized on.[183] At the same time, the concept of stress enabled scientists to define emotions in such a way that they could be identified through endocrinological changes and thus could be studied through animal experiments. Even though this did not reelevate the mouse to the measure of all things, it took away humans' monopoly on emotions and, in a sense, their special place in the cosmos, since scientists could now place mice and men on the same level of psychological evolution without running into too many barriers.[184]

With that, psychosomatics swept the rug from beneath a primary objection of hard-science-based oncology, namely: if cancer is the product of a complex life story involving a lack of motherly love and an embrace of fatherly authority, how

and Adaptation in the Twentieth Century (Rochester: University of Rochester Press, 2012); Patrick Kury, *Der überforderte Mensch: Eine Wissensgeschichte vom Stress zum Burnout* (Frankfurt: Campus, 2012).

[181] Roy R. Grinker and Fred P. Robbins, *Psychosomatic Case Book* (New York: Blakiston, 1954), 331.

[182] Nissim Mizrachi, 'From Causation to Correlation: The Story of Psychosomatic Medicine 1939–1979', *Culture, Medicine, and Psychiatry* 25, no. 3 (2001): 317–43, https://doi.org/10.1023/A:1011817010797.

[183] Alexa Geisthövel and Bettina Hitzer, 'Die Grenzen des Erfolgs. Endgültige Etablierung und das Verschwinden einer großen Antwort (1970–2000)', in Geisthövel and Hitzer, *Auf der Suche nach einer anderen Medizin*, 325–48.

[184] Kurt Bammer and Jürgen Wagner, 'Von Mäusen und Menschen', *Psychologie heute* 6 (1978): 40–3.

and why do animals and even plants get cancer? But if the emotional biography of a complicated human being only represented *one of many* stress factors that any living being—whether human, animal, or plant—could be subjected to, then the objection folds.

The potential for stress to be understood as a stimulus in animal experiments made it possible for oncologists in East Germany to conduct psychosomatic research without butting up against the ideological dictates of the GDR government, which, in the 1950s, had rejected 'bourgeois' psychoanalysis in favour of Pavlov's physiology.[185] However, after Stalin's death in 1953 and a medical scandal triggered by the death of a patient in Leipzig caused by a Pavlovian form of sleep therapy, the ruling SED party stepped back a bit.[186] They stopped requiring adherence to Pavlov in 1960 when the Gesellschaft für Ärztliche Psychotherapie der DDR (Society for Medical Psychotherapy of the GDR) was founded, which opened the doors for other models of psychotherapy. Still, working with the concepts of psychoanalysis and psychosomatics remained problematic.[187] Although a plurality of different psychotherapeutic methods slowly gained footing in the GDR, the state continued to surveil practitioners and exert pressure on them. At a 1971 conference, the SED party leadership tried to tighten the ideological and political strictures on psychotherapy and psychiatry. But a majority of attendees, many of whom were party members, insisted that medical integrity necessitated that therapists be able to participate in international—and thus Western-dominated—research.[188] After that, the SED dropped further attempts to directly influence psychotherapy in the GDR.[189]

While East German psychotherapy came closer to its West German counterpart as a consequence, marked differences persisted. Perhaps most notably, no studies on the psychology of cancer patients' personalities were conducted in the GDR, which is all the more remarkable because East German scientists had been carrying out experiments with personality tests since the late 1960s. But they remained restricted to illnesses that the international medical community had long agreed were psychosomatic in nature, including circulatory illnesses, eczema,

[185] Stefan Busse, '"Von der Sowjetwissenschaft lernen": Pawlowismus und Psychologie', *Psychologie und Geschichte* 8, no. 1/2 (1998): 150–73.

[186] Doreen Scholtz and Holger Steinberg, 'Die Theorie und Praxis der Pawlow'schen Schlaftherapie in der DDR', *Psychiatrische Praxis* 38, no. 7 (2011): 323–8, 324 and 326, https://doi.org/10.1055/s-0031%961276851.

[187] Marion Sonnenmoser, 'Psychotherapie in der DDR: Versunkene Welt', *Deutsches Ärzteblatt* PP [edition for psychotherapists] 3 (2009): 115–16.

[188] Michael Geyer, 'Ostdeutsche Psychotherapiechronik 1970–1979', in *Psychotherapie in Ostdeutschland. Geschichte und Geschichten 1945–1995*, ed. Michael Geyer (Göttingen: Vandenhoeck & Ruprecht, 2011), 245–56, 245–6.

[189] Winfried Süß, *Der 'Volkskörper' im Krieg. Gesundheitspolitik, Gesundheitsverhältnisse und Krankenmord im nationalsozialistischen Deutschland 1939–1945* (Munich: Oldenbourg Wissenschaftsverlag, 2003), 327.

and asthma.[190] Thus, in contrast to the FRG, East German psychotherapists did not venture into cancer psychosomatics.

There were probably a few different reasons for this.[191] First, considerably fewer resources were available to psychotherapists in the GDR, which pushed research to focus on illnesses that seemed more clearly to have a psychosomatic component. Another contributing factor was the decided emphasis of GDR health policy on research that could be directly translated into prophylactic and therapeutic means; from the short-term perspective, research in psychosomatic cancer research did not seem to promise much on this front. Third, psychotherapists in the GDR only had a limited range of peer-recognized journals to publish in, the most prominent being the *Zeitschrift für Neurologie, Psychiatrie und klinische Psychologie* (*Journal for Neurology, Psychiatry, and Clinical Psychology*) and the *Zeitschrift für Klinische Medizin* (*Journal for Clinical Medicine*). Both had narrow conceptions of what constituted scientific research and sound methodology, so that studies on the psychosomatics of cancer presumably would have had little chance of publication. And in all likelihood, the politicization of psychosomatic cancer research à la 1960s West Germany also played a role. Viewing cancer as the effect of too little or too much motherly love, as an outgrowth of the repression of negative emotions, and as a critique of an all too bourgeois society did not fit well with the image of actually existing socialism propagated by the SED.

In contrast, the concept of stress conflicted neither with the understanding of science and method dominant in East Germany nor with the party's hegemonic ideas about society and emotions. Because animal experiments on emotional stress stripped away the subjective dimension of inner psychic life and the narration of a life story, researchers could define stress as a predictable, evolved reaction to a particular stimulus. An example of this path was a 1964 experiment conducted by Theodor Matthes, head doctor and surgeon at the Robert Rössle Clinic in the Buch section of East Berlin. He staged a quasi-Darwinian situation of fear by placing rats, rabbits, and chickens in a ferret cage six times a day in fifteen-minute increments, but such that the ferrets could not hurt them. The test animals cowered away, which Matthes read as a sign of fear. Both the experimental group and the control group were injected with carcinogenic substances. The findings showed that the periodically terrified animals had better chances of survival: they got tumours less frequently and the tumours they did get were smaller and grew slower.[192] Matthes interpreted this as demonstrating that emotional stress could

[190] Michael Geyer, 'Psychosoziale Merkmale bei Herzinfarktgefährdeten—Untersuchung in einer großstädtischen Population 49- bis 59-jähriger Männer' (Habilitation diss., Medizinische Akademie Erfurt, 1978); K. Linser and H. Kleinsorge, *Die Hochseeklimakur. Grundlagen, Probleme sowie klinische und psychologische Ergebnisse bei endogenem Ekzem und Asthma bronchiale* (Leipzig: Barth, 1969).

[191] I would like to thank Michael Geyer (Akademie für Psychotherapie, Erfurt) for his helpful tips on this point.

[192] Theodor H. Matthes, 'Experimental Contribution to the Question of Emotional Stress Reactions on the Growth of Tumors in Animals', *Acta/Unio Internationalis Contra Cancrum* 20 (1964): 1608–10.

prevent or at least decelerate tumour growth, thus underscoring that the effects of stress need not be negative, but were rather contingent upon the individual's ability to process the stress and the nature of the event that caused it.

In the same vein, Howard B. Andervont, head of the laboratory of biology at the US National Cancer Institute, conducted experiments with mice that had a genetic predisposition to breast cancer. Andervont began by holding the mice together in cages. After he transferred them into individual cages without contact with other mice, their tumour rates climbed drastically.[193] The explanation for why stress had the opposite effect here was not that loneliness and isolation functioned differently than fear. Rather, Andervont believed that the deciding factor was that in Matthes's experiment, the intervals between the fifteen-minute fear sessions gave the animals a chance to recover their emotional equilibrium. Certainly, the stress forced them to adapt to their situation, but after they returned to their normal cages, they could relax; meanwhile, the intermittent release of hormonal reserves triggered by their instinct to defend themselves from the ferrets had an anti-cancer effect. In contrast, Andervont's mice never got a break, and their adaptation to the perpetual isolation ultimately spiralled into a pathological state.

This conclusion was supported by Soviet experiments that conditioned animals straight into neurosis by repeatedly offering them a stimulus and then denying them the satisfaction supposed to be provided by it. For instance, they allowed test mice to constantly see and smell food without being able to access it. These mice also developed chemically induced tumours earlier than their control group counterparts, which received just as much food as the test group, but did not always have unreachable food in front of them.[194]

Psychosomatic cancer researchers saw in these experiments confirmation of the conclusions that clinical psychologists in the 1950s had drawn from personality tests: the interaction of a neurotic personality and emotional stress increased the chances of tumour growth, while carcinogens and genetic predispositions played an exacerbating role. This was how the concept of stress entered both West and East German psychosomatic cancer research in the early 1960s.

The Risks of Diagnosing Society: The (In)ability to Mourn, Be Angry, and Feel Rage

This paradigm shift made the language of psychosomatic cancer research ripe for adaptation by those searching for a way to speak about contemporary experiences

[193] Howard B. Andervont, 'Influence of Environment on Mammary Cancer in Mice', *Journal of the National Cancer Institute* 4, no. 6 (1944): 579–81, https://doi.org/10.1093/jnci/4.6.579.

[194] Hans-Joachim Baltrusch and Kristen Austarheim, 'Psyche—Nervensystem—Neoplastischer Prozess. Ein altes Problem mit neuer Aktualität', *Zeitschrift für Psycho-somatische Medizin* 9, no. 4 (1963): 229–45, 244.

of loss and mourning. Evidence is provided by the West German media's reporting on the second conference of the New York Academy of Science on 'Psychophysiological Aspects of Cancer' held in May 1968. *Der Spiegel* tried to untangle the 'threads of fate' that wove together emotional dearth in early childhood with cancer in later life into the 'inability to express emotions'. In his weekly column in *Bunte*, Dr Fabian offered his readers some unusual advice. He showed them a photo of a woman sitting unhappily at the kitchen table, with shattered china on the floor—an iconic image of marital strife. But Dr Fabian was not warning them about the negative effects of marriage gone wrong. Instead, the photo's caption read: 'Smashed porcelain, channelled anger.' And defeated cancer? Nearly, at any rate, as his column concluded: 'Thus, if a person's everyday anger eats them up from the inside, they interrupt the body's defence against cancer, such that a cancerous tumour can more easily take root and spread in such an "introverted" person.'[195]

But between 1965 and 1980, the discourse on cancer and emotions in Germany was less focused on anger and more on repressed grief and fear, which situated it within a general psychosomatic conviction that the incapacity to acknowledge and express feelings was a fundamental aspect of psychosomatic illness.[196] It was this trend that turned conversations about the causes of cancer into an important medium of broader social debate, a point hit home by a 1977 article in *Der Spiegel*. Titled 'Cancer through Mental Anguish and Social Suffering?', the article, penned by an anonymous author, illustrated 'psychostress factors' with three photographs: two were images of sadness, one of which referenced experiences of war, flight, and occupation.

The first picture (Fig. 2) showed a soldier turning towards his crying wife—a farewell scene, as the caption 'Separation' makes clear. It could have represented all such scenes during the Second World War. From today's perspective, this seems to be the obvious interpretation, but whether readers in 1977 understood it this way is doubtful, because many would have noticed the man's badge of rank, which identified him not as a Wehrmacht soldier, but as an American GI.[197]

Thus, the photo is not first and foremost about a woman's sadness at seeing her husband, fiancé, or boyfriend off to war. Rather, it depicts the complicated relationship between a German woman and an American occupying soldier. It

[195] Dr Fabian, MD (W. E. J. Schneidrzik), 'Neue Waffe gegen den Krebs. Die Kobaltbombe', *Die Bunte* 14 (1968): 61.

[196] In expert literature, this syndrome is called alexithymia. Monica Greco, 'Homo Vacuus. Alexithymie und das neoliberale Gebot des Selbstseins', in *Gouvernementalität der Gegenwart. Studien zur Ökonomisierung des Sozialen*, ed. Ulrich Bröckling, Susanne Krasmann, and Thomas Lemke (Frankfurt am Main: Suhrkamp, 2000), 265–85; Cornelius Borck, 'Alexithymie oder wie der Mangel an Gefühl zur Krankheit wurde', in Geisthövel and Hitzer, *Auf der Suche nach einer anderen Medizin*, 415–33.

[197] Andrew Mollo, *The Armed Forces of World War II: Uniforms, Insignia and Organization* (London: Silverdale, 2002), 239.

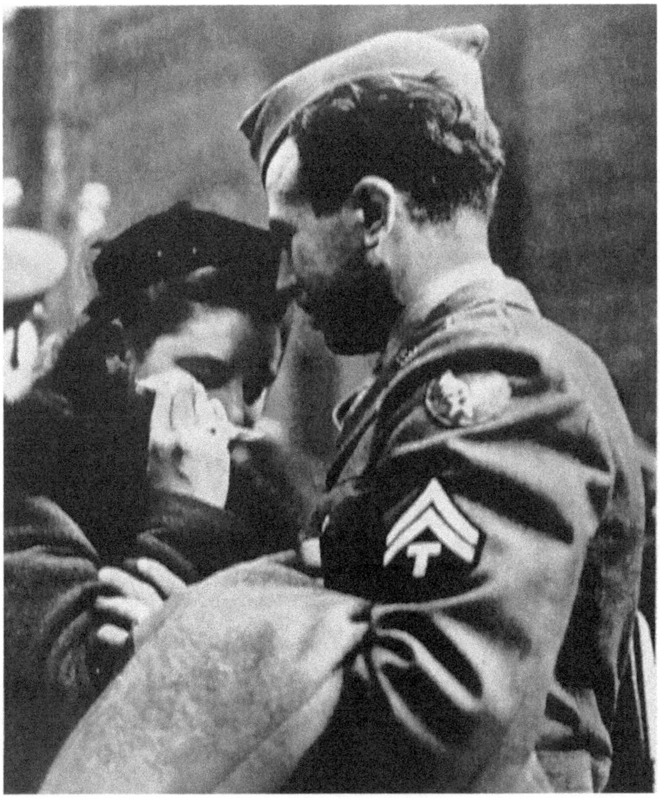

Fig. 2 Photo in an article on 'Cancer through Mental Anguish and Social Suffering?', *Der Spiegel* (1977).

thus evokes a situation in which it would have seemed expedient to suppress sadness about saying goodbye, since in post-war West Germany, the '*Fräuleins*' of American GIs were maligned as morally dubious women who should be ashamed of their intimate bond.[198]

The second image (Fig. 3) depicts death and mourning in a very specific way, showing a funeral procession moving through an oddly barren winter landscape. The photograph gives off a chilly air intensified by the fact that, though the mourners follow the coffin together, gestures of consolation or care are nowhere to be seen. The scene is not an explosion of grief, but the silent side of sadness experienced in emotional isolation.

Both photographs tapped into West German discourses about the past and present, which leaned on psychoanalysis and social psychology to support the claim that the repressed past lived on in the present. Here, too, Mitscherlich was a

[198] Annette Brauerhoch, *Fräuleins und GIs* (Frankfurt am Main: Stroemfeld, 2006).

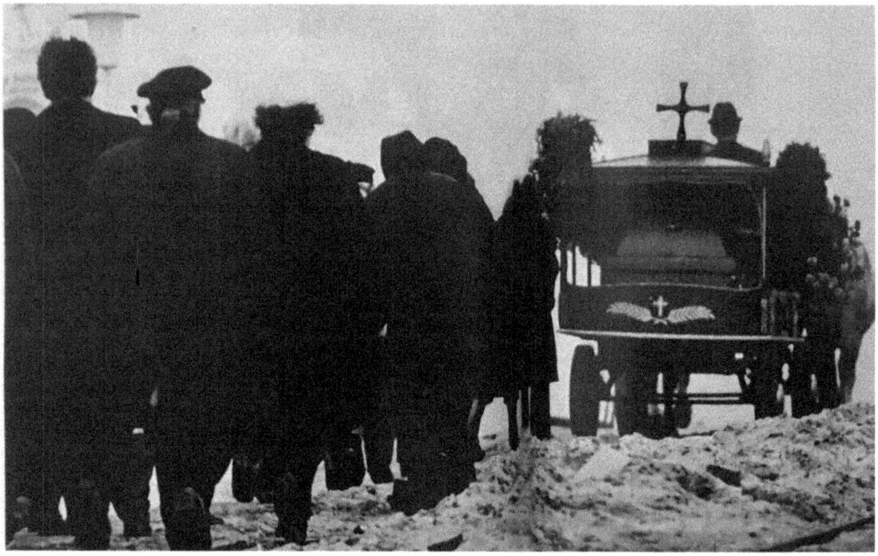

Fig. 3 Photo in an article on 'Cancer through Mental Anguish and Social Suffering?', *Der Spiegel* (1977).

name that played a key role. In 1967, Alexander Mitscherlich and his wife Margarete authored a book that criticized the German 'inability to mourn', diagnosing German society with repressed grief about the loss of the '*Führer*'. In 1979, Margarete Mitscherlich went a step further and asserted that individuals had a 'necessity to mourn', thus contributing to discussions on the repression of death and sadness in modern, rationalized societies, an issue that Norbert Elias would expound on only a few years later in his book *The Loneliness of the Dying*.[199] All of these writers shared a critique of a society they described as superficially friendly and unwilling to talk about unpleasant feelings and experiences.

As the author of the *Spiegel* article put it, cancer appeared to be the bitter price for the obsession with upholding decorum:

> Seemingly free of fear and without concern about stress; incapable of feeling aggressive emotions; ready to accept the authority of the state and conventions without complaint. Additionally, religious in the broad sense, with a tendency towards social engagement—a good person, who wouldn't gladly be one?

[199] Alexander Mitscherlich and Margarete Mitscherlich (1967), *Die Unfähigkeit zu trauern. Grundlagen kollektiven Verhaltens* (Munich: Piper, 1967); Margarete Mitscherlich-Nielsen, 'Die Notwendigkeit zu trauern', *Psyche* 33, no. 11 (1979): 981–90; Norbert Elias, *The Loneliness of the Dying*, trans. Edmund Jephcott (New York: Continuum, 2001).

> But who acts in such way may have already penned the text of their own death certificate: died of cancer, far before their time and as a victim of their own soul.[200]

The ever-growing deluge of psychological advice recommended that the healthy approach was to feel and openly grapple with sadness, fear, and rage.[201] At the same time, these emotions were more and more being lauded as signs of personal authenticity, political integrity, and critical thinking. This philosophy of emotions was reiterated again and again in the civil society movements of the late 1960s and 1970s. Aspects of it could be found in the alternative milieu's praise of emotional 'warmth', in the peace movement's politicization of emotions, and in Hans Jonas's redefinition of fear not as a dangerous, irrational feeling, but as an emotion that, in the face of new, threatening, hard-to-manage technologies, was to serve as the North Star of ethical, responsible future planning.[202]

The politicized reading of psychosomatics gradually supplanted mourning with rage as the emotion more likely to motivate people to take action, a point exemplified by a book that chose the name of the god of war for its title: *Mars*. The big title for a rather skinny book had an expressive author's name to stand beneath it: Fritz Zorn (*Zorn* is the German word for 'rage'), whose real name was Fritz Angst (*Angst* is the German word for 'fear'), chose a pseudonym that underscored his desire to transform his fear into rage. His fear was that of cancer, and it seized the young Swiss man when he learned that he had a malignant lymphoma in his throat and a low chance of survival. But it was overridden by the feeling of rage that seethed inside him when he began to grasp his cancer as the effect of his vapid bourgeois upbringing, which stamped out emotions in the striving for the superficial appearance of success and conformity:

> Although I still did not know that I had a cancer, I hit intuitively on the correct diagnosis in regarding the tumor as an accumulation of 'swallowed tears'. What this phrase suggested to me was that all the tears that I had not wept and had not wanted to weep in my lifetime had gathered in my neck and formed this tumor because they had not been able to fulfill their true function, which was to be wept. In strictly medical terms, of course, this poetic-sounding diagnosis is beside the point. But, seen in terms of the whole person, it expresses the truth. All the

[200] 'Krebs durch Seelenschmerz', *Der Spiegel*, 102.

[201] Maik Tändler, '"Psychoboom". Therapeutisierungsprozesse in Westdeutschland in den späten 1960er und 1970er Jahren', in *Das beratene Selbst. Zur Genealogie der Therapeutisierung in den 'langen' Siebzigern*, ed. Sabine Maasen, Jens Elberfeld, Pascal Eitler, and Maik Tändler (Bielefeld: transcript, 2011), 59–94; see also Tändler, *Das therapeutische Jahrzehnt*.

[202] See Hans Jonas, *Das Prinzip Verantwortung. Versuch einer Ethik für die technologische Zivilisation* (Frankfurt am Main: Suhrkamp, 1979); Häberlen, *Emotional Politics*; Biess, 'Die Sensibilisierung des Subjekts'; Sven Reichardt, *Authentizität und Gemeinschaft. Linksalternatives Leben in den siebziger und frühen achtziger Jahren* (Berlin: Suhrkamp, 2014).

> suffering I had swallowed and dammed up could no longer be compressed inside me. The pressure became too great, and the resulting explosion destroyed the body containing all that compressed pain.[203]

Author and literary scholar Adolf Muschg, who was given the terminally ill Fritz Angst's manuscript by a friend who ran a bookstore, wrote a foreword to the book in which he offered an interpretation of the author's self-questioning and anger at his own parents, which disturbed many readers:

> Yet this dying man's resistance, his rage . . . is not directed solely at the transcendental absurd. He is no less bold in his speculations on the concrete absurd as it manifests itself in our social institutions. He is no less harsh on the absurdities of his familial and social background . . . . He sees his death—or what little is left of his raging and outraged life—as a revolutionary attack on the status quo . . . . It is his death that will make what is deadly in this society visible and impossible to ignore.[204]

In Zorn's book, the private was not just political—as a beloved catchphrase of the 1970s had it—but potentially fatal. And it dissolved the old Cartesian dichotomy of mind and body. The new, psychosomatically defined human found themselves in a world whose every aspect impacted them immediately, from social change to the 'natural', yet polluted environment. This situation made cancer seem like a powerful existential and metaphorical expression of a world whose wholeness had been artificially divided up into relatively independent parts. And it made protesting against this modern world seem like a matter of life and death, both for the individual and for society.

This helps explain the success of *Mars*, which became a cult favourite of the civil society movements of the 1980s.[205] It also shines light on why Oswalt Kolle wrote about cancer in his *Bunte* reports before shortly thereafter reporting on the sexual revolution.[206] It gives context to why Hildegard Knef's 1975 autobiographical

[203] Fritz Zorn, *Mars* (New York: Knopf, 1982), 117–18.

[204] Adolf Muschg, Afterword to Zorn, *Mars*, 237–8.

[205] The book is now in its 25th edition. In 1978, *Mars* was translated into Swedish, Dutch, and Danish; in 1980 into French; in 1982 into English. In 1988, the brothers Alex and Daniel Varenne published a comic titled *Angoisse et Colère* that was based on Zorn's book and, interestingly, placed fear and rage on equal footing. Two examples of many contemporaneous reviews of *Mars* are Hellmuth Karasek, '"Mars": Ein dreißigjähriger Krieg im Frieden', *Der Spiegel* 15 (1977): 219; Hugo Leber, 'Der Zorn des Fritz Zorn', *Die Zeit* 23, 3 June 1977.

[206] Oswalt Kolle and Peter Schmidsberger, 'Millionen werden nicht an Krebs sterben, wenn . . . ', *Die Bunte* 32 (1966): 28–9, 53–4, *Die Bunte* 33 (1966): 56–8 and 60–2, *Die Bunte* 34 (1966): 44–7, *Die Bunte* 35 (1966): 28–30, 32 and 62, *Die Bunte* 36 (1966): 62–8, *Die Bunte* 37 (1966): 66–7, 69–70, 72–3; *Die Bunte* 38 (1966): 90–5, 97, *Die Bunte* 39 (1966): 92–6 and 98.

attack on the medical establishment and 'ashamed' society stoked up a furore.[207] Finally, it helps show why cancer even entered popular culture, as in Joe Jackson's 1982 song 'Cancer', with the chorus 'Everything gives you cancer'.

But the all-encompassing interpretation of cancer also attracted criticism, the most forceful of which flowed from the pen of American author Susan Sontag. In her 1978 book *Illness as Metaphor*, she asserted 'that illness is *not* a metaphor, and that the most truthful way of regarding illness—and the healthiest way of being ill—is one most purified of, most resistant to, metaphoric thinking'.[208]

Whether it is at all possible to think about the body and illness without metaphorical concepts continues to be discussed today. Theorists and historians of science tend towards the negative, particularly because all scientific models of these phenomena draw on concepts from other semantic spheres.[209] But Sontag's critique targeted not just those who sought to read a grander metaphorical significance into cancer, but above all the way in which they blamed the victim, an ethical failure that she saw psychosomatic research and theory as being particularly guilty of: 'Psychological theories of illness are a powerful means of placing the blame on the ill. Patients who are instructed that they have, unwittingly, caused their disease are also being made to feel that they have deserved it.' 'The view of cancer as a disease of the failure of expressiveness condemns the cancer patient: expresses pity but also conveys contempt.'[210]

Sontag's book sparked engaged discussion in West Germany, evidenced not least by the multiple print runs of the German translation.[211] Social movements, and in particular the women's movement, criticized psychosomatic theory's potential to stigmatize and blame as a symptom of male-dominated, paternalistic medicine. Special ire was reserved for the misogynistic stereotypes that defined many theories of the cancer personality, though they were more widespread in American research of the 1950s and 1960s than in West and East German psychosomatics. After all, the German psychosomatic tradition had stronger roots in medical anthropology, placing less weight on the concept of sex drives

[207] Hildegard Knef, *The Verdict* (New York: Farrar, Straus and Giroux, 1975). The book was first published in serial form in *Stern* magazine, supplemented with photos and an interview with the author in issues 19–27 (1975).

[208] Susan Sontag, *Illness as Metaphor* (New York: Farrar, Straus and Giroux, 1977), 3.

[209] Christina Brandt, 'Metapher', in *Literatur und Wissen: Ein interdisziplinäres Handbuch*, ed. Roland Borgards, Harald Neumeyer, Nicolas Pethes, and Yvonne Wübben (Stuttgart: Metzler, 2013), 21–8, 25–7; Christina von Braun, *Metapher und Experiment. Von der Virusforschung zum genetischen Code* (Göttingen: Wallstein, 2004).

[210] Sontag, *Illness as Metaphor*, 57, 48.

[211] In 1989, Sontag published an expanded, revised edition of her essay that also dealt with HIV/AIDS. In the new edition, Sontag admitted that it is impossible to speak about illness and the body without resorting to metaphors. See Susan Sontag, *Illness as Metaphor and Aids and Its Metaphors* (New York: Picador, 1991), 91: 'Of course, one cannot think without metaphors. But that does not mean there aren't some metaphors we might well abstain from or try to retire. As, of course, all thinking is interpretation. But that does not mean it isn't sometimes correct to be "against" interpretation.'

and more on social factors like guilt and behavioural norms. Theorists and practitioners of psychosomatics responded to Sontag's critique and admitted that it was justified, but they often played down the accusation of misogyny as a misunderstanding resulting out of the media's 'simplified' rendition of psychosomatic studies.[212]

But only few questioned the soundness of the notion that certain personality profiles had an inherent inability to perceive their own emotions and grapple with 'psycho-stress factors'. Quite the contrary. In a 1983 issue, *Psychologie heute* (*Psychology Today*)—a magazine that had been supplying an ever-growing number of interested laypeople with coveted psychological knowledge since 1974—asked its readers to answer a questionnaire that was supposed to reveal the probability that they would become seriously ill in the near future. The first block of questions on the two-page test revolved around the person's ability to express and perceive feelings.[213]

A lack of emotional expression and an inability to decipher one's own emotions were described as decisive in predicting illness. But there were two significant shifts from older assumptions about this causal connection. First, emotions and emotional styles were more and more treated as factors that predisposed people to engage in certain risky *behaviours*. Thus, the test inquired into sleep, work, free-time, and eating habits. Second, it was not just a test of people who were already sick. Rather, it was published with the intention of helping healthy people evaluate their risk for illness so that they could take steps to remain healthy and *prevent disease*. The double shift towards the identification of risky behaviour and the practice of disease prevention has developed into the dominant paradigm in medicine since the 1980s.[214]

Risk Factors and the Risks of a Scandal

The shift in Germany takes us back to Heidelberg, where this chapter began with the story of young Frau S. and her experiences at the women's clinic in the 1970s. In 1962, an institute was established there that stitched together many of the developments discussed thus far: The Institute for Social and Occupational Medicine of the Ruprecht-Karls University. It might be seen as West Germany's response to the Framingham Heart Study, the first longitudinal epidemiological study of chronic cardiovascular diseases.

[212] Magda Henle, 'Ist Krebs eine weibliche Krankheit?', *Psychologie heute* 4 (1982): 54–60, 56.

[213] Frauke Teegen, 'Krankheit: Was will uns der Körper damit sagen?', *Psychologie heute* 10 (1983): 65–72, 68. The questionnaire and the accompanying article were in advance of the publication of Frauke Teegen, *Ganzheitliche Gesundheit—Der sanfte Umgang mit uns selbst* (Reinbek: Rowohlt, 1983).

[214] Laukötter, 'Salutogenese'.

In 1948, over 5,000 residents of Framingham, Massachusetts, were selected as participants in the study; the only criterion was that they did not suffer from a cardiovascular condition at the time. In the following years, researchers collected data on their behaviour, particularly as it concerned a series of behaviours seen as being potentially risky, such as smoking. The goal was to establish statistically significant connections between these behaviours and the heart illnesses that arose over the run of the study. Initial findings were published in the 1950s. The study is still ongoing today, now in its fourth generation.[215] The Framingham Study represented a breakthrough for the idea that risky behaviours are a determining factor in the development of chronic illnesses.[216]

The first director of the West German institute for social and occupational medicine was Hans Schaefer, previously a professor of physiology at the University of Heidelberg who spearheaded the acceptance of the concept of stress in West German medicine.[217] In 1967, Schaefer and his assistant and later successor Maria Blohmke received a half-million Deutsche Mark grant from the Volkswagen Foundation to conduct a West German version of the Framingham Study on a smaller scale. They modelled how the interaction of environment, genetic disposition, and personality traits affected the body through emotions, stress, and risky behaviour.[218] Their model of risk factors exerted a lasting influence on West German conceptions of psychosocial stress and linked up with models prominent in American psychosomatic cancer research.

While Schaefer's research primarily focused on cardiovascular diseases, Blohmke's moved towards risk factors significant for cancer. At the same moment when doctoral candidate Michael Holm-Hadulla was conducting his test battery with cervical-cancer patient Frau S. at the Heidelberg women's clinic, Maria Blohmke was asking eighty female breast-cancer patients to respond to a series of questions about psychosocial risk factors. Part of a study at the Institute for Social and Occupational Medicine, her questionnaire, like Holm-Hadulla's, was an effort to identify a personality type characterized by an inability to express

[215] Gerald M. Oppenheimer, 'Becoming the Framingham Study 1947–1950', *American Journal of Public Health* 95, no. 4 (2005): 602–10, https://doi.org/10.2105/AJPH.2003.026419.

[216] Carsten Timmermann, 'Risikofaktoren. Der scheinbar unaufhaltsame Erfolg eines Ansatzes aus der amerikanischen Epidemiologie in der deutschen Nachkriegsmedizin', in *Das präventive Selbst. Eine Kulturgeschichte moderner Gesundheitspolitik*, ed. Martin Lengwiler and Jeannette Madarász (Bielefeld: transcript, 2010), 251–77.

[217] Carsten Timmermann, 'Appropriating Risk Factors: The Reception of an American Approach to Chronic Disease in the Two German States, c. 1950–1990', *Social History of Medicine* 25, no. 1 (2012): 157–74, 167, https://doi.org/10.1093/shm/hkr051; Hans-Georg Hofer, 'Labor, Klinik und Gesellschaft. Stress und die westdeutsche Universitätsmedizin (1950–1980)', *Zeithistorische Forschungen/Studies in Contemporary History* 11, no. 3 (2014): 382–405, 396.

[218] Hans Schaefer and Maria Blohmke, *Herzkrank durch psychosozialen Stress* (Heidelberg: Hüthig, 1977).

emotions and a tendency towards uncritical obedience, religiosity, and conformity.[219]

Blohmke's work is probably what inspired Ronald Grossarth-Maticek to come to Heidelberg. In the following years, he would provoke engagement with the topic in the media and self-help groups, but not without also bringing psychosomatic models of cancer into a degree of disrepute. Grossarth-Maticek studied in Belgrade and received his doctorate in sociology from the University of Heidelberg. In the spring of 1977, he submitted his habilitation (a book-length work required to be admitted as a professor in the German university system) to Heidelberg's department of psychology, which was based on data collected during a predictive study that he had conducted in Yugoslavia.

The study's sample was a group of 1,353 people who lived in the small Serbian town of Crvenka.[220] They responded to an eighty-eight-question survey that Grossarth-Maticek had himself developed. It centred on how they dealt with stress and their ability to express their psychological concerns. Grossarth-Maticek then analysed the answers in order to predict which respondent would be afflicted with which illness over the next ten years. He predicted that thirty-eight of them would get cancer—and in fact, ten years later, thirty-seven of those thirty-eight people had died of cancer, meaning he had an astonishing prediction rate of 97.3 per cent. But the habilitation committee was sceptical about this extraordinary number, a doubt underscored by the fact that Grossarth-Maticek had not supplied them with all the data from the study. Thus, they asked him to submit all data and predictions from a study that he had begun at the Heidelberg department of psychology in 1973. He obliged, but only after he had conducted a post-enumeration survey to validate the results; moreover, a plethora of data was missing here, too. The committee thus refused to accept the habilitation and Grossarth-Maticek retracted the manuscript.[221] But he continued the Heidelberg

[219] Irmgard Cramer, Maria Blohmke, C. B. Bahnson, M. B. Bahnson, H. Scherg, and M. Weinhold, 'Psychosoziale Faktoren und Krebs. Untersuchung von 80 Frauen mit einem psychosozialen Fragebogen', *Münchener Medizinische Wochenschrift* 119, no. 43 (1977): 1387–92. Michael Wirsching, assistant doctor at the Heidelberg Psychosomatic Clinic from 1973 to 1977 and head doctor at its division for psychoanalytic research and family therapy, also conducted a study on the psychosomatic origins of cancer around this time. So did Hans Becker, professor for psychosomatic medicine and psychoanalysis at the University of Heidelberg. See Michael Wirsching, 'Zur Psychosomatik des Brustkrebses—Stand der Forschung und neuere Entwicklungen', *Zeitschrift für Psychosomatische Medizin und Psychoanalyse* 25, no. 3 (1979): 240–50; Hans Becker, *Lebensgeschichte und Krankheitsverlauf bei Mamma-Karzinom-Patientinnen. Arbeitstagung 'Psychosoziale Einflüsse auf Entstehung und Verlauf von Krebserkrankungen'* (Heidelberg, 1981).

[220] On this point and the following, see Roderick D. Buchanan, *Playing with Fire: The Controversial Career of Hans J. Eysenck* (Oxford: Oxford University Press, 2010), 379–80.

[221] Thus, the department does not possess a copy of the manuscript. Psychologist Manfred Amelang, who sat on the habilitation committee, nevertheless retained his copy with the argument that he had annotated it. Buchanan's information is primarily based on statements made by Amelang, see Buchanan, *Playing with Fire*, 379.

study with 33,854 participants until 1978 and then conducted a follow-up study between 1988 and 1996.[222]

Grossarth-Maticek had two intellectual mentors who acquired him recognition in the scientific community. One was Helm Stierlin, who became professor of the new chair for psychoanalytic research and family therapy at the University of Heidelberg's psychosomatic clinic in 1974 and was thus a colleague of Holm-Hadulla's doctoral supervisor Walter Bräutigam. The other, who first met Grossarth-Maticek in 1980, was the influential psychologist Hans J. Eysenck. A German emigrant to Great Britain, Eysenck had made a name for himself in personality and intelligence research and had developed the important Maudsley Personality Inventory (MPI).[223]

In 1998, Grossarth-Maticek published a widely read study on cancer risk factors together with Stierlin, who had studied in Heidelberg and then gone on to spend nine years as the director of the family therapy division of the American National Institute of Mental Health, where his research focused on schizophrenia.[224] The book analysed a series of so-called predictive intervention studies conducted by the authors, in which participants first took a test to determine their personality type and risk of illness, and then underwent preventative therapy based on the results. Follow-up tests checked on whether the therapeutic interventions had led the person to change their behaviours as well as if and how this change/non-change correlated with them getting/not getting an illness and being cured/not being cured of it.

When the book was published, Hans J. Eysenck (1916–97) had already passed away. A few years previously, Eysenck and Grossarth-Maticek's work had been subjected to blistering criticism by other scientists, a scandal that shook the world of psychosomatic cancer research (though it hardly registered outside it).[225] Since the early 1960s, Eysenck had been studying the relationship between smoking and lung cancer. He concluded that the key risk factor was not smoking, but the extroverted personality incapable of properly grappling with stress.[226]

[222] Helm Stierlin and Ronald Grossarth-Maticek, *Krebsrisiken—Überlebenschancen. Wie Körper, Seele und soziale Umwelt zusammenwirken* (Heidelberg: Carl Auer, 1998), 18.

[223] On Eysenck's biography see Buchanan, *Playing with Fire.*

[224] Stierlin and Grossarth-Maticek, *Krebsrisiken* (1998).

[225] Buchanan, *Playing with Fire*, 361–408; David F. Marks, 'The Hans Eysenck Affair: Time to Correct the Scientific Record', *Journal of Health Psychology* 24, no. 4 (2019): 409–20; Anthony J. Pelosi, 'Personality and Fatal Diseases: Revisiting a Scientific Scandal', *Journal of Health Psychology* 24, no. 4 (2019): 421–39.

[226] For instance, in Hans J. Eysenck, *Smoking, Health and Personality* (New York: Basic Books, 1965). On debates on the cancer-causing properties of smoking, see Colin Talley, Howard I. Kushner, and Claire E. Sterk, 'Lung Cancer, Chronic Disease Epidemiology, and Medicine, 1948–1964', *Journal of the History of Medicine and Allied Sciences* 59, no. 3 (2004): 329–74, https://doi.org/10.1093/jhmas/jrh088, and on the debate in Great Britain in particular, Carsten Timmermann, 'As Depressing as It Was Predictable? Lung Cancer, Clinical Trials, and the Medical Research Council in Postwar Britain', *Bulletin of the History of Medicine* 81, no. 1 (2007): 312–34, https://doi.org/10.1353/bhm.2007.0012.

In 1962, Eysenck accepted financial support for his studies from the American Council for Tobacco Research. Originally called the Tobacco Industry Research Council, the trade group was established in 1954 by five of the six biggest American tobacco companies. It institutionalized their attacks against epidemiological studies on the carcinogenic properties of tobacco by means of scientific research.[227] In the years thereafter, Eysenck repeatedly applied for funding from the Council for Tobacco Research. Although he claimed that the source of his money did not influence the findings of his research, he initially did not disclose it.[228] His first largescale study carried out with money from the trade group was published in 1980 under the title 'The Causes and Effects of Smoking'.[229] The article emphasized both the role of genetics and of personality type in the emergence of lung cancer and was not received as a serious piece of research by other scientists. This was the context in which Eysenck met Grossarth-Maticek, who possessed data that seemed to support Eysenck's claim that there was a significant relation between personality type, stress management, and lung cancer.

After that, the two collaborated regularly. Grossarth-Maticek continued to lead the studies and supply data, while Eysenck commissioned his Heidelberg colleague Hermann Vetter and the statisticians working under him in London with statistically evaluating the data. Eysenck also made his mark on the interpretation of the data by foregrounding the importance of personality types.[230] But the data provided by Grossarth-Maticek was met with reservations, and Vetter ultimately published his doubts about their scientific validity.[231]

Even the researchers hired by the American tobacco industry voiced scepticism about Grossarth-Maticek's data. At the behest of Eysenck, the Council for Tobacco Research had granted an application of funds to Grossarth-Maticek under the condition that he allow his data to be analysed by a team of experts comprised of psychologist Charles D. Spielberger (University of South Florida), psychologist and former employee of the National Cancer Institute Bernard Fox (Boston University), and Henk van der Ploeg (Universiteit Amsterdam). Although all three were performing research on the psychosocial causes of cancer and the

[227] Buchanan, *Playing with Fire*, 369–70. [228] Ibid., 371 and 374.

[229] Hans J. Eysenck, *The Causes and Effects of Smoking* (Beverly Hills: Sage, 1980).

[230] Hans J. Eysenck, 'Personality as a Predictor of Cancer and Cardiovascular Disease, and the Application of Behaviour Therapy in Prophylaxis', *European Journal of Psychiatry* 1 (1987): 29–41; Buchanan, *Playing with Fire*, 385–6.

[231] Two of the key criticisms were, first, that only in 1987 did Grossarth-Maticek supply the complete data for his tests begun in Heidelberg in 1973, after all the data about the future illnesses of the subjects had been collected. Grossarth-Maticek responded to Vetter's protest by saying that he had already collected the pertinent data in 1972/3 and was only able to publish it later on. Later, he explained that the data had been falsely collected by a meanwhile deceased interviewer who had already known the illness rates of the subjects. Second, Grossarth-Maticek explained the study's absolute failure to predict any illnesses that developed after 1982 by saying that the code numbers given to test subjects to ensure anonymity had gotten mixed up and could thus no longer be properly matched, making the data useless. See Hermann Vetter, 'Some Observations on Grossarth-Maticek's Data Base', *Psychological Inquiry* 2, no. 3 (1991): 286–7.

physical effects of stress and anxiety, their evaluation was damning. Bernard Fox was the first to publish his assessment, in 1988.[232] Immediately thereafter, the trade group turned off the faucet on Grossarth-Maticek.[233]

Finally, in 1991, a group of prominent psychologists and doctors got together to articulate their doubts about the validity of Grossarth-Maticek's work in a special issue of the peer-reviewed journal *Psychological Inquiry*. Fox, Vetter, and van der Ploeg were joined by Heidelberg psychologist Manfred Amelang, who questioned the empirical basis of the 'Tales from Crvenka and Heidelberg', as he titled his article.[234] This criticism was seconded by American psychologist Lydia Temoshok, whose concept of the 'type C' personality had made her one of the biggest names in psychosomatic cancer research.[235] Only the epidemiologist Rainer Frentzel-Beyme—who was working at the German Centre for Cancer Research in Heidelberg at the time—defended Grossarth-Maticek on the grounds that conducting largescale epidemiological studies was extremely difficult and thus prone to error.[236]

But the critical voices did not let up. One year later, British psychiatrists Tony Pelosi and Louis Appleby published an analysis of the data in the *British Medical Journal*. They demonstrated that the configuration of risk factors articulated by Eysenck and Grossarth-Maticek had, by a wide margin, the greatest predictive power of any study ever published on the epidemiology of chronic diseases. Grossarth-Maticek and Eysenck's Type I personality was 121 times more likely to get cancer than other personality types. In short, the model was simply too good to be true. Moreover, they doubted that Grossarth-Maticek would have been able to complete the therapeutic measures at the foundation of the study with such a large number of test subjects in the purported timeframe.[237]

Surprisingly, however, this medical scandal was more or less ignored by the media. Perhaps it was just too complex to be moulded into a newspaper story.[238] But it cannot be ruled out that Grossarth-Maticek's critics feared that the scandal could irreparably discredit the entire field of psychosomatic cancer research in the eyes of the public. After all, the design of Grossarth-Maticek's studies in itself did

[232] Bernard H. Fox, 'Psychogenic Factors in Cancer, Especially Its Incidence', in *Topics in Health Psychology*, ed. Stan Maes, Charles D. Spielberger, Peter B. Defares, and Irwin G. Sarason (Chichester: Wiley, 1988), 37–55.

[233] Buchanan, *Playing with Fire*, 387.

[234] Manfred Amelang, 'Tales from Crvenka and Heidelberg: What About the Empirical Basis?', *Psychological Inquiry* 2, no. 3 (1991): 233–36.

[235] Lydia Temoshok, 'Assessing the Assessment of Psychosocial Factors', *Psychological Inquiry* 2, no. 3 (1991): 276–80.

[236] Rainer Frentzel-Beyme, 'Levels of Interest in an Epidemiological Approach of Identifying Psychomental Risk Factors for Cancer', *Psychological Inquiry* 2, no. 3 (1991): 290–93, 292.

[237] Anthony J. Pelosi and L. Appleby, 'Psychological Influences on Cancer and Ischaemic Heart Disease', *British Medical Journal* 304, no. 6837 (1992): 1295–8.

[238] Buchanan, *Playing with Fire*, 396–7. Only years later did an article on the debacle appear in *Der Spiegel*, Felix Kurz, 'Akademisches Schattenreich', *Der Spiegel* 37, 9 October 2002, 166.

not necessarily mark him as the 'pseudoscientific' outsider that he seemed to be in the eyes of many psychologists and doctors in 1991.

Psycho-oncology and Psycho-neuroimmunology

Grossarth-Maticek conceived of psychological matters—and above all a person's ability to grapple with 'negative' emotions—as one risk factor among many. Genetic disposition and exposure to carcinogens were among them, but he placed the greatest weight on psychic factors. He subsumed them all under the concept of stress, thus instigating a change in tack away from deciphering repressed trauma and early childhood relations and towards forms of self-regulation in stressful situations. His agenda was not about the search for hidden 'true' feelings, but about how emotions were lived out and modified by behaviour. From this perspective, denial could have positive effects, because the conscious decision to shut out 'negative' emotions like despair and to take a positive approach to oneself, one's feelings, and one's relationships seemed to him to itself be a form of betterment.[239]

But this about-face in the scientific conception of emotions was in no way an invention of Grossarth-Maticek. It took place within the broader rise of positive psychology represented by researchers like Martin Seligman, who in 1998 was elected president of the American Psychological Association with a sizeable majority.[240] American psychologist Daniel Goleman was another proponent of this shift; his book *Emotional Intelligence* gained him fame in Germany and around the world.[241] Fitting was thus the jolly declaration on the cover of a 1989 issue of *Psychologie heute* (*Psychology Today*): 'Have some illusions, no big deal!', with the corresponding article explaining: 'Repression and denial, the most common negative tactics for dealing with an uncomfortable reality, alter and distort this reality—illusions, in contrast, are just re-evaluations and interpretations of these facts in the most generous light possible.'[242] The loss of these illusions—and the concomitant loss of the 'necessary' belief of having one's life under control—was judged as a sign of declining mental and physical health.

In the end, Grossarth-Maticek was less interested in finding explanations for why people got cancer and more concerned with identifying practices that promoted health and curing, which were at the heart of the new concept of

[239] Ronald Grossarth-Maticek, 'Wer sich exponiert, ist gefährdet', *Psychologie heute* 6 (1978): 32–9, 37.

[240] Martin Seligman, *Learned Optimism* (New York: Pocket Books, 1990).

[241] Daniel Goleman, *Emotional Intelligence: Why It Can Matter More Than IQ* (New York: Random House, 1998) and Daniel Goleman, *Healing Emotions: Conversations with the Dalai Lama on Mindfulness, Emotions, and Health* (Boston: Shambhala, 1997).

[242] Heiko Ernst, 'Machen Sie sich ruhig Illusionen', *Psychologie heute* 9 (1989): 20–8, 27.

salutogenesis.[243] He prized therapeutic intervention that aimed at changing behaviours and relationships with the purpose of increasing the patient's well-being. The shift away from a search for causes and towards therapies based on 'coping' and 'quality of life' was also part of a larger movement facilitated by psycho-oncology, a new discipline that focused on how to support and care for cancer patients.[244]

As early as 1960, Lawrence LeShan predicted that psychosomatic research on cancer might have unplanned 'side effects', because when a doctor began conducting interviews and tests with a cancer patient that explored their biography, relationships, and emotions—as doctoral candidate Michael Holm-Hadulla had done with Frau S.—this affected both doctor and patient. LeShan wrote:

> If techniques are used which suggest to the patient that psychic factors are important in the disease process, he must not be left with a helpless feeling that he should be doing something about his emotions in order to reverse the development of the malignancy.... Thus if a relationship is built up in a series of interviews or in exploratory psychotherapy, it cannot be dropped when the patient becomes physically worse.... Once the psychotherapist starts the process, he must continue it to the very end.[245]

Psychosomatic research occasioned doctor and patient to reflect on emotions, analysed how emotions could serve a therapeutic function, and developed new ways to speak about them. Thus, whether the doctor wanted to or not, they were asked to take responsibility for the patient's mental health. In Germany East and West, the progression towards psycho-oncology gained footing later than in the United States, but it was well under way by the time Eysenck and Grossarth-Maticek were publishing their findings in the 1980s.[246]

Psycho-oncology continues to undertake psychosomatic research on cancer to this day. Today, however, most scientists do not believe that psychic factors can play a causative role in the genesis of cancer. The key question today is if and how they can influence the course of cancer, beginning with the initial appearance of isolated cancer cells all the way to the emergence of cancer and, later on, the therapeutic process. A large section of this research is concentrated on psychoneuroimmunology. The field's nascence is often traced back to experiments on rats carried out by psychologist Robert Ader and immunologist Nicholas Cohen in

[243] Stierlin and Grossarth-Maticek, *Krebsrisiken*, 91–2.

[244] Jimmie C. Holland and Julia H. Rowland, eds, *Handbook of Psycho-oncology: Psychological Care of the Patient with Cancer* (New York: Oxford University Press, 1989).

[245] Lawrence LeShan, 'Some Methodological Problems in the Study of the Psychosomatic Aspects of Cancer', *Journal of General Psychology* 63 (1960): 309–17, 313–14.

[246] Rolf Verres and Monika Hasenbring, eds., *Psychosoziale Onkologie* (Berlin: Springer, 1989). On the different developments in Germany and the United States see Hitzer and León-Sanz, 'The Feeling Body'.

1975. The two scientists conditioned the rats by feeding them sweetened water together with a medicine that weakened their immune system. When they later gave the rats unadulterated sweetened water, they observed that the conditioned rats were more prone to illness and more likely to die from it even without the poison. Thus, their bodies had clearly been conditioned to weaken their immune system's guard merely at the presence of the sugary water. After a series of further tests, Ader and Cohen concluded that the immune system could be influenced via the nervous system (in this case, through the sense of taste).[247]

Research in psycho-neuroimmunology thus rests on the assumption that stress, emotions, and psychic disposition can alter how the nervous system regulates hormones. In turn, this makes it possible to weaken or disable immune system functions, which are at least partially controlled by the nervous system. The idea is that such dysfunctions may potentially affect the growth of tumours or the likelihood that a tumour metastasizes.

In the 1970s, researchers had already begun studying tissues and conducting animal experiments in order to determine how the immune system and tumour growth mutually influenced one another on the level of the cell. But back then, the only medicine available that could be used to treat the link was the 'wonder drug' interferon, which had a relatively unspecific effect on the immune system. Since then, more and more immunological mechanisms have been discovered that can identify and destroy cancerous cells.[248] Still, the psycho-neuroimmunology of cancer only established itself as a dedicated field of research in the late 1980s.[249] The immune system—or, rather, the immune systems—are today no longer viewed exclusively as autonomous, self-regulating systems. But science remains far from achieving anything close to complete knowledge of the complex processes involved in immunological defences.

In Germany, a conference convened by Deutsche Krebshilfe (German Cancer Aid) in 1990 brought some of the most important figures of the 'older' psychosomatics like Claus Bahne Bahnson and Thure von Uexküll together with pioneers of psycho-neuroimmunology like American psychologist George F. Solomon.[250] Ever since, German oncological research has been more intensively engaged with psycho-neuroimmunology, transporting psychosomatics into what is now

[247] Robert Ader and Nicholas Cohen, 'Behaviorally Conditioned Immunosuppression', *Psychosomatic Medicine* 37, no. 4 (1975): 333–40. George F. Solomon laid the theoretical groundwork for the concept of psycho-neuroimmunology early on: George Freeman Solomon and R. H. Moos, 'Emotions, Immunity, and Disease: A Speculative Theoretical Integration', *Archives of General Psychiatry* 11, no. 6 (1964): 657–74, https://doi.org/10.1001/archpsyc.1964.01720300087011.

[248] F. M. Burnet, 'The Concept of Immunological Surveillance', *Progress in Experimental Tumor Research* 13 (1970): 1–27, https://doi.org/10.1159/000386035.

[249] Robert Ader, David L. Felten, and Nicholas Cohen, eds, *Psychoneuroimmunology*, 2nd rev. edn (San Diego: Academic Press, 1991).

[250] Deutsche Krebshilfe, 'Workshop "Psychoneuroimmunology in Relation to Cancer" vom 3.-7. Juni 1990 in Tutzing', *Onkologie* 13, no. 5 (1990): 393, https://doi.org/10.1159/000216803.

considered to be the avant-garde of oncology.[251] Few doctors and researchers today doubt that there is some kind of connection between emotions and tumour-growth via the immune system.[252] But it is contemporary common sense that the connection is neither simple nor particularly clear. Towards the end of his life, George F. Solomon wrote up some bits of wisdom that he had acquired in his life as a scientist. One of them was: 'Be wary of simple answers to complex questions.'[253]

[251] J. Hefner and H. Csef (2012), 'Psychoneuroimmunologie und Krebs. Neue Ergebnisse zu psychosozialen Einflüssen auf Tumorerkrankungen', *Best Practice Onkologie* 7, no. 1 (2012): 18–33, https://doi.org/10.1007/s11654-011-0374-x. For a general introduction, see Martin Bleif, *Krebs. Die unsterbliche Krankheit* (Stuttgart: Klett-Cotta, 2013), 158–89.

[252] How much this knowledge has established itself is attested to by the fact that has made its way into encyclopaedias. See, for instance, 'Krebs', *Brockhaus-Enzyklopädie*, 19th rev. edn (Mannheim: Brockhaus, 1990), 453–6.

[253] George Freeman Solomon, *From Psyche to Soma and Back: Tales of Biopsychosocial Medicine* (Bloomington, IN: Xlibris, 2000), 276.

3
Cancer Awareness

She looked as beautiful and confident as she always did onscreen. Only the hot pink blazer didn't belong to her normal outfit. She wore it as a tribute to the Pink Initiative. After all, she was supposed to be the smiling face of early detection during this Breast Cancer Awareness Month. This 1 October 2013 was reserved for a special event—the first mammogram live on TV was supposed to bring the awareness campaign to Americans with a bang.

In truth, she hadn't wanted this. She had a different topic she had wanted to talk about: How things were going for the widow of a man who, seven years ago, had shot five girls at an Amish school to get revenge on God for his daughter's premature birth and death a few moments after. How had this tragedy changed the woman's life?

When the producers of ABC called her while she was speaking with the widow, Marie Monville, she thought: Why me? I'm still young, in my early 40s; nobody in my family has died of cancer; I eat healthy, exercise regularly, have given birth to two children. None of the risk factors apply to me. But it was probably the point that someone who was not at risk got a mammogram without complications.

Her friend and colleague Robin Roberts, who had overcome cancer, ultimately convinced her. She said: 'You know what, Amy? If one life is saved because of early detection, it's all worth it.'

So, she put on her pink blazer and rode to Times Square, where the Mobile Breast Imaging Centre was parked. A large crowd of women with homemade signs and pink ribbons had already gathered. Robin Roberts was there, too, in a short, slim-cut pink dress that highlighted her thin, athletic figure. The broadcast switched to the young woman talking about how she had put off the mammogram over the past year because she had never found the time and thought it wasn't so pressing, even though she knew how important it was for women over 40. In the talk round on Good Morning America beforehand, Robin said: 'We're hearing the word stronger and you are being so strong today.... We have made a real commitment to bring you what you need to know to be healthy and to be informed.' Robin's optimistic outlook was clear: she said not 'what you need to know to find out if you are healthy', which is the purpose of the mammogram, but 'what you need to know to be healthy'.

When she entered the 'mammovan', women outside cheered. The mammogram itself was, of course, not broadcast live. She was only shown in front of the x-ray machine. The camera then showed her again after it was all over and she was hugging her colleague. Robin smiled and said: 'I gotta tell you, she was so nervous this morning, she is so happy right now, I can just see the relief.' Both laughed. It was so easy and now she felt so good. Even though she did not yet have the results, in her eyes the worst was over.

On 11 November 2013, she, a host of Good Morning America, was featured as a guest on the show. Her husband sat alongside her—he had been on a trip while she got the live mammogram because they had been so sure. But that was a mistake, as she explained to the audience, because the mammogram revealed a tumour. She was going to have a bilateral mastectomy. She did not yet know if chemotherapy would be necessary.

This story could have come out of an American television show about a beautiful, successful TV journalist. Indeed, in the summer of 2013, Showtime aired the final season of the tragicomic television series *The Big C*, which followed how the life of fictional character Cathy Jamison was turned topsy-turvy after she was diagnosed with 'malignant melanoma'. But this story is not that of a TV character, but of a real woman. Her name is Amy Robach. Millions of viewers of *Good Morning America* watched as she glowingly exited the 'mammovan' and then again when she revealed her diagnosis on air.[1] Robach continued working as the show's host while undergoing therapy, despite having a double mastectomy, eight sessions of chemotherapy, radiation treatment, and reconstructive surgery. She talked on television about how she was doing, and together with her husband, *Melrose Place* actor Andrew Shue, she talked about how the diagnosis and the ensuing therapy had placed a strain on their marriage. In September 2015, she published a book titled *Better*, in which she wrote about her experiences and lessons learned.[2]

Some aspects of this story are decidedly American. There is probably no other country in the world where people talk so much about cancer, and breast cancer in particular. And there is certainly no other country with such intense campaigns for mammogram screening backed up by self-help groups of breast cancer survivors, who have made pink their colour. Although the German Bundestag

[1] 'ABC News' Amy Robach Reveals Breast Cancer after On Air Mammogram', *Good Morning America News*, 12 November 2013, https://www.youtube.com/watch?v=K2g6OzkEkKQ; 'BREAST CANCER: Good Morning America Reporter Amy Robach Diagnosed after On Air Mammogram', *NewsBreaker*, https://www.youtube.com/watch?v=Qy9jXuT7J5E; 'Amy Robach Diagnosed with Breast Cancer', *ABC News*, http://abcnews.go.com/GMA/video/amy-robach-breast-cancer-diagnosis-mammogram-air-change-20848609. The beginning scene is based on these snippets as well as information that Amy Robach gave in later interviews.

[2] Amy Robach, *Better: How I Let Go of Control, Held On to Hope, and Found Joy in My Darkest Hour* (New York: Ballantine Books, 2015).

initiated a mammography programme in 2002 open to all women between 50 and 69, it is not taken advantage of nearly as much as its counterparts in the United States. In Germany, the sceptics who doubt that mammograms are useful at all are many and they are loud.[3]

But Amy Robach's story illustrates a trend that has also taken hold in Germany. This chapter studies its genealogy in the history of early detection and preventive care in the twentieth century. On the one hand, it is the history of the expansion of early detection. The first early detection measures and campaigns were developed in the early twentieth century. They aimed to educate people to recognize and seek medical attention for symptoms that were at once typical of cancer, yet highly unspecific. French historian Patrice Pinell describes this as an attempt to turn patients into the guardians of their own health.[4] But with the rise of early detection measures in the second half of the twentieth century—first and foremost the Pap smear—the 'guardian patient' has gradually been supplanted by a new ideal. The prevention-minded patient is supposed to attend regular check-ups *before* any symptoms appear and practice various techniques of self-care.[5]

On the other hand, it is the history of the emotions that campaigns engaged in order to reach this goal. And it is the history of the feelings people felt about their body during a time when medical discourse and public health campaigns increasingly depicted it as a risk factor. This history was defined by the conflation of early detection and prophylaxis, so that the former often seemed like an instance of the latter.[6] While Amy Robach's friend Robin Roberts praises the mammogram as a way to stay healthy, what goes unspoken is that the real challenge is not the examination, but facing its potential result: a cancer diagnosis. Nevertheless, this is the emotional attitude that many early detection campaigns in contemporary Germany try to impart.

A particularly illustrative example are the Felix Burda Foundation's campaigns, which, since 2001, have been recommending men undergo colonoscopies as an effective form of early detection. In 2008 and 2009, they ran a series of television ads depicting famous people dancing to James Brown's soul classic 'I Feel Good' (Fig. 4). Accompanying billboard ads explained: 'Do you feel good too? You might

[3] P. C. Gøtzsche and K. J. Jørgensen, 'Screening for Breast Cancer with Mammography', *Cochrane Database of Systematic Reviews* 6 (2013), https://doi.org/10.1002/14651858.CD001877.pub5; Gerd Gigerenzer, 'Towards a Paradigm Shift in Cancer Screening: Informed Citizens Instead of Greater Participation. Germany Aims to Stop Nudging the Public on Screening', *British Medical Journal* 350, no. 2175 (2015), https://doi.org/10.1136/bmj.h2175.

[4] Pinell, Naissance d'un fléau, 301.

[5] Martin Lengwiler and Jeannette Madarász, 'Präventionsgeschichte als Kulturgeschichte der Gesundheitspolitik', in Lengwiler and Madarász, *Das präventive Selbst*, 11–28; Ulrich Bröckling, 'Dispositive der Vorbeugung: Gefahrenabwehr, Resilienz, Precaution', in *Sicherheitskultur. Soziale und politische Praktiken der Gefahrenabwehr*, ed. Christopher Daase, Philipp Offermann, and Valentin Rauer (Frankfurt am Main: Campus, 2012), 93–108.

[6] In German, both are often to referred to as 'Vorsorge', literally 'pre-care', which suggests that early detection could prevent cancer.

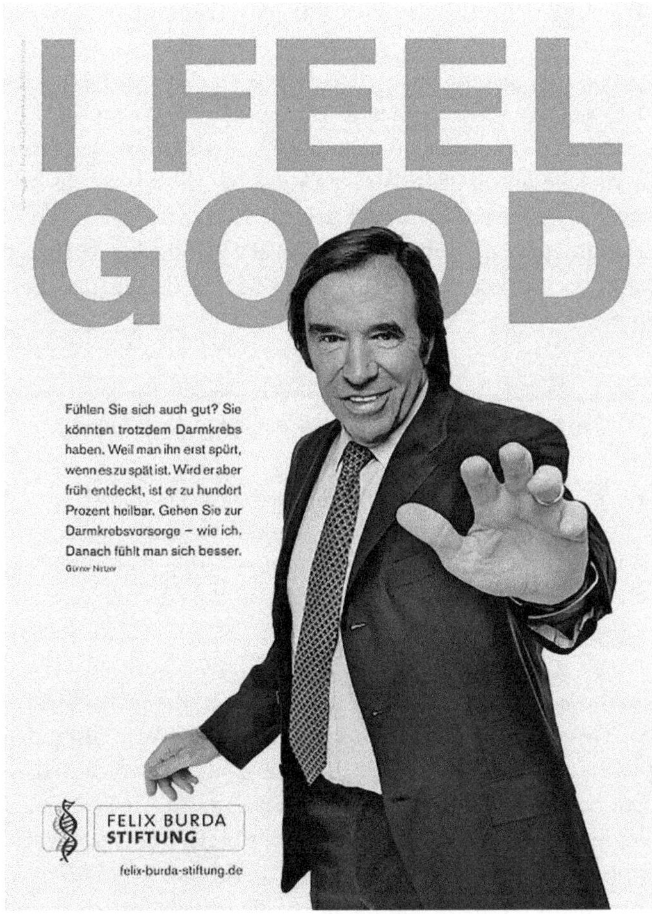
I FEEL GOOD
Fühlen Sie sich auch gut? Sie könnten trotzdem Darmkrebs haben. Weil man ihn erst spürt, wenn es zu spät ist. Wird er aber früh entdeckt, ist er zu hundert Prozent heilbar. Gehen Sie zur Darmkrebsvorsorge – wie ich. Danach fühlt man sich besser.
FELIX BURDA STIFTUNG
felix-burda-stiftung.de

Fig. 4 Advertisement of the Felix Burda Foundation (2009).

still have colon cancer. Because you only feel it after it's too late. But if it's detected early, then it is up to 100 per cent curable. Get a colonoscopy like I did. You'll feel better.'

Feeling good thus has two sides. As an 'intuitive' visceral feeling it can be misleading. Perceiving health as 'life in the silence of the organs', as French philosopher and doctor Georges Canguilhem once defined it, can be risky.[7] In contrast, feeling good is seen as justified when it is the result of preventive practice. Still, whether the patient really feels better after a check-up depends on the findings. Because even if the chances of recovery were as high as the campaign promises, nobody is going to 'feel good' when they find out they have cancer.

[7] Georges Canguilhem, 'New Reflections on the Normal and the Pathological', in *On the Normal and the Pathological*, trans. Carolyn R. Fawcett (Boston: Reidel Publishing Company, 1978), 141–80.

Amy Robach's story demonstrates how this part of the story is often left out by public health campaigns.

What emotions do people feel when observing their own bodies? Why do people need to observe their bodies in the first place? What kind of emotions need to be activated in order to get people of different genders and social backgrounds to take an 'appropriate' approach to their physical health? These are the questions that have occupied cancer awareness campaigns for over a century. But ultimately, a seemingly simple development laid the groundwork for all of them: the notion that cancer could be cured and that there was thus reason for hope.

Hope: The Invention of a Curable Disease

> 'Cancer!' spoke my inner voice. It penetrated me. How could such a terrible thing happen to my yet young wife? The affliction was considered by the science of the time to be incurable; after the subtle onset of suffering that outdid everything human, death was the inevitable end. I knew this disease very well. With shudders I thought of its grim final stage.[8]

These are the thoughts of the fictional doctor Franz, the protagonist of Theodor Storm's 1887 novella *A Confession.*[9] He examined his wife after she expressed vague complaints and believed to have discovered uterine cancer. His suspicion is confirmed, but he feels totally helpless against the illness. He is incapable of doing anything to cure it, nor can he palliate his wife's bouts of severe pain. In the end, he gives in to her wishes and lets her drink a liquid that kills her.

Hopelessness drove Franz to end the life of his wife and patient, a hopelessness rooted in his experience as a doctor and his trust in the authority of medical science. Storm set the story in the early 1850s. But the doctor's 'confession' to his friend Hans does not conclude with his admission that he acted against the Hippocratic Oath by terminating his patient's life. He continues that soon thereafter, he was called to aid another woman with uterine cancer. His duty as a doctor wrests him out of his mourning state and leads him to read some medical journals, where he comes across an article on the 'abdominal illnesses' of women. The narrator elaborates: 'Then came a sentence that seared into me as with burning letters: "Up until now"—I read two and three times again—"one has held this

[8] Theodor Storm, *Ein Bekenntnis. Novella Medici*, ed. Walter Zimorski (Hamburg: Diplomica, 2017), 37.

[9] The novella was first published in October 1887 in *Westermanns Illustrierten Deutschen Monatsheften*, see Yahya Elsaghe, '"Die Krankheit unserer Marschen". Zur Verdrängung der Krebsangst in Theodor Storms Novelle "Ein Bekenntnis"', *Zeitschrift für Germanistik* 20, no. 3 (2010): 508–21, 508, https://doi.org/10.3726/92130_508.

ailment for absolutely incurable; but in the following, I will expound upon a procedure that enabled me to give three of five women their lives and families back to them."'[10]

With the patient's permission, Franz performs the dangerous operation on her and is successful. The confession ends with the doctor's bitter realization that he had given in to hopelessness too soon. He had ceased to act as a doctor and failed to read the article on the potentially life-saving operation, which had been published when his wife was still alive. He tries to pay penance for the guilt he feels by leading a life of self-imposed loneliness and absolute dedication to his occupation. It is the guilt of a man who abandoned his hope in science.

Storm composed this exceptionally touching rejection of hopelessness at a time when the issue had existential significance for him. In early 1887, he was diagnosed with stomach cancer. The diagnosis threw him into such intense despair that a colleague as well as his brother, who was himself a doctor, both asked for a second opinion. They convinced the physician to say that the diagnosis was a false alarm and that Storm was suffering from an affliction of the abdominal aorta that was indeed life-threatening, but not 'hopeless'. *A Confession* was written in the period between the first and second diagnosis.[11]

Storm clearly placed weight on rendering as realistically as possible the hope for a cure on which the entire novella hinges. The passages from the medical article that the protagonist reads are almost word-for-word quotations from an article published by professor of gynaecology Wilhelm Alexander Freund.[12]

As Storm's novella indicates, the last third of the nineteenth century was, for many oncologists, a time of game-changing discoveries and a new type of hope. Indeed, doctors had been operating on cancer since the early modern period. But these were exceptional cases in no way approaching standard treatment for cancer patients of all ages and social backgrounds.[13] Operations were only possible for those who had a certain degree of wealth, as they were conducted at the patient's home and nurses had to be hired to take care of them during the lengthy recovery process.

At a time when reliable anaesthesia was not available and the principles of aseptic surgery had yet to be discovered, operating on cancer represented unimaginable torture and had many serious risks. Large stomach operations were simply not possible. And those who did survive other surgeries usually died soon thereafter from relapses or metastases. Thus, up until the mid-nineteenth century, very few people could be cured of cancer. This is why the instances of success attracted so much attention. For example, in 1811, 58-year-old

[10] Storm, *Ein Bekenntnis*, 48.
[11] Elsaghe, '"Die Krankheit unserer Marschen"', 517–21.
[12] Wilhelm Alexander Freund, 'Eine neue Methode'.
[13] Javier Moscoso, 'Exquisite and Lingering Pains: Facing Cancer in Early Modern Europe', in *Pain and Emotion in Modern History*, ed. Rob Boddice (London: Palgrave Macmillan, 2014), 16–35; Marjo Kaartinen, *Breast Cancer in the Eighteenth Century* (London: Routledge, 2013).

English author and former lady-in-waiting Frances 'Fanny' Burney decided, after considerable hesitation, to have her breast amputated after the pain caused by her tumour became unbearable. The operation was conducted by seven doctors and she was awake the entire time. Three months later, she recollected the traumatic experience in a long letter to her sister.[14] She lived for twenty-nine years after the operation. Her letters were posthumously published between 1842 and 1846, meaning that the details of her case might have been known to English-speaking persons in the Germanophone countries.

The state of medicine made going to the doctor early not particularly advisable. When people did, they were treated with cauterizing compresses and tonics. This all began to change around the time when Storm was working on his novella, which documented the swing from medical hopelessness towards hope.

Progress in anaesthesia and surgical techniques represented a knickpoint. In 1847, a person was etherized in Germany for the first time. The method spread like wildfire. This anaesthetic technology, which was constantly being altered, was what first enabled invasive operations—Frances Burney's mastectomy had 'only' lasted twenty minutes.[15] The feared risk of infection could only be somewhat brought under control after Louis Pasteur and Joseph Lister discovered that bacteria are omnipresent. In 1864 and 1867, respectively, they developed antiseptic and aseptic methods for sanitizing surgical instruments and spaces. These discoveries, too, were quickly integrated into Germany's internationally well-connected medical practice.

Accordingly, in the late nineteenth century, forms of cancer that had been considered inoperable until then, such as stomach cancer, could be operated on for the first time. Moreover, doctors developed surgical procedures for some of the most common types of cancer that then became 'standard protocol', a few of which are still practiced in modified form today.[16] Only when the vision of a cure won over elite surgeons could early detection even be declared a desirable project.[17] The enthusiasm of surgeons was fuelled by the optimism that took hold of medicine as a whole in the late nineteenth century. That bacteria cause illnesses had just been discovered, and the microscope had become a standard tool of medical research, enabling scientists to study paths of transmission and develop vaccines. Some diseases that had theretofore been counted among the deadliest, such as diphtheria, splenic fever, rabies, and tetanus, were minimized into

[14] Fanny Burney, *The Journals and Letters of Fanny Burney (Madame D'Arblay)*, Vol. 6: *France 1803–1812, Letters 550–631*, ed. Joyce Hemlow (Oxford: Oxford University Press, 1975), 596–616.

[15] Wilfried Witte, *Unerhörte Leiden: Die Geschichte der Schmerztherapie in Deutschland im 20. Jahrhundert* (Frankfurt am Main: Campus, 2017).

[16] Erwin H. Ackerknecht, 'Zur Geschichte der Krebsbehandlung', *Gesnerus* 37, no. 3/4 (1980): 189–95; Michael Schmiedebach, *Geschichte der operativen Chirurgie*, vol. 1 (Heidelberg: Kaden, 2000), 157–226.

[17] Georg Winter, 'Die Bekämpfung des Krebses im Königreich Preussen', *Zeitschrift für Krebsforschung* 10, no. 3 (1911): 343–64, 343, https://doi.org/10.1007/BF02365516.

avoidable ones. New hygienic practices also made it possible to inhibit the spread of other diseases like cholera.

These discoveries engendered enormous interest in illness prevention. Advances in sanitation and hygiene did have a preventive effect by encouraging healthy lifestyles and diets, the construction of clean, well-lit, adequately ventilated living quarters, the provision of parks in cities, and the installation of modern plumbing. But preventive healthcare sought to hinder particular illnesses by educating people about how they were transmitted and how they could change their behaviour to avoid being at risk. The first public health campaigns of this sort targeted widespread sicknesses for which neither effective medicine nor vaccines had yet to be found; namely, tuberculosis and sexually transmitted diseases like gonorrhoea and syphilis.[18]

The campaigns against tuberculosis in particular served as a model for the health professionals who met in Berlin on 18 February 1900 to establish the Comité für Sammelforschung auf dem Gebiete der Krebsforschung (Committee for General Cancer Research).[19] One of its main goals was to spread the hope that cancer could be cured to a lay audience, a hope previously only harboured by a small group of doctors. The association also sought to develop new methods of early detection.

Thus, a 1911 publication of the Internationale Hygiene-Ausstellung (International Hygiene Exhibition) in Dresden declared as its goal 'to show that cancer, when it is detected early enough and operated on, is curable'. 'Detected early, curable' would become the mantra of a century of early detection campaigns. The postulate's countless iterations were printed in pamphlets and on posters. But behind these three simple words is a whole history of shifting notions of what 'early' means, how to identify cancer, what exactly cancer is, and what should be considered 'cured'. Above all, however, ideas changed about what inhibits early diagnoses, how these barriers can be demolished, and how people who might have cancer or be at risk of getting it can be brought to embark upon the sole path of hope: the one that leads to the office of a qualified medical doctor.

When the International Hygiene Exhibition in Dresden opened its doors on 6 May 1911, scores of visitors flooded the space to get a look at the 'encyclopaedic knowledge' about the body and health. The exhibition kicked off the first largescale public health campaign of the Deutsches Zentralkomitee zur Erforschung und Bekämpfung der Krebskrankheit e.V. (German Central Committee for

[18] Lutz Sauerteig, 'Geschlechtskrankheiten, Gesundheitspolitik und Medizin im 20. Jahrhundert: Europäische Entwicklungen im Überblick', *Sexuologie. Zeitschrift für Sexualmedizin, Sexualtherapie und Sexualwissenschaft* 19, no. 3/4 (2012): 111–18; Anja Laukötter, 'Medien der Sexualaufklärung: Forschungsstand und Forschungsperspektiven', *NTM: Zeitschrift für Geschichte der Wissenschaften, Technik und Medizin* 20, no. 3 (2012): 225–32, https://doi.org/10.1007/s00048-012-0075-8.

[19] Atzl and Helms, *Die Geschichte der Deutschen Krebsgesellschaft*, 14–15; Matthias Kaiser, 'Zur Geschichte des Deutschen Zentralkomitees zur Erforschung und Bekämpfung der Krebskrankheit (1900–1933)' (PhD diss., University of Greifswald, 1988).

Researching and Fighting Cancer), as the association was now called. The exhibition also revealed that over the committee's first ten years of existence, it had succeeded in inscribing cancer onto the agenda of health policymaking, because an entire section of the health exhibit was dedicated to cancer. But the gain was limited. In the eyes of the committee's members, state funding of oncological research remained inadequate, and they had still been unable to communicate 'knowledge' about the short window of curability to broad swathes of the population.

Thus, the group started putting pressure on political representatives. Oncologist Vinzenz Czerny demanded that the government build fewer 'murderous "dreadnoughts"' and pump more money into cancer research.[20] Statistical studies revealed the increase in cancer cases and documented the high costs of treating and caring for cancer patients. Other reports analysed the loss of productivity that followed when workers debilitated by cancer were forced to leave their stations. Thus, cancer posed a problem for the 'human economy', a central concept for the founder of the Dresden Hygiene Museum, Karl August Lingner, who adopted it from sociologist Rudolf Goldscheid.[21] The exhibition was intended to move cancer out of the confines of private life and to initiate a public, fact-based conversation on it. The ultimate goal, however, was to spur people to voice their concern that they might have cancer to their doctors early on.

Accordingly, the exhibition foregrounded openness and objectivity. The curators selected medical, scientific imagery and language as the right media to communicate this attitude, situating it in a visual narrative that depicted the new techniques of science as revealing the secrets of the body, making visible the invisible. The idea was to hook visitors into the exhibition by arousing their curiosity about the body's functions.[22]

The cancer section of the exhibit foregrounded objects of knowledge produced in the laboratory, approaching them with an almost encyclopaedic level of detachment without harping too much on the desired outcome that people act in the

[20] HMS Dreadnought was the name of a British battleship that was built in 1906. It became the prototype of modern ships of war; in contrast to previous models, it only had high-calibre guns. The Czerny quote comes from a special issue of the popular *Illustrirten Zeitung* published on the occasion of the health exhibition: Vinzenz Czerny, 'Hygienische Zeitfragen. I. Krebsforschung', *Illustrirte Zeitung*, 1911, 19.

[21] Martin Roth, 'Menschenökonomie oder der Mensch als technisches und künstlerisches Meisterwerk', in *Der Gläserne Mensch—Eine Sensation. Zur Kulturgeschichte eines Ausstellungsobjekts*, ed. Rosmarie Beier and Martin Roth (Stuttgart: Hatje, 1990), 39–67, 59–64; Jochen Fleischhacker, 'Menschen- und Güterökonomie. Anmerkungen zu Rudolf Goldscheids demoökonomischen Gesellschaftsentwurf', *Wissenschaft, Politik und Öffentlichkeit. Von der Wiener Moderne bis zur Gegenwart*, ed. Mitchell G. Ash and Christian H. Stifter (Vienna: Facultas, 2002), 207–29, 216.

[22] Sybilla Nikolow, '"Wissenschaftliche Stillleben" des Körpers im 20. Jahrhundert', *Erkenne Dich selbst! Strategien der Sichtbarmachung des Körpers im 20. Jahrhundert*, ed. Sybilla Nikolow (Cologne: Böhlau, 2015), 11–43.

name of early detection.[23] Among the 488 displayed objects were a number of anatomical models, including wax casts, or moulages—real moulds of patients' body parts that had a strong reality effect. There were also representations of microscopic images that showed various local malignant tumours in humans, animals, and plants and that offered a peek into laboratory experiments.

The objects depicted advanced tumours that, from today's perspective, seem frightening, jarring, and disgusting. Later exhibitions only featured such items when they could be contrasted with images of successful treatment. The 1911 exhibition did work with such juxtapositions, but not many. Seemingly, the organizers viewed the potential evocation of fear of cancer as unproblematic. The presented objects were solely intended to generate fascination for and trust in medicine and allow people to see what a cancerous tumour looked like.

A smaller subsection of the exhibit documented the first-ever public health campaign in Germany to specifically promote early detection of cervical cancer. Between 1903 and 1907/8, professor of gynaecology Georg Winter developed the campaign for the German province of East Prussia and its capital city Königsberg. Evidence of the campaign's success was provided in the form of tables, curves, and graphs, which visualized how it led to an increase in the number of women who went to the doctor shortly after symptoms appeared. Complicated calculations were supposed to prove how many women's lives had been saved by the early detection campaign and the early operations occasioned by those important doctor's visits.[24] The tables suggested a clear-cut connection between early detection, early operation, and cure, as if every woman whose cervical cancer was caught early were saved. Georg Winter knew that this was not true, and he admitted elsewhere that many other types of cancer only caused symptoms so late that only half of the cases could be operated on despite early detection measures.[25] Thus, in contrast to the exhibition's claims, cervical cancer only had limited value as a general model for how early detection campaigns should be conducted.

Nevertheless, on 10 March 1911, at the invitation of the Central Committee for Researching and Fighting Cancer, Winter gave a detailed account of his campaign. He listed three hurdles that stood in the way of effective early detection. First was doctors' inability to diagnose cervical cancer, as many dispensed with 'internal' gynaecological examinations with a speculum, even though this was the only way to reliably identify potential early symptoms. Second, Winter assumed that many women were not aware that some common, usually harmless symptoms could actually be signs of an onset of cervical cancer; as a consequence, he thought they

[23] Ludmilla Jordanova, 'Objects of Knowledge: A Historical Perspective on Museums', in *The New Museology*, ed. Peter Vergo (London: Reaktion, 1989), 22–40.

[24] Gruppe Krebs, *Sonder-Katalog der Gruppe Krebs der wissenschaftlichen Abteilung der Internationalen Hygiene-Ausstellung in Dresden 1911* (Dresden, 1911), 14.

[25] Winter, 'Die Bekämpfung des Krebses', 349.

would pay little attention to them. Third, Winter believed that women who suspected they might have cancer only ever went to the doctor very late because they trusted 'quacks' more than doctors in matters of cancer treatment or believed that cancer was not curable.[26]

Winter's campaign thus targeted two groups: doctors, who he thought should be better trained in the methods of early detection, and laypeople, who he wanted to teach about early symptoms of cancer and the chances of overcoming it through early operations. A third important group for Winter were midwives and nurses, because he observed that petit-bourgeois and underclass women sought out advice from them more often than from doctors. He thought that they should fill the role of pointing potential cancer patients on the right path.

But biting criticism alleged that his widescale press campaign stoked the populace's fear of cancer.[27] The essence of the remonstrations concerned the emotions that critics believed people should feel towards their bodies and how they should perceive their bodies. Should they view it as a complex, delicate marvel and thus recognize the necessity to properly care for it and protect it from risks that might cause tuberculosis or sexually transmitted diseases? Or should they trust their subjective feeling of health, be 'strong', and not complain about 'every little ailment'?

But the producers of early detection campaigns wanted to teach people to take *certain* 'ailments' seriously, even if they felt like they were healthy. They sought to cultivate awareness of the potentially hidden threat in people's by all appearances healthy bodies and a mindfulness towards one's body that matched this potential danger.[28] However, Winter warned against the kind of unrelenting self-observation that never let the body be quiet even in a healthy state, a thought captured in his statement: 'The main idea of this education is that the sick person should always be aware of the possibility of cancer when certain symptoms or findings appear. He should in no way allow fear of cancer to lead him to constantly check his body for lumps and suspiciously surveil all his bodily functions. He should only focus on disruptions and then let the doctor determine their significance.'[29]

Winter had no doubt that people could be brought to adopt this kind of rational, well-defined fear of cancer, because he believed that they were too robust to fall prey to nervous, round-the-clock self-observation. His concern was more that his fellow citizens wallowed in 'indolent dullness' and did not pay attention to their body at all or never found the time amidst the business of everyday life.[30] Precisely this assessment convinced Winter that fear was his friend and that it

[26] Ibid., 344, 346, and 353. [27] Ibid., 351.

[28] *Krebs-Merkblatt zur Aufklärung des Volkes über die Krebskrankheit*, Bundesarchiv Berlin-Lichterfelde BArch R 86/850.

[29] Winter, 'Die Bekämpfung des Krebses', 359. [30] Ibid., 358.

posed no danger if it could be acted upon. He thought that if healthy people were aware of the available treatments and chances of recovery, their 'rational' fear would help them overcome their hesitation and evoke an equally 'rational' response, which is to say, going to the doctor and asking for a diagnosis. Similarly, he reasoned that when a person went to the doctor and was told they did not have cancer, their fear would dissipate at once.[31]

Thus, Winter subscribed to a concept of fear that was dominant in the late nineteenth century. It held that fear, so long as it did not become all-consuming, was an appropriate, rational emotion because it could motivate people to act and could, without exception, be overcome through education. The idea that fear could be traumatic and enduringly alter a person's perspective on life was not yet prevalent. Advice books for parents as well as children's and young adult literature of the time discussed fear without judging it as inherently morally negative, while little time was expended on how people experienced fear. Decisive for all these texts was simply that children and young adults overcome their fears. Stories illustrated this normative viewpoint with exemplary protagonists, while guides offered tips and tricks on how to raise children who could adhere to it.[32] The period's psychology of emotions, represented by thinkers like Wilhelm Wundt and William James, thought that fear had an evolutionary function, making animals aware of dangers and initiating the fight-or-flight response.[33]

With the turn of the century, voices warning about the dangers of fear multiplied. Now, childrearing guides and children's and young adult literature detailed the potentially lasting negative effects of fear. Some advice books acknowledged that parents' expectations that their children overcome their fear, especially when forced through 'test situations' like locking them in the cellar, could damage their children's emotional development. This insight into the psychic mechanisms of fear owed much to psychoanalysis, which was on the ascent.[34]

These opposing ideas defined the debate over the first pamphlet on cancer published by the Central Committee for Researching and Fighting Cancer. Designed by Berlin-based doctor Alfred Pinkuß, it was distributed throughout all of Prussia in 1911.[35] Criticism focused neither on the text-heavy layout nor on the information selected. Instead, detractors complained that it burdened readers with the premonition that they might have a hidden illness, that it fractured their intuitive feelings of wellness, and that it thus might lead them to fear the worst at the sight of even the most minimal symptoms. For example, Dr Kroenig, head

[31] Ibid., 351–2. [32] Hitzer, 'Jim Button's Fear', 174–5.

[33] Claudia Wassmann, 'The Science of Emotion: Studying Emotions in Germany, France, and the United States, 1860–1920' (PhD diss., University of Chicago, 2005).

[34] Hitzer, 'Jim Button's Fear', 176–7.

[35] *Krebs-Merkblatt zur Aufklärung des Volkes über die Krebskrankheit*, ed. Dr Alfred Pinkuß (Berlin: Deutschen Zentralkomitee zur Erforschung und Bekämpfung der Krebskrankheit e.V., 1911), Bundesarchiv Berlin-Lichterfelde BArch R 86/850. In 1911, the pamphlet was already on its second print run. In 1921, it was republished with significant revisions, BArch R 1501/111968, 38–41.

gynaecologist of Freiburg, Lörrach, and Waldshut, warned the State of Baden's interior ministry against using the pamphlet: '... in my personal opinion, such a pamphlet will only succeed in creating an army of hypochondriacs and whip up already anxious persons into even more self-observation. A person artificially pushed into such fear of cancer loses the desire to live and work. It will produce more harm than the somewhat earlier consultation with a doctor will help.'[36] Thus, Kroenig did not believe that people would only experience fear of cancer when actual symptoms appeared. He perceived fear as a paralyzing emotion that, to be sure, would drive the hypochondriac to the doctor's office, but at the cost of permeating all other aspects of their life and extinguishing the individual's vitality. 'Normal mortals', in his eyes, were not equipped to face the knowledge that their lives were constantly in danger. He did not share the committee's optimism that early detection would significantly increase opportunities to treat cancer and accused the pamphlet's author of raising unfounded hopes that would predictably be proven false and thus erode trust in medical doctors.[37]

The members of the committee and the responsible persons at the Imperial Office of Health took these concerns seriously. They did not contest that the pamphlet could cause fear. However, in their assessment, the desired effect of earlier diagnosis and treatment of cancer outweighed the burden that the fear of cancer placed on the populace, which they thought was less dramatic than Kroenig depicted it.[38] Their evaluation was to have lasting consequences, setting German public health on a course that diverged from that travelled by countries like the Netherlands and Great Britain, which, for reasons similar to Kroenig's, did not carry out any early detection campaigns for laypeople until the 1950s. They restricted themselves to providing information for doctors, midwives, and nurses, encouraging them to keep their ears open for complaints about potential early symptoms and schedule patients for an exam when they heard them.[39] In contrast, public health in France and the United States tracked closer to Germany. Both countries' lead doctors trusted that people's emotional fortitude would keep them from falling into a spiral of anxiety about cancer, and their early detection campaigns even drew on Georg Winter's as a predecessor worthy of imitation.

[36] Bernhard Kroenig, head gynaecologist for Freiburg, Lörrach, and Waldshut, Letter to the Ministry of the Interior in Karlsruhe, Freiburg, 18 February 1913, BArch R 1501/111967, 190–2.

[37] Ibid.

[38] President of the Imperial Health Department, transcribed by Dr Hamel, Letter Concerning the Krebs-Merkblatt, Berlin, 21 May 1913, BArch R 1501/111967, 208–12.

[39] Elizabeth Toon, '"Cancer as the General Population Knows It": Knowledge, Fear, and Lay Education in 1950s Britain', *Bulletin of the History of Medicine* 81, no. 1 (2006): 116–38, https://doi.org/10.1353/bhm.2007.0013; Stephen Snelders, Frans J. Mejiman, and Toine Pieters, 'Cancer Health Communication in the Netherlands 1910–1950: Paternalistic Control or Popularization of Knowledge?' *Medizinhistorisches Journal* 41, no. 3 (2006): 271–89.

Shame, Disgust, and Fear: How to Communicate Knowledge

In the 1920s, the economic conditions of public health programmes changed, which had effects on early detection campaigns. Around the same time, film had its breakthrough and psychologists' ideas about educating the public shifted. Health policy came to place greater emphasis on personal responsibility and moral duties.

In the Weimar Republic, the inflation of the early 1920s and the currency reform of 1923 threw many people into dire straits, and the events hit the provision of medical care hard, too. The number of beds in some hospitals was well below actual needs, a problem that hospital administrations sought to resolve by finding ways to release patients as early as possible. Adequately treating cancer patients was difficult under these circumstances, because they generally needed intensive care over a long period of time and often had little chance of being definitively cured.

Early detection campaigns did not escape unscathed, either. In the previous decades, cancer had often been depicted as an illness of old age, an assumption propped up on the correlation between rising cancer cases and increased life expectancy. Lean coffers put a damper on both public and private expenditures for fighting cancer, while confronting diseases like syphilis and tuberculosis, which overwhelmingly affected younger people, seemed more pressing. Moreover, cancer treatment was expensive, especially when radium was used—because there are no stores of the metal in Germany, it had to be purchased on the international market.

This helps explain why campaigns of the 1920s emphasized that people between 30 and 60 years of age could get cancer, too, and why they placed even more focus on cervical cancer than had already been the case in the previous decade. Women in this age group—precisely when society needed them to become mothers and care for their children—were the most likely to be diagnosed with cervical cancer.[40] Similarly, men in their 40s and 50s—when they were needed in the workforce—were the most likely to get stomach cancer. Other forms of cancer that were difficult to detect early and that primarily afflicted older people remained mostly unmentioned in the early detection campaigns of the decade.

Campaigns and exhibitions produced by the Dresden Hygiene Museum in the 1920s and early 1930s continued to channel their energy into communicating information about early symptoms and forms of early treatment. But their faith in knowledge's potential to stimulate action waned as many doctors realized that

[40] Transcription of a meeting of the presidium of the Imperial Committee for Fighting Cancer, 30 January 1932 in Berlin, BArch B142/412, 256–66. A detailed graphic at the travelling 'Kampf dem Krebs' exhibition, produced by the Dresden Hygiene Museum, claimed that people ages 45 to 60 constituted the primary risk group: DHMD 2001/247.65.

ignorance was often not the reason that people shied away from the doctor's office. Rather, many patients reported that they decided against early treatment despite suspecting that they might have cancer. Some even made this decision after consulting with their general practitioner or gynaecologist, because the doctor, too, had doubted they could be cured and thus only bolstered their existing scepticism towards conventional medical treatment.[41]

Organizers of health campaigns surmised that doctors' 'hopelessness' derived from their everyday experience that, for the most part, only patients who had been unsuccessfully treated or were dying returned to their practices, while cured patients might only come back years later. This distorted their reporting and, by extension, statistics, which then seemed to reaffirm doctors' prejudices.[42] But oncologists, radiologists, and surgeons also had to admit that around 80 per cent of cancer patients were inoperable when they arrived and that the long-term rates of recovery of patients that had been operated on or undergone radiotherapy remained meagre.[43] And yet, they sustained hope that these rates could be boosted through early detection.

So long as concrete evidence proving that early detection increased recovery rates was lacking, though, general practitioners and gynaecologists could not be won over. Their primary counterargument against early treatment were the 'mutilations' caused by operations. Some places tried to get around doctors' reluctance by opening dedicated care centres. In 1929, Baden's Landesverband zur Bekämpfung des Krebses (State Association for Fighting Cancer) erected central 'Examination and care stations for the prevention and fighting of tumorous illnesses'.[44] Similar care stations in Berlin predated the First World War.[45]

The counselling centres were supposed to downplay many doctors' dearth of hope by cutting them out of the equation altogether. A number of the centres did not have the word 'cancer' in their names, instead opting for the more innocuous term 'tumour', since tumours can be benign. Even the choice of name was intended to boost hopes that the suspicious lump or persistent bleeding might be traceable to a harmless tumour, not a cancerous one.[46] A series of pamphlets published by the centres sought to evoke expectations that an exam would bring

[41] Ferdinand Blumenthal, 'Die Bekämpfung des Krebses', *Blätter des Deutschen Roten Kreuzes* 7, no. 10 (1928): 3–9, 7. BArch R 1501/126318, 75.

[42] Anton Mißriegler, 'Krebsbehandlung durch den Hausarzt', *Hippokrates* 25 (1936): 661–4, 661–2.

[43] Transcription of a meeting on the founding of an East Prussian committee on fighting cancer, Tuesday, 17 November 1931 at the Landeshaus, BArch R 36/1391.

[44] Meeting of the working committee of Baden's State Association for Fighting Cancer, Mannheim, 9 November 1929, UAH H-III-051/2.

[45] Design of a care station for cancer patients by Ernst von Leyden, presented on 15 July 1904 to the Royal Charité directorship, HU Archiv Charité-Direktion, 955, 2–4; Draft on the organization of an institute for cancer research at the Charité, Berlin, 22 December 1914, HU Archiv Charité-Direktion, 950, 117–19, 117.

[46] Meeting of the working committee of Baden's State Association for Fighting Cancer, Mannheim, 9 November 1929, UAH H-III-051/2.

relief, reassurance, and comfort, much like the strategy pursued decades later by the 'Feel Good' campaigns with their smiling faces.[47]

At the same time, counselling centres were designed to be more accessible than clinics, thus ensuring that people with concerns could get an examination in their area without investing a lot of time or having to bear travel expenses. The free provision of diagnostic and preventive care accorded with the principles of a number of other social and health services that were being experimented with during the Weimar period. In particular, information centres run both by private organizations and by the state underwent a boom.

These kinds of services were supposed to help people overcome emotional barriers to treatment. While the producers of the first early detection campaigns did discuss these hurdles, they were given greater weight in the run of the 1920s. One of the feelings seen as particularly important was what Alfred Pinkuß had labelled in 1911 as 'false shame'.[48] The campaigns against venereal diseases homed in on it so intensively that one of the first health education films on STDs was named after it. But campaigns promoting measures to detect cancer early considered 'false shame' a serious problem, too.

They connected false feelings of shame most explicitly with cervical cancer. Pinkuß, a gynaecologist, referenced Winter's experience that many women shied away from gynaecological examinations performed with a speculum, particularly when they were suffering from bleeding and discharge—typical symptoms of cervical cancer. He thus argued that campaigns had to chip away at the perception of this condition as 'unclean' so that women would no longer feel a need to conceal it. He also implored campaigns to teach women not to feel embarrassment about the examination, which doctors did not yet conduct as a matter of routine.[49] The 'embarrassment' associated with the exam did not rest exclusively on its intrusive nature. Rather, it had a bad reputation because, until that point, it had generally been carried out when there was reason to suspect that the patient had a venereal disease. In Imperial Germany and the Weimar Republic, the state forced sex workers to routinely submit to gynaecological examinations. The women's social reform movement of the era criticized these compulsory measures as dishonouring, shameful, and coercive.[50] But early detection campaigns never explicitly mentioned this context. Instead, discussions on gynaecological checks for cervical cancer merely stated that a 'trustworthy doctor' would help their patient 'get past the embarrassing aspect of the exam' by using objective language to strip it of its

[47] *Krebs-Merkblatt* (1911), 7; *Krebs-Merkblatt* (1921), 4. [48] *Krebs-Merkblatt* (1911), 10.

[49] Sabine Hering and Gudrun Meierhof, *Die unpässliche Frau. Sozialgeschichte der Menstruation und Hygiene*, 2nd edn (Frankfurt am Main: Mabuse, 2002), 29–50 and 55–98.

[50] Bettina Hitzer, 'Prostitution in Berlin 1869: Eine Spurensuche', in *Zwischen Tanzboden und Bordell. Lebensbilder Berliner Prostituierter aus dem Jahr 1869*, ed. Michael Häusler and Bettina Hitzer (Berlin: Be.Bra Wissenschaft, 2010), 7–64, 19–20.

association with lasciviousness.[51] The campaigns' schematic representations of the cervix thus served to train people to take a fact-based, desexualized perspective on female sex organs.

But feelings of 'false shame' among people who suspected they may have cancer were not just a problem when it came to cervical cancer. Many people concealed that they had cancer because they believed that it was contagious. Newspaper reports seemed to support this notion.[52] Health education thus highlighted that cancer did not pose a danger to others, which was supposed to signal that people did not need to hide their own cancer out of fear of stigmatization or shame.

Other campaigns tried to evoke fear for certain ends, however. Still, organizers were well aware that fear was a complex ally that could not be allowed to get too strong lest it turn into paralysis.[53]

Public health professionals also came to recognize that knowledge, images, and fascination alone would not suffice to change people's everyday approach to their own bodies. In 1926, Martin Vogel, the head of the Dresden Hygiene Museum, criticized the traditional style of health campaigns:

> The form of our educational programmes generally has an abstract, theoretical character, which is often the reason for their weakness and much-maligned ineffectiveness. They do not touch on the recipient's lifestyle, do not say anything about practical matters or the learned knowledge's immediate use value, and of course, we know from research on education that only that which we ourselves have experienced affects us viscerally and influences our lifestyle.[54]

So, how to communicate knowledge about cancer that affected people 'viscerally' and made an impact? Certainly, in a general exhibition on health, the 'immediate use value'—a concept Vogel borrowed from reformist pedagogy and psychology—of ideas could be transmitted through objects that visitors themselves could touch and move. But in an exhibition on cancer?

The conundrum demanded experimenting with strategies that might enable visitors to experience cancer for themselves, at least in some fashion. Two techniques that stirred up emotions in different ways filled the gap. First were visual representations of cancerous tumours in very high resolution. They aimed

[51] *Krebs-Merkblatt* (1911), 10.

[52] 'Der Krebserreger entdeckt?', *Dresdner Neueste Nachrichten* 167, 19 July 1925; 'Der Krebserreger—eine deutsche Entdeckung? Haben die Engländer deutsche Arbeiten benutzt? Ein Gelehrtenstreit', *Berliner Tageblatt* (morning edition), 362, 2 August 1925; 'Der Krebserreger entdeckt?', *Volkszeitung Dresden* 136, 13 June 1924. All articles can be found in Hauptstaatsarchiv Dresden [HSTA D] 10702, no. 1318.

[53] Bruno Gebhard, 'Der Krebs und seine Bekämpfung. Eine Sonderschau des Deutschen Hygiene-Museums', *Hygienischer Wegweiser* 12 (1929): 307–9, 309; Fritz de Quervain, 'Ist Krebsfurcht schlimmer als Krebs?' *Hygienischer Wegweiser* 12 (1929): 303–4.

[54] Martin Vogel, 'Das Experiment von Framingham', *Hygienischer Wegweiser* 1, no. 2 (1926): 21–5, 21.

to get under visitors' skin by triggering shock and disgust. Second, the representation of cancer patients was personalized through narratives. Stories were supposed to allow visitors to identify with the protagonists and thus feel the same emotions that they did. At the same time, they were framed with moral language intended to force visitors to reflect on these emotions.

Moulages played a crucial role in the first strategy. The three-dimensional wax models have been around since the Renaissance and began being employed in the nineteenth century to represent symptoms of illness. The models are created by making a plaster cast of a body part and then covering it with wax after it dries. Finally, the wax relief is painted in the presence of the patient to recreate the colour and form of the symptom as realistically as possible; in some cases, hair was even placed on the models. The Dresden Hygiene Museum further accentuated the lifelike impression of their moulages by appending them to a model of the patient's body cast with a cloth coated in wax.[55]

Professors of medicine used moulages in their seminars, but by the end of the nineteenth century, they were being exhibited at fairs and cabinets of curiosities. Health educators caught on to their potential pedagogical value after realizing that they attracted large numbers at popular events.[56] This spurred reformist entrepreneur Karl August Lingner—owner of the Odol mouthwash company and initiator of the Hygiene Museum—along with his colleagues, Drs Eugen Galewsky and Arthur Schloßmann, to display moulages for the first time at the 1903 exhibition 'The Fight against Widespread Diseases'. At the 1911 Hygiene Exhibition, moulages were featured in the sections on tuberculosis, venereal diseases, and cancer.[57] In contrast with real anatomic samples, the moulages gave viewers a chance to see different types of tumours. That they could simultaneously frighten and interest people was encapsulated in the nickname given to the section on venereal diseases: 'Galewsky's chamber of horrors', after curator and dermatologist Eugen Galewsky, whose collection provided many of the wax models.[58] Thus, organizers knew early on about the ambivalent emotions elicited by moulages, but they seriously began debating their use in the 1920s. One main criticism was the severity of visitors' emotional, visceral reactions. For instance, Martin Vogel stated that there were enough people who 'could not tolerate the sight of such things (sometimes even normal models!) and faint'. Lampooned by

[55] Thomas Schnalke, *Diseases in Wax—The History of the Medical Moulage*, trans. Kathy Spatschek (Berlin: Quintessenz, 1995), 15–24; Thomas Schnalke, 'Die Medizinische Moulage—ein historischer Überblick', in *Wachs—Moulagen und Modelle*, ed. Susanne Hahn and Dimitrios Ambatielos (Dresden: Verlag des Deutschen Hygiene-Museums, 1994), 13–28.

[56] Hahn, 'Die Medizinische Moulage', 39. See Hahn's book in general for a history of the moulage.

[57] Gruppe Krebs, *Sonder-Katalog der Gruppe Krebs*.

[58] Lutz Sauerteig, 'Lust und Abschreckung: Moulagen in der Geschlechtskrankheitenaufklärung', in Hahn and Ambatielos, *Wachs*, 47–68.

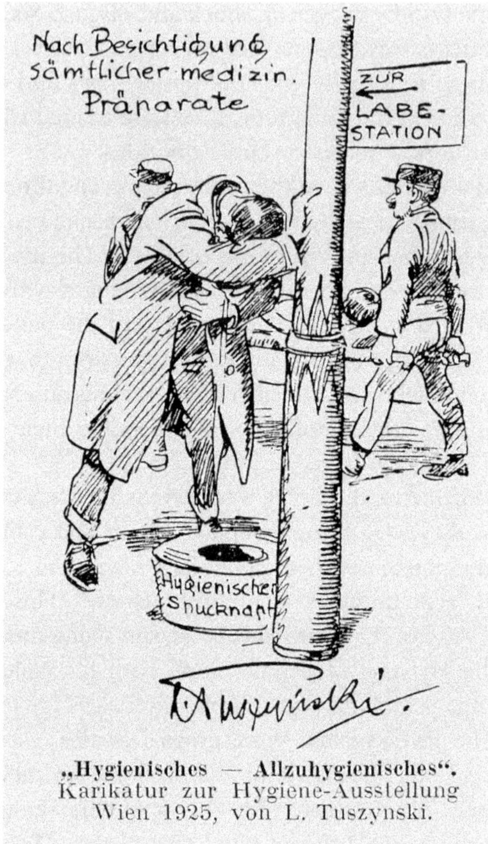
Nach Besichtigung sämtlicher medizin. Präparate
ZUR LABE-STATION
Hygienischer Spucknapf
„Hygienisches — Allzuhygienisches".
Karikatur zur Hygiene-Ausstellung Wien 1925, von L. Tuszynski.

Fig. 5 Cartoon parodying the *Internationale Hygiene-Ausstellung* (1911).

cartoonists (Fig. 5), the effect stood in marked contradiction to the exhibitions' aim of improving and maintaining visitors' health.[59]

Thus, moulages evoked a sort of excitement about being scared and disgusted, simultaneously attracting and repelling visitors. This posed an issue for their intended educational effect, because it blurred the boundary between scientific exhibition and carnival funhouse. Moreover, without proper guidance, the powerful emotional jolt could impede the long-term behavioural changes desired by the exhibitions' organizers.

To elide these issues, the exhibition curators strained themselves to clearly situate the moulages within a scientific context, presenting them as the doctor's perspective. The at least partial success of this strategy is evidenced by favourable newspaper reviews of the first largescale exhibition at the Hygiene Museum after

[59] Martin Vogel, 'Wie veranstaltet man hygienische Ausstellungen?', *Hygienischer Wegweiser* 1, no. 1 (1926): 1–36, 12.

the end of the First World War. Put on in 1922, the exhibit 'Humans' also grappled with their illnesses.[60]

Yet while the deployment of moulages in exhibits on venereal diseases and tuberculosis uninhibitedly aimed at evoking disgust in order to warn against the dangers of infection, matters were more complicated when it came to cancer for the simple reason that visitors could not necessarily protect themselves from it by changing their behaviour. To rein in the fear and disgust evoked by cancer moulages, Bruno Gebhard developed multiple strategies. In 1930, he designed the cancer section of the Dresden Hygiene Museum's first permanent exhibition and, in 1931, he curated the museum's travelling exhibition 'Kampf dem Krebs' (Fight Cancer), which initially drew a lot of traffic and ran for multiple years. His first step for these exhibits was to employ considerably fewer cancer moulages than in the 1911 display on cancer. Those he did choose to show were overwhelmingly of early-stage tumours, which Gebhard thought were less frightening. Most of the moulages from the 1911 exhibition were of late-stage tumours, because doctors at the time had been more interested in forming models of such 'remarkable' tumours rather than of 'unspectacular' ones.

But Gebhard also concocted another strategy to mitigate fear and disgust. He placed moulages of healed body parts alongside the moulages of tumours. He often opted for wax models of skin cancer, since it could often be cured with radiotherapy without leaving behind visible scars. The 'Fight Cancer' exhibition (Fig. 6) contained a typical example of this approach.

That such a large tumour could be made to disappear was an impressing testament to the potential of treatment, even if it was certainly the exception and not the rule. And even in this specific instance, it was unclear whether the cancer had been totally cured or whether metastases had already formed that would end the patient's life. In effect, Gebhard's depiction of skin cancer fed hopes that had no application to other forms of cancer.[61] Further, by demonstrating that serious cancers previously considered untreatable were now being cured, he consciously stirred up hopes that similar 'breakthroughs' could happen for different types of cancer. This, too, nudged visitors to draw the intended conclusion: it was always beneficial to go to the doctor early on.

The strategy not only neglected to mention the potential side effects and complications associated with surgery and radiotherapy. Although Gebhard knew better, it depicted them as harmless and painless. This point highlights

[60] Dr Popitz, 'Der Mensch (Ausstellung des Deutschen Hygiene-Museums)', *Leipziger Volkszeitung* 225, 26 September 1922; 'Die Ausstellung "Der Mensch"', *Chemnitzer Allgemeine Zeitung* 5, 7 January 1923.

[61] Thus, in 1931, Ferdinand Blumenthal complained that while patients often refused to go through with an operation out of fear, many believed that every form of cancer could be cured with radiotherapy without serious side effects. See Ferdinand Blumenthal, 'Krebsfilm, Krebsaufklärung, Krebsbekämpfung', *Sonderdruck. Medizinische Klinik* 1 (1931): 38–9, 39, BArch R 86/2584.

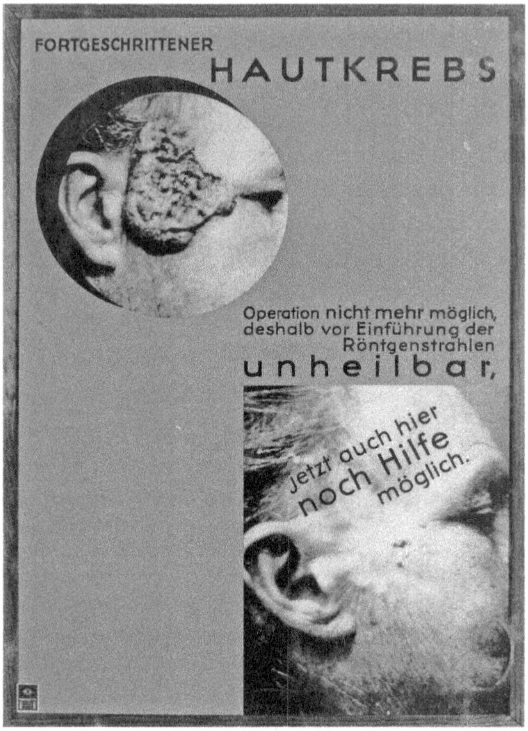

Fig. 6 Image from the travelling exhibition 'Kampf dem Krebs' (Fight Cancer, 1931).

that the purpose of the campaigns was not primarily to communicate factual information about cancer, but to cultivate a certain form of hope. And hope, the curators held, could not be relativized. They inflated chances of recovery just as much as they trivialized the dangers of treatment. Discussing the real prospects of therapy and its limits seemed off the table, because doctors and curators alike feared this would diminish trust in doctors' capabilities. Thus, although Gebhard's use of moulages created the illusion of 'realism', it was just one tool in a calculated strategy that played fear and hope against one another.

Ferdinand Blumenthal, head of the Berlin Centre for Oncological Research at the Charité hospital, encouraged doctors to remain optimistic and campaigners to print in bold and italics statements about the high chances of recovery in pamphlets. Like Gebhard, he was against telling patients the facts about the risks and benefits of treatment and for exaggerating reasons for hope.[62] Many doctors were well aware that many exhibition visitors were familiar with the dark side of cancer treatment from the travails of friends and family. But they hoped that by

[62] Ferdinand Blumenthal, 'Die Organisation der Krebsbekämpfung', *Strahlentherapie* 42 (1931): 809–20, 811–12.

foregrounding the expertise of doctors and researchers through scientific artefacts, campaigns would help dismantle people's tendency to see future possibilities through the lens of past experiences.

The Time to Decide: Happy Endings and Not So Happy Endings

In the late 1920s, campaigners were looking for a way to 'hammer into people's brains' the necessity of early detection. They discovered a dimension of fear well suited to the task, one that gave a different weight to the decision for or against going to the doctor's office early on. It was moral fear, which they constructed in formulaic narratives that imbued the decision with a specific emotional connotation.[63]

Posters with rudimentary before-and-after narratives had already promoted recovery as a real possibility. New scripts told of the choices made by those who got cured and those who missed their chance, casting cancer fatality as a consequence of the individual's false choice against rushing to the doctor when the first signs of cancer arose. This storyline shifted responsibility to the patient and them alone. At the same time, it increased the heft of responsibility and gave it a moral overtone by presenting it not only as a duty towards oneself, but also towards one's family and '*Volk*'. Exhibition curators and campaign producers propagated this sentiment through all the media at their disposal, including picture stories, theatre, and film.

The year 1927 ushered in theatre's use as a medium of health education, when the Deutsche Bühne für Volkshygiene (German Theatre for Public Health) was established in Kassel. Its founders took inspiration from the new conviction that, in contrast to 'abstract' lectures and 'scientifically illustrative' posters, dramatic narratives about health and illness would 'hit a nerve' and might even bring a grown man to tears.[64] Vividly transmitting knowledge that would compel people to act seemed to require the kind of emotional identification that would leave a lasting impression on the hearts and minds of visitors and audience members. This pedagogical theory focused on the 'psyche of the masses' and the 'everyday man'. It thus represented a stark departure from the driving ideas of pre-First World War campaigns, which sought to implant knowledge through fascination, astonishment, and to a lesser degree deterrence through fear.[65]

[63] '"Zu spät!" Die Schallplatte im "Kampf dem Krebs"', *Volkszeitung Berlin*, 23 February 1932, HSTA D 13658, no. Z 2, vol. 2, 74.

[64] Dr Schadendorf, 'Die Bühne im Dienste der Volkshygiene', *Hygienischer Wegweiser* 5, no. 2 (1930): 50–2, 51; Dr Schadendorf, 'Die Bühne im Dienste der Volksgesundheit', HSTA D 13686, no. 106, 23–4.

[65] Schadendorf, 'Die Bühne im Dienste der Volkshygiene', 51. A similar earlier text is Curt Thomalla, 'Hygiene und soziale Medizin im Volksbelehrungsfilm', *Zeitschrift für Medizinalbeamte* 35 (1922): 589–610, 591–2.

An illustrative example of this approach was the didactic play *Die Tragödie des Arztes* (*The Tragedy of the Doctor*); composed with Ferdinand Blumenthal as scientific advisor, it premiered in 1930. Although attendance data has not been preserved, newspaper reviews attest to its success.[66] The play generated suspense through the tragic helplessness of its protagonist, a competent doctor and loving husband who is unable to save his wife from her fatal cancer because she waited too long before revealing her illness to him. Coming 'too late!', as cancer awareness campaigns of the time repeated, initiated the tragedy's unstoppable momentum and acquired a particularly desperate significance for the dying wife.[67] Having to bear responsibility for the inevitability of one's own death was thematized even more unforgivingly in the series of tableaus *Tragödie der heilbaren Krebskranken* (*Tragedy of the Curable Cancer Patient*), which was staged in 1930 at the Second International Hygiene Exhibition in Dresden (the sequel to the 1911 exhibition, not to be confused with the permanent exhibition of the Hygiene Museum erected in 1930). In contrast to a live stage play representing the bitter end of a 'foolish' woman, the revolving series of five tableaus repeated the same story over and over: while she could have been cured at the beginning, the cancer patient embarked upon the 'path of folly'. Opting to forego a visit to the doctor, she instead listened to friends' advice and went to the 'quack'. The ending, shown again and again, is preordained: death.

Although the story did not have a happy end, it attracted droves. '"Land of Laughter" a hundred times is nothing in comparison', wrote a reviewer with reference to Franz Léhars's popular operetta, which also told of the sad fate of a woman who, against all 'sound' advice, makes a gut decision, though with a less drastic outcome than the Dresden tableaus.[68]

These cancer narratives demonstrate that there were many reasons why women were often the target audience of early cancer awareness campaigns. On the one hand, when younger, more 'productive' women were afflicted with cervical cancer, it could be diagnosed relatively early and treated relatively well. On the other, historically older gender stereotypes depicted women as more emotional and thus more easily deceived than men. These stereotypes held that women were thus more susceptible to the promises of alternative 'quack' therapies and the 'foolish' choice to not undergo surgery or radiotherapy.[69]

[66] Head Regional Official Sägmüller, 'Die Krebsbekämpfung in Baden', *Monatsschrift für Krebsbekämpfung* 3 (March 1933): 109–19, 112.

[67] The text of the play, penned by a duo going by the name Müller Manger and Schrank-Telfan, is unfortunately lost. A rough sketch of its plot can be pieced together from reviews: '"Die Tragödie des Arztes". Uraufführung durch die "Bühne für Volkshygiene" im Staatlichen Schauspielhaus, Berlin', *Die Medizinische Welt* 12 (1930): 422 and *Münchener Medizinische Wochenschrift* 11 (1930): 471, both in HSTA D 13686, no. 106, 6+7; Schadendorf, 'Die Bühne im Dienste der Volkshygiene'.

[68] 'Kleine Blicke in die große Ausstellung', *Dresdner Anzeiger* 243, 25 May 1930, 5–6, HSTA D 10702, no. 1317.

[69] Ute Frevert, 'Defining Emotions: Concepts and Debates over Three Centuries', in Frevert et al., *Emotional Lexicons*, 1–31, 30.

Produced by the Dresden Hygiene Museum, the 1931 'Kampf dem Krebs' travelling exhibition employed a piece with a similar narrative, this time with the fates of two male characters. After reviewing how the men had the same childhood, adolescence, and early parenthood, their lives diverge when the man in the first plotline has a doctor check on his symptoms, while the other man avoids the doctor's visit. The former lives to a 'ripe old age', while the latter succumbs to an 'untimely death' (Fig. 7).

Here, too, the timespan during which the all-important decision can be made is brief, and after this moment, everything is predetermined—there's no turning back. The use of such parallel narratives with one happy end and one irreversibly fatal conclusion distinguished German early detection campaigns from their American counterparts, which tended to opt for conversion narratives. These stories related how an initially irrational person—here, too, almost always a woman—abandoned their erroneous ways and went to the doctor just in the nick of time.[70] In contrast, the narratives in German cancer awareness campaigns always had one protagonist sail the wrong river and end up on the rocks. They never forewent depicting death as the consequence of a single wrong decision and

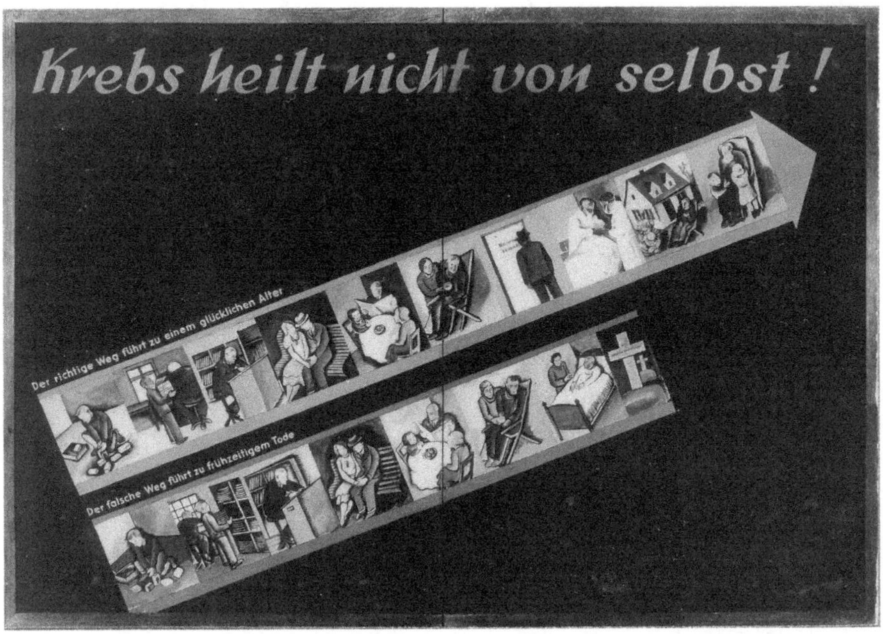
Krebs heilt nicht von selbst!
Der richtige Weg führt zu einem glücklichen Alter
Der falsche Weg führt zu frühzeitigem Tode

Fig. 7 Image from the travelling exhibition 'Kampf dem Krebs' (Fight Cancer, 1931).

[70] David Cantor, 'Choosing to Live: Cancer Education, Movies, and the Conversion Narrative in America, 1921–1960', *Literature and Medicine* 28, no. 2 (2009): 278–332.

thus sent the message that the time to decide did not last for long and could not be recovered once it did.

Hustle and bustle also dominate the first scene of the film *Krebs* (*Cancer*), which premiered in 1930.[71] The film combines narrative and explanation, like the film *Falsche Scham* had done with venereal diseases a few years before and like three older films put out by the American Cancer Society (*Reward of Courage*, 1921; *A Fortunate Accident*, 1925; *This Great Peril*, 1929).

Krebs dispensed with telling the story of an individual patient to communicate knowledge and stimulate emotional identification, thus setting it apart from the stage play and the series of tableaus discussed above. The film begins with a rapid sequence of images of illness in order to illustrate the hectic acceleration of time, breathlessness, and drama brought on by cancer. The first image, of a woman in agonizing pain, segues into a chopped-up montage crammed into a relentless rhythm by the repetitive interjection of the intertitle 'Cancer'. The images contain the story of a woman suffering from cancer whose terrified husband calls an ambulance, which brings her to the hospital to be operated on. How the story 'ends up' and why the woman waited until now to undergo surgery is left open. The initial sequence does not tell the well-known story of the 'foolish' cancer patient. A visual onslaught of fear and pain, of images of advanced tumours, surgery, and radiotherapy, it was intended to overwhelm viewers.[72]

In the run of the 1930s, however, the Reichsausschuss für Krebsbekämpfung (Imperial Committee for Fighting Cancer) voiced reservations about using images of malignant tumours to shock viewers. In 1935/6, it put out a 'very gentle' film that only showed cartoon images of tumours, divesting them of their urgent corporeality and displacing them into the realm of scientific abstraction.[73] *Krebs* had no such misgivings and intentionally robbed viewers of 'respite'.[74] It bolted out of the gates with drama and horror to set the emotional stage for the information transmitted in the rest of the story.

[71] Originally just titled *Krebs* (*Cancer*), it was renamed *Kampf dem Krebs* (*Fight Cancer*, like the exhibition) in, at the latest, 1933. It was produced by the Dresden Hygiene Museum together with the Verlag wissenschaftlicher Filme (Scientific Film Production Company). See Bruno Gebhard, *Kampf dem Krebs* (Dresden: Deutscher Verlag für Volkswohlfahrt, 1933), 52.

[72] Rudolf Neubert, 'Der erste Film aus der Produktion des Gesundheitsdienstes', *Hygienischer Wegweiser* 5, no. 11 (1930): 292.

[73] The 1,018-metre-long sound film was titled *Kampf dem Krebs* (not to be confused with the other film of the same title) and was supposed to be screened after lectures. Despite intensive research, I was not able to find a copy of the film. However, one of the three censor's cards (dated 26 August 1936) required at the time has been preserved; it gives a brief synopsis of the film. See Bundesarchiv Filmarchiv B.43197. It was described as 'very mild' and 'tactful' in 'Reichsausschuss für Krebsbekämpfung, Mitteilungen des Reichsausschusses für Krebsbekämpfung. Bericht über eine außerordentliche Tagung der Reichsarbeitsgemeinschaft und des Reichsausschusses für Krebsbekämpfung in Berlin', *Zeitschrift für Krebsforschung* 46, no. 1 (1937): 306–12, 310, BArch B 142/412, 308, RS-311.

[74] Neubert, 'Der erste Film', 292. See also, Anja Laukötter, '"Anarchie der Zellen". Geschichte und Medien der Krebsaufklärung in der ersten Hälfte des 20. Jahrhunderts', *Zeithistorische Forschungen/Studies in Contemporary History* 7, no. 1 (2010): 55–74, 68.

After the first minute, the film switched to a calmer rhythm. The main part revolved around the focal points of earlier campaigns by thematizing cancer statistics, cancer research, early diagnosis, different forms of treatment, and self-examination. Like its predecessors, the film promoted curability and advised the audience to go to the doctor early. But the film had three novel elements. It significantly expanded the appeal to self-examination, asserted a stronger, different type of connection between individual responsibility and one's duties towards family and society, and politicized cancer. The film did not just list these things side by side, but placed them in a complex, polysemous relation to one another.

The Morality of Self-Examination in the Health-Obsessed National Socialist State

Self-examination and early detection were two topics that acquired a new verve in 1920s health discourse. Past campaigns had focused on raising awareness about early symptoms of cancer and encouraging men and women to go to the doctor if they had them. But the more women who really did make a doctor's appointment when suspicious symptoms appeared, the clearer it became that so-called early symptoms could sometimes appear during a later stage of cancer.[75] In the beginning of the 1930s, an increasing number of doctors seconded this finding. Many pleaded with public health officials to promote regular examinations regardless of whether symptoms were present. Everyday citizens voiced similar demands. Particularly in the first half of the 1930s, general interest in cancer rose, a point evidenced by the consistently high attendance of the travelling exhibition 'Kampf dem Krebs' over multiple years, which regularly had to close its doors due to overcrowding.[76]

Two self-examination techniques for detecting breast and cervical cancer early rose to prominence: checking the breasts by looking and feeling for irregularities (Fig. 8), and keeping a menstrual calendar. While doctors debated calls for women to examine their breasts every month (in the United States, it took another thirty years for breast self-exams to be advertised prominently), they greeted campaigns promoting menstrual calendars.

[75] Health Commissioner Dr Hartkopf, Cologne, 'Alte und neue Wege zur Bekämpfung der Krebskrankheit', *Kölnische Zeitung* 467, 4 July 1924, HSTA D 10702, no. 1318.

[76] See, for instance, Letter from Max Liebecher, Dresden, to Reichskanzler Adolf Hitler, 8 February 1934. The letter demands not only that screenings be offered for women free of charge, but that they be made mandatory. The exhibition was a success. In 1932, 51,000 people visited at Berlin's Europa Haus; in 1933, a copy of the travelling exhibition was made so that it could be put on at two places at once. See Protocol of the Managing Committee of the Hygiene Museum, Dresden, 21 March 1932, 2 December 1932, and 27 March 1933, HSTA D 13686, no. 52: 84, 91, and 92.

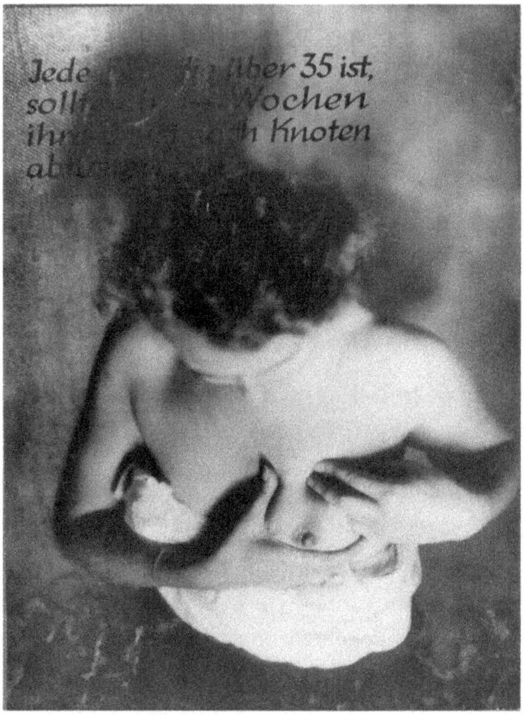

Fig. 8 'Every woman over 35 should check her breast for lumps every 4 weeks.' Poster from the traveling exhibition 'Kampf dem Krebs' (Fight Cancer, 1931).

Some doctors feared that monthly self-exams would train women to hypochondriacally stress about every little bodily abnormality.[77] But another factor may have been doctors' perception of self-exams as a trespass on their medical authority and an—albeit very minor—delegation of a doctor's work to medically 'untrained' women.[78] Perhaps, too, the public call for women to touch their own breasts discomforted doctors, a profession dominated by men.[79]

[77] See Ferdinand Blumenthal, 'Krebsfilm, Krebsaufklärung, Krebsbekämpfung', *Medizinische Klinik* 1 (1931): 38–9. On Germany being 'ahead' of the American campaigns, see Proctor, *The Nazi War on Cancer*, 29.

[78] The travelling exhibition from 1931, the revised version from 1939, and the exhibition 'Ewiges Volk' (The Eternal People) from 1937 all warned against the female friend's 'bad' advice to go to a 'quack healer' and the trivialization of symptoms, just like the series of tableaus from the 1930 International Hygiene Exhibition had done.

[79] It is probably not far-fetched to draw a connection here to the near obsession with adolescent boys' masturbating. Particularly intense in Imperial Germany, but living on well into the Weimar Republic and Nazi Germany, doctors, social hygienists, teachers, and theologians branded masturbation as extremely detrimental to young men's health. On the history of masturbation in the eighteenth and nineteenth centuries, see Jürgen Martschukat and Olaf Stieglitz, *Geschichte der Männlichkeiten* (Frankfurt am Main: Campus, 2008), 149–51.

In contrast, menstrual calendars easily found their place in an era when the quantification of the body was becoming part of standard medical practice, while at the same time constituting the foundation of scientific epistemes and racial pseudoscience. This general epistemic shift encouraged people to take a more objective perspective on their own bodies and see them as complex structures in need of constant maintenance. This position necessitated not just paying attention to signs of illness and pain but also keeping tabs on bodily parameters. Posters began comparing the human body with machines and cars.[80] But the machine metaphor was less about actually conceptualizing the body as a machine—which would have clashed with the National-Socialist obsession with the body's 'naturalness'—and more about training people to take a matter-of-fact, emotionless view of their bodies. For instance, when the 'Kampf dem Krebs' exhibition was revised in 1939, a new poster asserted that the 'many-sidedness of natural experience' fundamentally distinguishes the living body from the image of 'man as machine'.[81] This is the context in which campaigns started pushing men and women alike to get regular check-ups after their fortieth birthday.

In 1929, twenty-four life insurance companies coalesced to form the Zentrale für Gesundheitsdienst in der Lebensversicherung (Centre for Healthcare Provision in Life Insurance), a clearinghouse established to pay the costs of regular check-ups at doctors of the patients' choice for the roughly 600,000 people they insured. Dr Gottfried Frey—then head of the medical division of the Reichsgesundheitsamt (Imperial Health Department) and later head of the Reichsarbeitsgemeinschaft für Krebsbekämpfung (Imperial Working Group for Fighting Cancer)—praised the initiative and argued that Germany's public health insurers should imitate it.[82] The Reichsausschuss für Krebsbekämpfung, which was established in 1931 by the Reichstag and was also led by Frey, took up the idea in its discussions on a general law for cancer care.[83]

The members of the Reichsausschuss generally agreed that free screenings for women were a good thing. But they debated whether men should be offered free exams for stomach and colon cancer. In the end, the idea was nixed with the argument that cervical cancer and breast cancer were easier to diagnose, that they had greater economic relevance, and that they were more consequential for the

[80] See a poster from the 'Kampf dem Krebs' exhibition (1931) that depicts a mechanic repairing a car: DHMD 2001/247.79. The same poster was also used in the exhibition 'Die Frau als Gattin und Mutter' (Woman as Wife and Mother, 1933), DHMD 2001/246.165. The revised version of the exhibition 'Kampf dem Krebs' (1939) showed in its place a worker next to a machine (perhaps a printing press) under the title 'Gesundsein ist Pflicht' (Being Healthy Is a Duty), DHMD 2001/248.21.

[81] See the corresponding poster from the 1939 version of 'Kampf dem Krebs', DHMD 2001/248.37.

[82] Director Dr Frey, Imperial Department of Health, 'Hygienische Volksbelehrung', *Vossische Zeitung* 456, 27 September 1929, 10, HSTA D 10702, no. 1317.

[83] On discussions on the law for cancer care, see Atzl and Helms, *Die Geschichte der Deutschen Krebsgesellschaft*, 59–60, and Proctor, *The Nazi War on Cancer*, 43–4.

Nazis' racist ideology since they affected 'women of childbearing age'.[84] Moreover, it seemed smart to target women in particular with cancer screenings because of the hope that they, as 'guardians' of their families' health, would set an example for their husbands, sons, and brothers, who would then perceive early detection as something unremarkable and thus be more willing to accept it when the programme was expanded to men in the future.[85]

These discussions thus fused early 1930s health discourse with Nazi policy on science and health. East Prussia developed into a kind of model region with the help of aforementioned gynaecologist Georg Winter (1856–1946), who was now retired.[86] Participation in East Prussia's early detection programme was voluntary. However, once the National Socialist Women's League and local authorities began promoting it, helping organize events and providing general support, the campaign started exerting moral, social, and political pressure on women to undergo an exam. Using the cudgel of law was out of the question, since compulsory exams, which some people supported, would have conflicted with existing statutes.[87] Nevertheless, the high costs of treating cancer motivated louder calls to make exams obligatory. The 'Kampf dem Krebs' exhibition, begun in 1931, featured a poster that cut straight to the chase: 'How many losses does cancer cause the German economy every year?' The poster's background showed a large apartment building, while the foreground text calculated that the 120,000 people diagnosed with cancer annually cost 500 million Reichsmarks in lost earnings, care, sick pay, and treatment. It translated this sum into the 30,000 housing units that the state could have built with the money—a stark political statement in the context of the Weimar Republic's permanent housing crisis, which was exacerbated by the Great Depression.[88] Considering the consistently low cure rates, it is unclear if and to what extent early detection exams would have actually reduced these costs. And the notion that the saved money would have been spent on housing was likewise anything but certain. Still, the poster suggested both claims held.

The 1931 exhibition visualized another type of 'damage' caused by cancer that probably held more significance in the eyes of many visitors. Two posters depicted children whose mother or father had died of cancer. The posters claimed that the tragedy could have been avoided if the parents had only gone to the doctor sooner.

[84] Article by the deputy chairperson of the Imperial Committee, 12 November 1933, BArch R 36/1389.

[85] A. Läwen, 'Propaganda, Laienaufklärung und Reihenuntersuchungen im Kampfe gegen den Krebs in Ostpreußen', in Meetings of the German Imperial Working Group for Fighting Cancer at the Conference in Munich on 12 and 13 May 1939, *Monatsschrift für Krebsbekämpfung* 7 (1939): 1–48, 7–20, BArch B 142/412, 320–44.

[86] Atzl and Helms, *Die Geschichte der Deutschen Krebsgesellschaft*, 60.

[87] 'Verhandlungen der Deutschen Reichsarbeitsgemeinschaft für Krebsbekämpfung auf der Tagung in München am 12. und 13. Mai 1939', *Monatsschrift für Krebsbekämpfung* 7 (1939): 1–48, 13, BArch B 142/412, 320–44.

[88] DHMD 2001/247.14.

These scenes stimulated parents' fears by implying that the untimely deaths had robbed the children of their futures and put them in the care of heartless individuals. Visitors in Königsberg, Munich, Minden, and Leipzig saw an image of two children with their heads down sitting at the odd table out during dinner time while their visibly wealthy foster parents reprimanded them. The citation read: 'The orphaned children are now pushed around by strangers, their mother died of uterine cancer at age 44.' Things did not seem to be going much better for the hardworking boy shown on the second poster, whose fate was narrated: 'The boy has the ability to learn a useful skill, but he has to help earn money because his father died of cancer at age 41.'[89]

Alongside hammering on visitors' moral and emotional duty towards their children, the exhibition also drilled in their duty towards the '*Volk*'—not just in the sense of potential economic costs, but in the sense of damages caused to the healthy, resilient '*Volkskörper*', or 'body of the German people'.[90] The exhibition propagated the notion that staying healthy was every individual's duty towards the 'body of the German people', and early detection examinations were part of fulfilling it, as a revised version of the exhibition energetically proclaimed in 1939.[91] The move situated early detection examinations firmly within the numerous regulatory measures implemented as part of National-Socialist public health policy, which was first explicitly formulated in 1936. It subordinated the health of the individual under the health of the racially defined 'people' or '*Volk*' and commanded every person to maintain and guard their health for the good of the whole. Illness and weakness, in turn, were branded as 'anti-social'.[92]

The plethora of directives and images must have amplified already existing fears of a rarely curable disease like cancer, but the early health campaigns also increasingly addressed the fear of cancer. Already in 1930, the cancer section of the Second International Hygiene Exhibition relieved visitors with the all-caps maxim: 'Thou shalt have no fear of falling ill with cancer.'[93] The travelling 'Kampf dem Krebs' exhibition picked up the torch: 'Fear makes everything worse, even cancer. Courageous, deliberate action makes everything better, even cancer.'[94] On the surface, the poster simply advertised 'courageously' going in for a check-up and changing one's lifestyle instead of 'anxiously' avoiding such prudent actions.

[89] Both posters are from the 1931 version of 'Kampf dem Krebs', DHMD 2001/247.1+2.

[90] Thorsten Hallig, Julia Schäfer, and Jörg Vögele, 'Volk, Volkskörper, Volkswirtschaft—Bevölkerungsfragen in Forschung und Lehre von Nationalökonomie und Medizin', in *Das Konstrukt 'Bevölkerung' vor, im und nach dem 'Dritten Reich'*, ed. Rainer Mackensen and Jürgen Reulecke (Wiesbaden: VS Verlag für Sozialwissenschaften, 2005), 388–428; Süß, *Der 'Volkskörper' im Krieg.*

[91] 'Gesundsein ist Pflicht', DHMD 2001/248.21. See Thomas Beddies, *'Du hast die Pflicht, gesund zu sein!' Der Gesundheitsdienst der Hitler-Jugend 1933–1945* (Berlin: Be.bra Wissenschaft, 2010).

[92] Eckart, *Medizin in der NS-Diktatur*, 171–3.

[93] Ernst John, 'Das Wunder, das wir selber sind. Ein Gang durch die "Internationale Hygiene-Ausstellung", Dresden 1930', *Grüne Post* 24, 15 June 1930.

[94] DHMD 2001/247.93.

At the same time, these recommendations were embedded in an emotional logic that was touted as a necessary part of 'mental health'. After 1933, the Deutsche Seelenheilkunde (German Psychotherapy) movement integrated this brand of emotional self-control into its ideas about a healthy, productive inner life. The theory was captured well by journalist and psychologist Charlotte Köhn-Behrens. In 1940—the first year of the Second World War—she wrote in the popular magazine *Gartenlaube* (The Garden Arbour) that being frightened by a particular situation was completely normal. Fear was a 'natural', evolutionary reaction to danger and getting cancer was a legitimate danger. But reflexive fear, according to her, could turn into cowardice when a person repressed it and failed to confront it. She saw the end result of this fear of fear itself in 'war neurosis' and 'nervous types'. This stood in diametrical opposition to the 'hero' who transformed 'his instinctive fear into mental-spiritual courage and braveness' because his knowledge of his own strength enabled him to overcome himself.[95]

The logic of fear, cowardice, and courage gained widespread acceptance, which helps explain why past concerns that early detection campaigns would stir up unjustified fears of cancer fell to the wayside. Now, the programme of early detection found a partner in the concept of preventive care. Every exhibition, film, and lecture started advancing the idea that a 'healthy' lifestyle could prevent cancer. This meant not smoking, limiting one's consumption of alcohol, meat, and preserved, chemically treated foods, regularly exercising, wearing loose-fitting clothes, and practicing good bodily hygiene. The extent to which such lifestyle choices could actually mitigate the risk of cancer was still a matter of speculation at the time, as there were no studies that established any clear links. One exception, however, were serious findings about the carcinogenic effects of tobacco consumption. In 1929, Dr Fritz Lickint had published one of the first epidemiological studies seeking to establish a statistically robust connection between smoking and lung cancer. Lickint's research culminated in a monumental 1939 article on 'Tobacco and Organism', which used statistical data to prove the connection between smoking and all cancers of the 'smoke path', i.e. of the lips, tongue, mouth, jaw, throat, trachea, and lungs.[96]

Tobacco was not only suspected of causing cancer, though. Lickint and others conducted epidemiological analyses of other harmful effects of smoking, from heart disease to female infertility, male impotence, and foetal defects. Like alcohol consumption, processed foods, and lack of exercise, smoking was also considered detrimental in the eyes of eugenicists. They asserted that people who did not adhere to the widely propagated rules of a healthy lifestyle were revealing their

[95] Charlotte Köhn-Behrens, 'Das Kapitel von der Angst', *Die Gartenlaube* 17 (1940): 246.

[96] Fritz Lickint, 'Tabak und Tabakrauch als ätiologischer Faktor des Carcinoms', *Zeitschrift für Krebsforschung* 30, no. 1 (1929): 349–65, https://doi.org/10.1007/BF01636077; Fritz Lickint, *Tabak und Organismus* (Stuttgart: Marquardt, 1939).

inability to fulfil their responsibilities towards the 'body of the people'. But beyond allegedly betraying personal weakness, National Socialist public health policies increasingly treated tobacco and alcohol consumption as evidence of an inherited inclination towards addiction and thus as a visible sign of 'inferior' genetic makeup or genetic degeneration.[97]

Metaphors politicizing and militarizing the image of cancer further amplified this form of stigmatization. This development was neither new nor was it specifically German, as similar trends appeared in France and the United States.[98] Indeed, Rudolf Virchow himself was one of the first to draw parallels between state and cellular organisms and described cancerous cells as parasitic degenerates in the cell state.[99] In the early 1930s, producers of anti-cancer campaigns adapted this epistemic metaphor, while in political discourse, the metaphorical denigration of opponents and 'enemies of the people' as cancerous tumours became common. The 1930 film *Krebs* followed suit. In it, cartoons illustrated how black cancer cells branched out like spiders in healthy tissue (Fig. 9). An intertitle narrated: 'Uncontrollably, the cancer cells eat into the healthy tissue and destroy it.'

After 1933, cancer cells were not just described as anarchic, revolutionary, or 'degenerated'. They were increasingly called 'Jewish'. Frankfurt-based radiologist and SS member Hans Holfelder brought this antisemitic metaphor to its extreme in a 1936 lecture at the University of Frankfurt medical school, where he showed

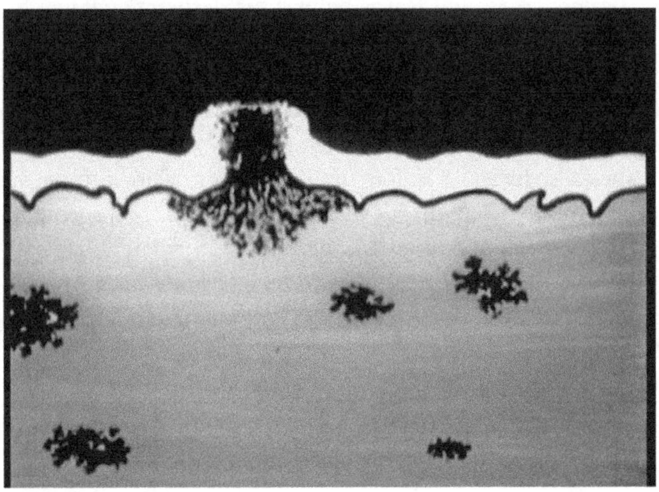

Fig. 9 Still from the film *Krebs* (*Cancer*, 1930).

[97] Proctor, *The Nazi War on Cancer*, 189.
[98] Pinell, *Naissance d'un fléau*, 268–70 and 312–17; Proctor, *The Nazi War on Cancer*, 49.
[99] Virchow, *Die Cellularpathologie*, 408. See also Johach, *Krebszelle und Zellenstaat*.

students a slide that depicted cancer cells as Jews and the x-rays attacking them as Nazi stormtroopers.[100]

The metaphor of cancer as 'Jewish' took on another dimension in the run of the 1930s. As the New German Medicine—with its opposition against 'Jewish', 'mechanistic' medicine—lost political support and academic medicine regained its status as the foundation of Nazi public health policy, campaigns against 'quackery' in cancer treatment came to be infused with antisemitism. A pointed example of this was the UFA-produced sound movie *Jeder Achte* (*Every Eighth*, 1941).[101] The film was directed by Walter Ruttmann, who had made a name for himself as an experimental filmmaker with the 1927 feature *Berlin—Die Sinfonie der Großstadt* (*Berlin: Symphony of a Metropolis*). Hans Auler, at the time head of the Berlin university clinic for cancer patients, served as scientific advisor for the seventeen-minute opening short film, which was premiered in September 1941 in Munich as part of the Reichswoche für den deutschen Kulturfilm (Reich Week for German Cultural Cinema).

But scientific explanations faded to the background in it. With the exception of the initial scene, in which a professor of medicine presents his students with a highly condensed model of cellular order and disorder, the film alternates between two parallel plotlines: the story of the 'rational' Frau Hoffmann, who, after finding a lump in her breast, immediately goes to the doctor, gets treatment, and, in the end, happily and healthily departs the hospital with her husband and children, and the story of the mechanic Herr Weber, who sells away his tools in order to pay various 'healers', dies, and leaves behind his desperate wife with nothing to her name.

The imitable role model—blonde, careful, neatly dressed—is remarkably unworried. She goes to the doctor without a bit of hesitation, gets examined, and undergoes radiotherapy without showing any signs of discomfort or fear. Ultimately, she is reduced to a foil for the doctor, who lectures her and the audience about methods of diagnosis and treatment in his responses to her questions. He assumes the role of the paternalistic, friendly, absolutely certain doctor. In contrast, Herr Weber commands much more screen time. Close-ups of his body and face visualize his doubts, fears, hesitation, and his resulting recklessness and lack of consideration for his wife. A gloomy, threatening atmosphere shrouds Weber's lengthy visits with the many 'healers', whose shifty eyes and hidden gestures betray their greedy, fraudulent nature. Although none of the

[100] British doctor Richard Doll, who had attended the lecture in 1936 as a student, discussed the slides with historian Robert Proctor in 1997. See Proctor, *The Nazi War on Cancer*, 46–8 and 291. It was probably part of Holfelder's lectures for students and doctors on 'Diagnostics and therapy of cancer with in-person patient case studies', which he began holding together with surgeon Victor Schmieden in the 1935/6 winter semester. See the digitized course catalogues contained in the University of Frankfurt's archives: http://publikationen.ub.unifrank furt.de/solrsearch/index/search/searchtype/collection/id/17036/start/100/rows/100/sortfield/year/sortorder/desc, last accessed 27 March 2017).

[101] Bundesfilmarchiv B 55709.

'healers' in the film are explicitly labelled as Jewish, Ruttmann so clearly characterized them with antisemitic stereotypes that most viewers would have immediately identified the 'healers' as 'Jews'. At the end of the short film, Weber dies and the National-Socialist state ensures 'justice' by prosecuting and convicting the last 'healer' that he visited.

But the film's denunciation of alternative medicine did not enjoy unanimous support, neither from the audience nor from Nazi health policymakers. Joseph Goebbels had supported the production of the film. But he only allowed it to be publicly screened after Rudolf Hess, one of the most dedicated adherents of alternative medicine among the Nazi Party's heavyweights, had flown off to England on his ill-fated, unauthorized peace mission, after which he fell out of Hitler's favour. In the flight's wake, Goebbels unleashed a wave of arrests, and on 16 July 1941, 'occult' methods like divining rods, hypnosis, and shields against earth rays were banned. Goebbels then personally ordered that *Jeder Achte* be shown before a 'hit film'.[102] The choice ended up being Helmut Käutner's love drama *Anuschka*, which was also about lies and deception; it premiered on 27 March 1942.[103]

Reich Health Leader Leonardo Conti and his deputy Kurt Blome, who became the plenipotentiary for oncological research in 1943, spoke out against the film and pled 'for the time being to abstain from all explanations about fighting cancer' because 'knowledge about the cause and treatment of cancer are still very meagre'.[104] They even mustered support from the Reich Chancellery under Martin Bormann's leadership. But all to no avail, as the film continued to play. Soon, however, the Munich division of the SD (Security Service) reported that people did not like the film because 'curing cancer is not so simple as it is depicted in the film', but above all, because of how it hyperbolically cast practitioners of alternative medicine as 'medieval witches'.[105] Goebbels countered the Munich dispatch with more positive SD reports from other parts of the country. But Conti and Blome also criticized the film's 'clumsy' representation of cancer treatment.[106] The preserved archival records make it impossible to determine whether the film was ultimately pulled.

The conflict between Goebbels, Conti, and Blome demonstrates that some important Nazi public health officials questioned the utility of early detection measures as such. A particularly strong signal was sent by Conti and Blome's recommendation that early detection campaigns be shut down so long as certain

[102] Elke Fröhlich, *Die Tagebücher von Joseph Goebbels. Sämtliche Fragmente*, part 1, vol. 4 (Munich: de Gruyter, 1987), 651. See also the handwritten note—probably by Goebbels himself—on the letter: Direktor Pro. Dem Herrn Minister, Berlin, 27 February 1942, BArch NS 18/349, 198.

[103] Note for Party Comrade Tießler, 17 July 1942, BArch NS 18/349, 196–7.

[104] Ibid.

[105] Büro Tießler, Letter to Party Comrade Guszmann about Section Pro, Berlin W. 8, 24 July 1942, BArch NS 18/349, 195.

[106] Note for Party Comrade Bühler, Berlin, 28 January 1943, Ti/Sp/As, BArch NS 18/349, 190; Note for Party Comrade Tießler, 17 July 1942, BArch NS 18/349, 196–7.

knowledge about cancer's causes was lacking. It contradicted every public statement made by health authorities over the previous years as well as the Nazis' aggressive early detection and prevention campaigns. But the broader context of the recommendation clarifies it. Around 1938/9, National-Socialist health policy shifted towards the medical care of healthy or easily treatable men and women important for the war economy. People considered seriously ill, untreatable, suffering from a hereditary illness, or 'racially inferior' were, with ever increasing radicality, shut out, denied care, and, in the end, murdered. For instance, at the time when Kurt Blome made his statement against 'fighting cancer', he was taking part in the development of plans to send the SS x-ray division—under the leadership of aforementioned radiologist Hans Holfelder—to hunt down Polish tuberculars with the aim of forcing them into a ghetto and killing them. The plan was, however, cancelled out of concerns that it would be impossible to conceal it from local residents.[107]

The strategies and goals of 'fighting cancer' in the 1930s explicitly thematized fear, setting them apart from their predecessors. Public health discourse in late Weimar and the Nazi era conceived of fear as a 'natural' emotional reaction that had to be confronted 'courageously' in order to contain it in rational concern rather than letting it spiral into cowardice. At the same time, campaigns intentionally stoked fear by casting moral blame on cancer patients for their illness and ultimately stigmatizing cancer with the language of eugenics. Cancer patients were maligned as people of weak character who had failed to take care of their own health, had ducked away from necessary early detection measures, had allowed themselves to be seduced by 'Jewish' quacks, and had allowed a disease to grow inside themselves that indicated that their body was anarchic and their blood 'degenerate'.

National-Socialist public health policy spun cancer patients into this web of morality, emotion, and biological racism, making their status ever more precarious. State functionaries publicly declared that healthy 'Germans' were the most valuable people. The consequence, by no means secret, was the sterilization and murder of people considered hereditarily ill or 'life not worth living'. Doctors, health officials, and others debated the extent to which the lives of those suffering from illnesses with little or no chance of being cured were 'worth living'. Supporters of euthanasia had long been enthralled by this question, which was spelled out by the author Gerhard Hoffmann—penname Ernst Mann—in the 1920s. His writings advocated creating 'selection committees' of doctors tasked with rounding up and 'eliminating' all people afflicted with 'incurable,

[107] Ernst Klee, 'Kurt Blome', in *Das Personenlexikon zum Dritten Reich. Wer war was vor und nach 1945*, 2nd edn (Frankfurt: Fischer, 2003), 54. On Holfelder, see Klee, *Das Personenlexikon*, 267 and Süß, *Der 'Volkskörper' im Krieg*, 292–310.

transmissible, and heritable illnesses like tuberculosis, inheritable venereal diseases, cancer, leprosy, mental illnesses, physical deformities'.[108]

When Hoffmann wrote this passage in 1922, the position was considered extreme and, in 1933, Conti still rejected it. But, in 1938, Gerhard Wagner, then Reich Health Leader, published his maxim that the 'productivity of the German human must be conceived as a biological value' and that medicine must 'turn away' from the 'cult of the sick'.[109] In the same year, Karl Kötschau, who had worked as leader of the Reichsarbeitsgemeinschaft für eine Neue Deutsche Heilkunde (Reich Working Group for a New German Medicine) until 1937, explained:

> While the practice of protection and care that has until now been custom has only enabled us to prolong suffering and palliate discomfort, the struggle with nature only gives us two decisive possibilities: either to prevail or to perish. A nice solution and release for a hopelessly lost sick person. I'm thinking here of cancer patients, tuberculars, rheumatics, and people afflicted with other chronic diseases.... The disabled or future disabled person—so long as he has not yet reached retirement age—must be trained to be productive and healthy, even if this accelerates an adverse outcome of his illness. In other words, a decision is to be induced: either productivity or natural elimination.[110]

These discussions were carried out in public and later realized in the Aktion T4 euthanasia programme. That the mass killings were no secret was underscored by the public protests of Münster bishop Clemens August Graf von Galen in the summer of 1941. Galen asserted that the logical conclusion of the claim that all unproductive people should be killed would lead to the killing of those unable to work, those with incurable illnesses, and 'decrepit' old persons.[111]

After Galen's sermons of objection, the centralized murder of mentally and physically ill people under the T4 campaign was cancelled. But the Nazi regime continued to kill disabled people and 'indirectly' end the lives of many others by depriving them of food or refusing them medical treatment. Those targeted included people with tuberculosis and diabetics, whose food and insulin rations were shortened and who were forced to perform hard labour in full knowledge of the devastating effect it would have on their health. Under the guise of a therapeutic experiment, medical journals debated 'reducing' the food allowed to cancer

[108] Ernst Mann, *Die Erlösung der Menschheit vom Elend* (Weimar: Fink, 1922), 67.

[109] Gerhard Wagner, 'Gesundes Leben—Frohes Schaffen', *Ziel und Weg* 8 (1938): 549–55, 551 and 555.

[110] Karl Kötschau, *Der Einfluß des Christentums auf Stellung und Einstellung des Kranken* (Nuremberg: Schriften des Vereins Deutsche Volksheilkunde e.V, 1938), 35–6. See also Süß, *Der 'Volkskörper' im Krieg*, 294.

[111] Bischof Clemens August Graf von Galen, *Akten, Briefe und Predigten 1933–1946*, Vol. 2: *1939–1946*, ed. Ludwig Löffler (Mainz: Ferdinand Schöningh, 1988), 876.

patients to the 'minimum needed for survival'.[112] Increasingly, people deemed 'infirm seniors', among them cancer patients, were 'evacuated' to special, under-supplied care centres after Allied bombs started hitting hospitals in 1943. Available archival sources do not give an answer as to how many people were targeted by these measures, how many died, and whether any of the 'infirm seniors' were directly murdered.

Thus, in the 1920s, and even more in the 1930s, early detection examinations constituted a technology on the precarious edge between making live and letting die, to borrow Foucault's words. Originally promoted as a way to identify cancer while it could still be treated, they were now conceptualized by proponents of euthanasia as an instrument to separate the dying from the healthy to 'let' them die faster. Though the National Socialists' effort to 'fight cancer' did not explicitly articulate this relationship, it was not unknown to the population. SD reports from the last years of the war note that 'infirm seniors' refused to take their medicine out of fear that it might be spiked. Prosecutors at the 1947 Nuremberg Doctors' Trial inquired into whether 75,000 'infirm seniors' were murdered in the last years of the Nazi regime, though the investigation ultimately did not yield answers, as it was overshadowed by other issues in the run of the trial.[113] Nevertheless, the suspicion that such events did occur should be considered as important context when studying the history of the early detection of cancer in the early years of the Federal Republic of Germany and the German Democratic Republic.

Socialist Optimism and West German Morality

In the first years after the war, cancer dropped on the public health priority list in both the Soviet and the Western Allied occupied zones, as fears were fixed on infectious illnesses like tuberculosis, typhus, dysentery, and venereal diseases. The reconstruction and reorganization of the health system seemed the most pressing issue for all the occupying powers. The Western forces, and first and foremost the Americans, initially conceived of this project as another aspect of the broader efforts at denazification and democratic re-education. In the Soviet occupation zone, government returned to the public health tradition of the Weimar Republic and aligned itself with Soviet ideas. 'Prophylaxis' had been a key concept of Soviet health politics before the Second World War, and it was elevated to the categorical imperative of early East German health and welfare policy to such a degree that it was defined as being identical with the construction of a new socialist society.

[112] Süß, *Der 'Volkskörper' im Krieg*, 295–6; Robert Jütte, *Medizin und Nationalsozialismus. Bilanz und Perspektiven der Forschung*, 2nd edn (Göttingen: Wallstein, 2011), 214–55; K. R. Roques, 'Diät gegen Tumoren', *Deutsches Ärzteblatt* 26, no. 42/3 (1941): 371–3, 373. See also Madarász, 'Die Pflicht zur Gesundheit', 155–6.

[113] Süß, *Der 'Volkskörper' im Krieg*, 300–2 and 308.

'The best prophylaxis is socialism' read the epigraph at the beginning of Alfred Beyer and Kurt Winter's 1953 book *Lehrbuch der Sozialhygiene* (*Textbook of Public Health*). The motto was inscribed on the walls of many East German hospitals up through the 1980s.[114]

Prophylaxis had two core pillars in East Germany. The first was prevention through behavioural changes, which comprised, in particular, the improvement of working conditions and work safety measures. The other was illness prevention for all. The right to free medical care was enshrined in the GDR constitution, a right that was actualized through the creation of a universal social insurance system. It was not without compulsion, though, as East German citizens were legally required to get vaccinated against smallpox and diphtheria; vaccinations against tetanus, whooping cough, tuberculosis, and polio, on the other hand, were available but not obligatory. Compulsory vaccinations were temporarily abolished in 1954, but as GDR citizens gradually stopped getting them, they were reimplemented in the mid-1960s. In addition, all citizens had to undergo regular check-ups and violations were punished with fines. The exams' purpose was to screen for tuberculosis, but doctors also used them to look for signs of lung cancer.[115]

The socialist state, with its principles of peace and 'life', championed prophylaxis as a political mission, and early detection campaigns became one tool in the box. The first East German campaigns stuck to a tradition dominant in Germany since the turn of the century by focusing on cervical cancer. But the Cold War motivated East German public health officials to situate the issue in a different political context by redefining the role of women and mothers in the socialist state. Robert Ganse, head doctor at the women's clinic of the Dresden-Friedrichstadt hospital, explained:

[114] Alfred Bayer and Kurt Winter, *Lehrbuch der Sozialhygiene* (Berlin (GDR): Verlag Volk und Gesundheit, 1953). See Arndt, *Gesundheitspolitik im geteilten Berlin*; Gabriele Moser, *'Im Interesse der Volksgesundheit...' Sozialhygiene und öffentliches Gesundheitswesen in der Weimarer Republik und der frühen SBZ/DDR. Ein Beitrag zur Sozialgeschichte des deutschen Gesundheitswesens im 20. Jahrhundert* (Frankfurt am Main: Verlag für Akademische Schriften, 2002), 151–201; Ulrike Lindner, *Gesundheitspolitik in der Nachkriegszeit. Großbritannien und die Bundesrepublik Deutschland im Vergleich* (Munich: Oldenbourg, 2004); Wolfgang Woelk, 'Zur Geschichte der Gesundheitspolitik in Nordrhein-Westfalen und in der Bundesrepublik Deutschland', in *Geschichte der Gesundheitspolitik in Deutschland. Von der Weimarer Republik bis in die Frühgeschichte der 'doppelten Staatsgründung'*, ed. Wolfgang Woelk and Jörg Vögele (Berlin: Duncker & Humblot, 2002), 285–312, 33–44; Sabine Schleiermacher, 'Prävention und Prophylaxe in BRD und DDR. Eine gesundheitspolitische Leitidee im Kontext verschiedener Systeme', in *100 Jahre Sozialhygiene, Sozialmedizin und Public Health in Deutschland*, ed. Udo Schagen and Sabine Schleiermacher (Berlin: Institut für Geschichte der Medizin, 2005), 1–7, 1–2. On the American Zone of Occupation, see Ellerbrock, *Healing Democracy*. On health policy in the British Zone of Occupation, see Woelk, 'Zur Geschichte der Gesundheitspolitik'; Jenny Linek, *Gesundheitsvorsorge in der DDR zwischen Propaganda und Praxis* (Stuttgart: Franz Steiner, 2016), 26–38.

[115] Malte Thießen, 'Vorsorge als Ordnung des Sozialen: Impfen in der Bundesrepublik und der DDR', *Zeithistorische Forschungen/Studies in Contemporary History* 10, no. 3 (2013): 409–32, 414, 417; Jeannette Madarász, 'Prävention chronischer Herz-Kreislauf-Krankheiten. BRD, DDR und Großbritannien im Vergleich, 1945–1990', *Prävention und Gesundheitsförderung* 5, no. 4 (2010): 313–18, 314, https://doi.org/10.1007/s11553-010-0259-9.

> The state's most valuable asset is its mothers and children. The task of gynaecologists is to prevent around 20,000 women a year from falling victim to this terrible illness [cervical cancer] and being torn from their families, and we do everything in our power to fulfil it.... But all of our efforts are dependent on the peaceful development of our fatherland. Preventive medicine is tightly bound to the maintenance of peace. Our medical work only makes sense if we do everything we can to ensure that our accomplishments are not destroyed by atomic bombs. War is the worst enemy of doctors and our children and mothers. The doctors' fight against cancer and other diseases would be incomplete if it were not tied to the fight against the violent destruction of human life.[116]

The statement turned cancer into the biological cipher of the threat of nuclear winter, describing the protection of 'life' against both as an interlinked task. This helps explain why the older military metaphor of the 'fight' against cancer fell out of use in East German health policy, which instead placed an accent on the 'peaceful' prevention of cancer. Concomitantly, an appeal to the socialist joy of life supplanted the open mobilization of fear characteristic of past early detection campaigns.

The first cancer awareness film produced by DEFA, East Germany's state-owned studio, helped facilitate this shift. Between 1957 and 1962, the starkly titled *Rechtzeitig—eine Mahnung des Lebens* (*In Time—A Warning for the Living*) was screened at workplace health events and as part of the travelling exhibitions 'Wie werde ich 100 Jahre alt?' (How Can I Live to Be 100?) and 'Gesund leben—lange leben' (Live Healthy—Live Long).[117] The emotional tenor of the nineteen-minute sound film's opening sequence is the polar opposite of the opening sequence of the 1930 film *Krebs* discussed above. The first two minutes depict not the pain and agony of cancer, but children living in happiness. A voiceover speaks the first words of the film: 'Happy children. They deserve all our love, all our care. Their health must be looked after.'[118] A slow succession of scenes shows a nurse weighing and swaddling a new-born, and babies, schoolchildren, and prepubescent boys

[116] Dr Robert Ganse, MD, 'Die hauptsächlichen Krebserkrankungen der Frau (Dresden: Deutsches Hygiene-Museum Dresden, undated [1956/7]), 13–14. This paragraph was added to the second, 1957 edition of a booklet that was first published in 1952. Titled *The Most Important Female Cancers*, it was one of the Hygiene Museum's bestselling booklets in the 1950s. In 1954 alone, 57,000 copies were sold. See Susanne Roeßiger, 'Die Krebskampagnen des Deutschen Hygiene-Museums', *'Rechtzeitig erkannt—heilbar'. Krebsaufklärung im 20. Jahrhundert*, ed. Stiftung Deutsches Hygiene-Museum (Dresden: Sandstein, 2002), 21–31, 28, DHMD 2001/287.

[117] Travelling exhibitions 'Wie werde ich 100 Jahre alt' and 'Gesund leben—lange leben', 1959, Dokumentation, Zusammenstellung, Zeitungsartikel, Begleitvorträge/Ankündigungen, Fotografien von Ausstellungstafeln, HSTA D 13658, no. Au 163 b and DHMD 2001/1656.

[118] This stands in marked contrast to the synopsis printed in the publications of the Hygiene Museum, which describes the first scene as one of shock and horror. However, what ended up being the actual initial sequence is followed by a flashback to a time when disease—first the plague, then cancer—spread fear. Why the actual initial sequence does not appear in the synopsis is confounding,

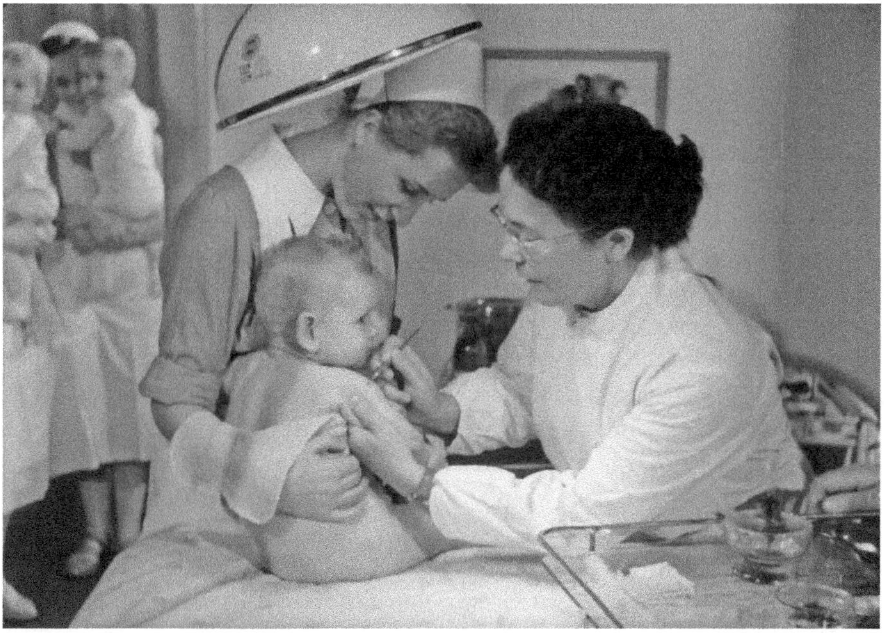

Fig. 10 Still from the film *Rechtzeitig—eine Mahnung des Lebens* (*In Time—An Admonition for Life*, 1956).

being vaccinated and measured (Fig. 10). The camera repeatedly zooms in on the innocent, trusting faces of the children as well as on the parents' and caretakers' gestures of attention. The conclusion of the opening sequence emphasizes the humanitarian mission of the socialist state by portraying a white doctor vaccinating a black man in an unspecified African country.

The sequence thus tells a story of logical progression, in which educating children to take prophylactic measures for granted—and, in particular, the specific type of illness prevention represented by vaccination—naturally blossoms into them regularly going to the doctor to get checked for cancer symptoms. Habituating people to accept routine exams and procedures as normal distinguished this type of early detection from the anxious observation of the body.

By depicting prophylaxis as a collective practice involving doctors, nurses, and everyday citizens, the film shifted focus away from the individual body, pain, tumours, and potential death. Only a single image shows a tumour, and even it is a photo of an early-stage skin tumour, which must have appeared fairly harmless in comparison with the devastating images that had featured in previous campaigns.

since it distinguishes the film from all previous films on cancer in Germany and from many in the United States being produced around the same time. See Susanne Roeßiger, 'Bewegte Bilder', in Stiftung Deutsches Hygiene-Museum, *'Rechtzeitig erkannt—heilbar'*, 132.

Instead, the film framed going to an early detection exam as an act of solidarity. Taking responsibility for oneself and the health of one's neighbours assumed a different shape here than in the National Socialists' lectures about the duty of the individual towards the 'body of the German people'. The film cast early detection as just one step on the way to retaining the health of socialist society, promoting international understanding, and working towards peace.

One of the film's storylines symbolizes this concept of mutual responsibility. A woman cured of breast cancer sits in the cafeteria recounting her experiences and convinces two colleagues to visit the doctor together. Their friendly walk contrasts starkly with the close-ups of the first woman's solo trip to the doctor, which was accompanied by dramatic music. While she went by herself after developing serious concerns that she might have symptoms of cancer, her colleagues walk at ease—and, for good reason, one might say, neither is found to have cancer. The motif of a hopeful march into a better future is one that the film repeats again towards it end, when a long procession of women moves past the camera as if in a parade (Fig. 11).

Fear does appear in the film, for sure, but it is coloured as an emotion no longer in tune with the times. Perhaps fear was justified in a 'dark' past dominated by the plague and other diseases, as a few iconic medieval stereotypes shown after the film's initial sequence seem to suggest. But fear, it emphasizes, is superfluous in

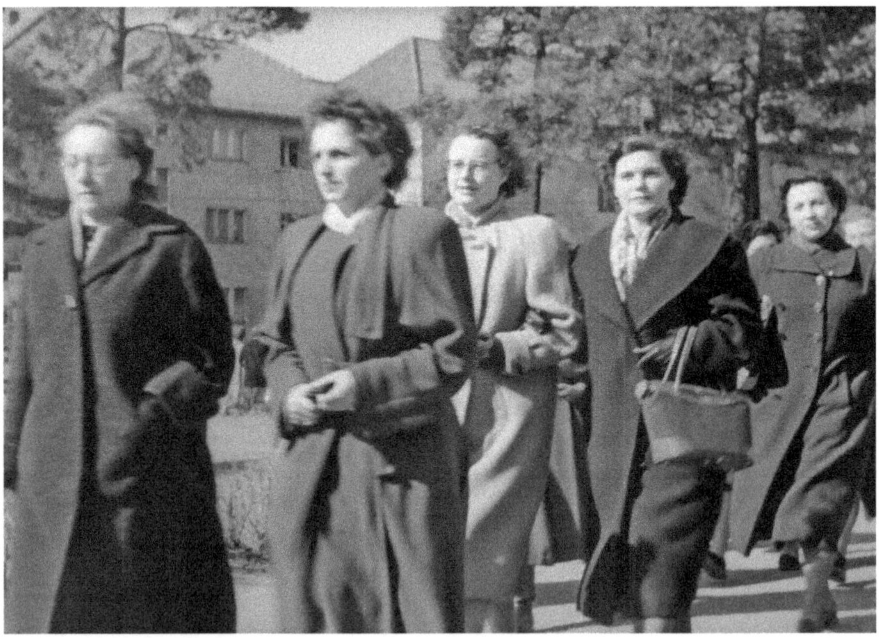

Fig. 11 Still from the film *Rechtzeitig—eine Mahnung des Lebens* (*In Time—An Admonition for Life*, 1956).

the present and future of a state constructed on the foundation of scientific progress, well-planned healthcare, and mutual solidarity.

This political interpretation of fear defined the practice of socialism itself as the very embodiment of joy in life and work. Years later, East Germany's television series *Wegweiser Gesundheit* (*Health Guide*) aired an episode on emotions that echoed this sentiment with the words: 'In our society, there is no place for fear, pessimism, discontent, because desire and reality are identical.'[119] The film *Rechtzeitig* also celebrated the identity of desire and reality by proclaiming—contrary to all evidence—that: 'Everyone could be saved if they got an early detection exam once a year.'[120] The movie marked the first time in the history of early detection exams that they were championed as a practice that liberated people from fear and anxiety, a point underscored when the doctor tells the former cancer patient that she should spread the message to other women: 'A doctor's visit is worth it. It brings clarity. And how liberating is the knowledge that you're healthy.'[121]

Indeed, the GDR's health officials exerted themselves to enable all women to attain such 'knowledge' about their bodies. In July 1952, three years after the state's founding, its legislature decreed that care centres for cancer patients be constructed in all cities with more than 100,000 residents. One of the centres' primary duties would be to provide all women over 25 years of age with annual early detection exams for breast and cervical cancer. In addition, local nurses' offices, the new polyclinics, and factories with a high number of women workers were ordered to offer early detection check-ups.[122] The policy represented an effort to universalize something that had been discussed since the 1920s and sporadically realized in isolated regions of the German Empire: the institution of accessible treatment encumbered neither by long distances nor long waits. But in contrast to models that had preceded it, East Germany's programme was intended to regularly screen women regardless of whether they showed potential symptoms. The practice was not altogether unfamiliar, as x-ray tests for tuberculosis had been implemented in Germany in 1938 and were resumed by the GDR in the early 1950s.

The 'just-in-case' early detection exams (*Vorsichtsuntersuchungen*) were so popular that demand for them rapidly outpaced availability. After one of the first talks that he held in 1952 at the VEB Projektierung Sachsen (Publicly Owned Enterprise for Planning, Saxony), aforementioned gynaecologist Robert Ganse

119 Scene from a film from the series *Wegweiser Gesundheit* with the title 'Emotionen', 17 July 1975, HSTA D 13658, F VIII, no. 17.

120 Author's transcription of the film *Rechtzeitig—eine Mahnung des Lebens* (1956).

121 Author's transcription of the film *Rechtzeitig—eine Mahnung des Lebens* (1956).

122 Susanne Roeßiger, 'Bildappell und schnelle Botschaft. Plakate', in Stiftung Deutsches Hygiene-Museum, *'Rechtzeitig erkannt—heilbar'*, 78; Dr E. Bisch, Görlitz, 'Krebsprophylaxe der Frau', *Alles für Deine Gesundheit* 7 (1956), HSTA D 13658, no. Z 7.

stated: 'The effect was that the women became uproarious because exams could temporarily not take place.... Because our informative message went well beyond the means of the exams and the clinic could not keep up with the rush, a catastrophic situation arose and turned a good thing into its opposite.'[123]

In consultation with the director of Dresden's Museum of Hygiene, Ganse made a spur-of-the-moment decision to talk about health topics unrelated to cancer at the following events in order to avoid drawing attention to the inadequate number of clinics. The discrepancy between far-reaching, utopian plans and their insufficient realization on account of a dearth of resources was a problem that plagued East German health policy until the state's demise in 1990. In the 1950s, though, the heavily politicized prophylaxis efforts amplified the problem. Still, prophylaxis was not just a principle that East German leaders employed to legitimize the political system. By preventing expensive therapies and care for seriously ill persons, prophylaxis saved money, which is why work to set up a sufficient number of clinics continued.[124]

In order to relieve the overtaxed clinics, the government raised the age when women were supposed to get a yearly exam to 30.[125] However, the greatest challenge facing the expansion of early detection clinics was many gynaecologists' lack of the specialized training needed to perform colposcopies on symptomless women. While the procedure was policy in the GDR, it was uncommon in most other countries, which generally conducted biopsies only on women with existing symptoms.

The colposcope was invented in 1925 by Hans Hinselmann, a gynaecologist and head doctor of the Altona hospital in Hamburg.[126] The instrument allowed doctors to examine the cervix close-up and detect even the smallest abnormalities. But before 1945, colposcopies were not standard practice in Germany. One reason was that many doctors thought examining the cervix with a speculum and the naked eye was just as effective; another was that the necessary preparatory treatment with iodine and acetic acid was time-consuming.[127]

The GDR's focus on prophylaxis led it to embrace colposcopies, despite the complicated nature of the procedure. Beyond enabling doctors to identify alterations of the cervix before symptoms appeared, the colposcopy had an additional advantage over speculums and biopsies: it created distance. Although public health campaigns only indirectly noted this, discussions of colposcopies in leaflets

[123] Quoted in Susanne Roeßiger, 'Krebskampagnen', 28.

[124] Madarász, 'Prävention chronischer Herz-Kreislauf-Krankheiten', 314; Thießen, 'Vorsorge als Ordnung des Sozialen', 414–15.

[125] Susanne Roeßiger, 'Informationen für alle. Broschüren und Merkblätter', in Stiftung Deutsches Hygiene-Museum, *'Rechtzeitig erkannt—heilbar'*, 78.

[126] On Hinselmann's role in concentration camp 'experiments' on colposcopy, see Jutta Hübner, 'Kolposkopie ohne Menschlichkeit', *Hamburger Ärzteblatt* 66, no. 4 (2012): 34–5.

[127] Iodine and acetic acid make altered cells visible: in contrast to healthy cells, the acetic acid turns altered cells white; iodine turns healthy cells brown, while the altered cells remain the same colour.

and newspaper articles emphasized that the colposcope did not enter the body and did not cause pain.[128] Drawings underscored the distancing factor by placing the doctor's eye far away from the patient's body (Fig. 12). Although colposcopies also required the use of a speculum so that the lens could reach the cervix, and were thus invasive in a certain sense, the doctor could only see the patient's intimate region through the optical instrument. The articles and their visual accompaniment thus suggested that colposcopies were supposed to help women overcome their 'false shame', which might have otherwise inhibited them from undergoing an exam that seemed less urgent because of the lack of symptoms.

The brochures' focus on the technical details of the colposcopy pushed into the background the reason why the procedure was performed in the first place—as a measure to 'prevent' cancer. Old analogies with car inspections framed colposcopies as part of a 'rational', scientific, technological approach to the body, which was being checked and measured more and more at work, school, and elsewhere. This all fit with the growing acceptance of the idea that everything from social structures to human life could be planned, regulated, and controlled. This idea

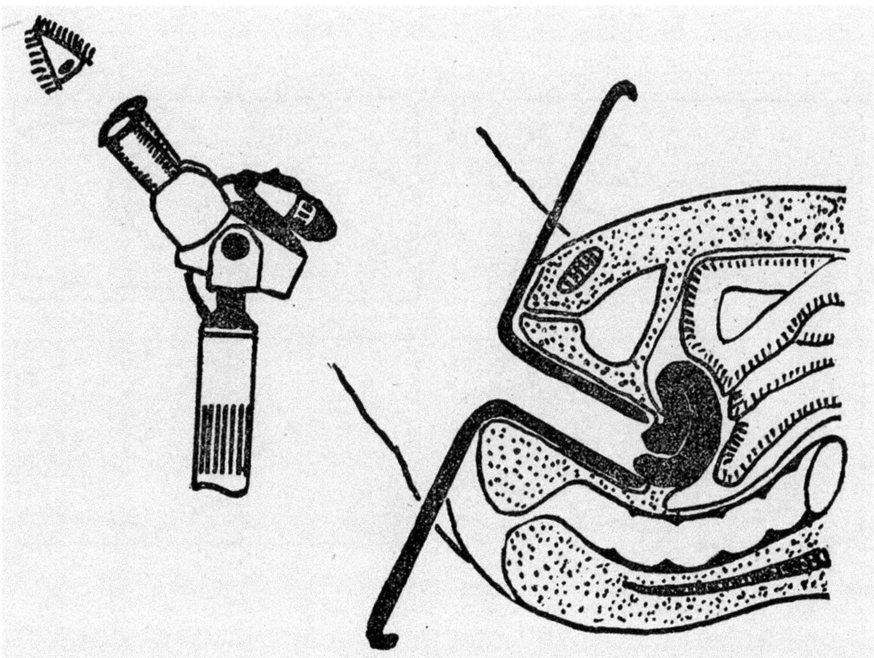

Fig. 12 Illustration, *Alles für Deine Gesundheit* (Everything for Your Health, 1956).

[128] Dr E. Bisch, Görlitz, 'Krebsprophylaxe der Frau', *Alles für Deine Gesundheit* 7 (1956), HSTA D 13658, no. Z 7.

found practical expression in the endeavour to turn formalized rationality completely stripped of emotions into the guiding principle of society.[129]

This model shaped publications about another type of early detection for women propagated in the GDR: breast self-examinations. In contrast to most other countries, public health campaigns in Germany had been promoting breast self-examinations since the 1930s.[130] However, they only stated *that* women should check their breasts for lumps, without ever explaining *how* they should do it, neither in print materials nor in films' fleeting images of women examining their breasts. But in the 1950s, leaflets, pamphlets, and articles in East Germany described in detail how women should perform the monthly routine, often visualizing it with schematic drawings that reduced a woman to the structure of her body (Fig. 13). Such informative materials were intended to train every woman to become their own 'screening assistant' and empower them to examine their own bodies and thus save the costs of a doctor's visit, as the articles frankly admitted. But they admonished women to rush to the doctor for diagnosis if they did find anything abnormal.

East German health policy dispatched the image of the 'foolish', overly anxious woman who listened to the 'false' advice of friends, and it also did away with the

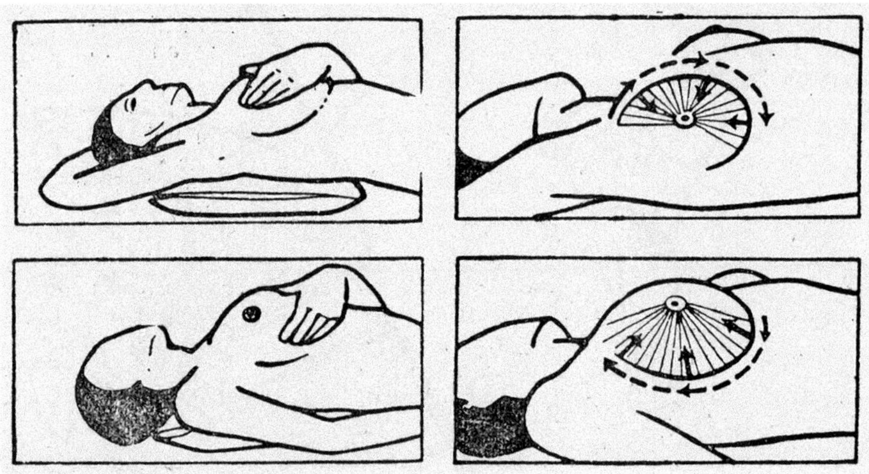

Fig. 13 Guide to breast self-examination (1959).

[129] Thomas Etzemüller, 'Social Engineering', *Docupedia-Zeitgeschichte*, 11 February 2010, http://docupedia.de/zg/Social%5Fengineering); Michael Hagner, 'Vom Aufstieg und Fall der Kybernetik als Universalwissenschaft', in *Die Transformation des Humanen. Beiträge zur Kulturgeschichte der Kybernetik*, ed. Michael Hagner and Erich Hörl (Frankfurt am Main: Suhrkamp, 2008), 38–71; Erickson et al., *How Reason Almost Lost Its Mind*.

[130] For example, the United States, where self-examination was only seriously propagated after 1945; however, as soon as the decision was made to promote it there, films were produced to demonstrate the technique. See Gardner, *Early Detection*, 110–20.

associated strategy of moral blame. Its campaigns supplanted her with the new ideal of a woman who was well informed, who acted prudently, and whose advice others could trust. All this took place in a political context in which successful prophylaxis was considered a barometer of the health system's success. Accordingly, the government could count on the collaboration of the collective. The consequences of public pressure could hurt, and it was well known that the state could take punitive measures against people who failed to get vaccinated or undergo the mandatory x-ray check for tuberculosis. As such, it seems plausible that women saw it necessary to comply, even without the threat of sanctions or reproach.

But like contemporaneous campaigns in other countries, the GDR's remained silent about the uncertainty of diagnostic methods, an issue that medical professionals were discussing heatedly. Around this time, a screening method that could detect potential issues earlier than other tests became standard practice. Named after its inventor George Papanicolaou, the Pap smear revived with increased urgency an unresolved question from the 1920s: do all abnormal cells indicate cancer or always develop into cancer? West Germany initiated an early detection scheme in 1971 that provided the test free of cost, while East Germany made it available in 1972 with the Berliner Zytologieprogramm (Berlin Cytology Programme). However, women could get the test in both states before these dates.

Two factors explain the late adoption of the cytopathological test. First, the cell sample had to be carefully assessed under a microscope. Conducting the test once or twice a year as part of regular check-ups would overwhelm medical labs. The United States resolved the issue by creating a new (women's) occupation, the cytology technician, and many other countries followed suit. Still, it took a while until enough cytology technicians could be trained. The second issue was of a more fundamental nature: nobody really knew exactly what 'unhealthy' cells detected in a Pap test meant.[131] Were they signs that the patient had cancer? Or at least some kind of precancerous condition? Or did they indicate cell alterations that could potentially, but not necessarily, lead to cancer, and that thus might simply disappear on their own? Comparisons of the number of abnormal screens with epidemiological statistics on cervical tumours supported this hypothesis, since the former was many times greater than the latter.[132] They suggested that most abnormal cells would *not* develop into malignant cancer.

Further research studied women whose Pap tests revealed a 'carcinoma in situ'. The concept was controversial because its name begged the question as to whether detected cell changes, their loss of differentiation, and their atypical growth

[131] See Löwy, *Preventive Strikes*, 127–30.

[132] John E. Dunn, Jr, 'The Relationships between Carcinoma in Situ and Invasive Cervical Carcinoma: A Consideration of the Contribution to the Problem to be Made from General Population Data', *Cancer* 6, no. 5 (1953): 873–86, https://doi.org/10.1002/1097-0142(195309)6:5%3C873::AID-CNCR2820060506%3E3.0.CO;2-Q.

patterns should be viewed as precancerous alterations only distinguishable from cancerous tumours because they did not spread past a particular area of tissue and thus had not become 'invasive' (thus the term 'in situ', or 'in its place'). These studies divided the women into three groups. The first were treated as if they had an invasive tumour, either by performing a hysterectomy—that is, the surgical removal of the uterus and the surrounding lymph nodes—or radiotherapy. The second group received a more 'conservative' treatment: only their cervix was partially or wholly removed through an operation or cervical conization. The third group of women received no treatment at all, but regularly came in for check-ups in short intervals.

The studies showed that in many cases, 'carcinoma in situ' never developed into full-fledged cancer. All of the women who submitted to the most 'radical' treatment remained free of cancer well past their 50s, while some women from the other two groups later suffered from cervical cancer. The lead researchers were surprised to learn that despite the thorough check-ups, a few women from the third group were later diagnosed with and succumbed to advanced, untreatable tumours. Making predictions about if, why, and when a 'carcinoma in situ' would turn into invasive cancer thus seemed an impossible undertaking. But simply performing hysterectomies or radiotherapy on all women found to have a 'carcinoma in situ' of the cervix was not a riskless option either. Removal of the uterus would force young women to forego having (more) children. Moreover, in one study, two of eight women died of the effects of the drastic operation, while many women who underwent radiotherapy suffered from severe side effects, such as burns, necrosis, and incontinence.[133]

In the face of such uncertainty and despite the risks, a majority of oncologists in the 1950s—in West Germany and in East, in the United States and in the United Kingdom—elected to operate on or irradiate every case of 'carcinoma in situ' on the cervix (the laser therapy that has become prevalent since the 1980s did not yet exist). Findings of dysplasia were often treated with less damaging methods. But a series of studies demonstrated that different cytology technicians—and even different pathologists—could interpret the same Pap smear differently. While one saw only a simple dysplasia, another might see 'carcinoma in situ'.[134] Consequently, the function of Pap smears evolved in the 1960s into a sort of pre-screening the results of which had to be verified through colposcopies or biopsies. Still, doubts about where to draw the line between dysplasia and 'carcinoma in situ' remained.

Women who underwent early detection exams at the polyclinics and counselling centres, though, rarely caught wind of these debates and uncertainties.

[133] Olaf Petersen, *Precancerous Changes of the Cervical Epithelium* (Copenhagen: Danish Science Press, 1955), 102.

[134] Löwy, *Preventive Strikes* (2010), 129–30.

Informative literature published not only in the GDR but also in other countries around the world suggested that doctors could make clear diagnoses with the existing technologies. Things were similar for other types of cancer. A lump in the breast or prostate, altered tissue in the colon or stomach lining—how to distinguish between harmless dysplasia, precancerous cells, and manifest and potentially fatal cancer remains a topic of discussion among medical professionals even today.

The unwarranted certainty propagated by early detection campaigns often pushed doctors to fabricate the appearance of confidence with an act of interpretive simplification. By suppressing the complexities involved in diagnosis, public health campaigns tacitly accepted the danger that cancer patients might blame themselves for their own fate because they went to the doctor 'too late', even though having gone to the doctor earlier would not have necessarily meant that cancer would have been found. While self-blame was implicit in East Germany's campaigns, however, it was a central feature of those in West Germany.

The Moralizing Strategy of West Germany

Initially, early detection campaigns in the Federal Republic of Germany revolved around the metaphor of war that had been used frequently in the past. However, they defined getting precautionary examinations solely as the responsibility of an individual towards themself and their family, discarding all reference to the 'population' or the 'body of the people'.

Moralizing strategies thus blended continuity and discontinuity with the preceding decades, a point particularly apparent in health officials' discussions on the appropriate film for early detection campaigns. Wilhelm Hagen, head of the Interior Ministry's health division, believed that the existing films were defunct. Commenting on Walter Ruttmann's 1941 film *Jeder Achte*, he stated that it would be 'purposeful if [this] film in particular disappears from the screen'.[135]

Producing a new film was not yet on the table, the main reason likely being the high costs. Health was not an issue that occupied the concerns of the federal government much, as responsibility for it was delegated to the federal states. In contrast to the GDR, West Germany did not have a Ministry of Health in the 1950s, but only a health division housed within the Ministry of the Interior. Moreover, in the early 1950s, West Germany's health policy focused on curative medicine. Consciously distancing themselves from the politicized preventive medicine and eugenics of National Socialism, health officials rejected the centralized administration of prophylactic care.[136]

[135] Referat IV 3: Note on the educational film 'Krebs', Bonn, 8 June 1953, BArch B 142/410, 159.
[136] Madarász, 'Prävention chronischer Herz-Kreislauf-Krankheiten', 313.

Thus, in order to have a film ready quickly and inexpensively, the Zentralausschuss für Krebsbekämpfung und Krebsforschung (one of the many rebrandings of the German Central Committee for Researching and Fighting Cancer first founded in 1900) acquired the screening rights for a film that had been produced during the war by the Schweizer Krebsliga (Swiss Cancer League). Titled *Krebs ist heilbar* (*Cancer is Curable*), it premiered in 1953.

Like Ruttmann's 1941 film and films commissioned by the American Society for the Control of Cancer before the war, *Krebs ist heilbar* combined live action with animation. Integrated into the plot of the film are lectures of a professor of medicine, positioning viewers into the role of medical students. They learn directly from an expert, with the film suggesting that the knowledge communicated is just as comprehensive and scientific as that imparted at a real medical school. The content and the metaphors employed to communicate it are hardly distinguishable from those of the German films from 1930 and 1941 discussed above. They were based on dichotomies like order and anarchy, responsibility towards community and anti-social behaviour. Like its predecessors, the Swiss film offered radical solutions: 'These cancer cells must be exterminated, all of them.'[137] Even if the film contained no Nazi images of 'Aryan Germans' and explicit antisemitic stereotypes, it designated cancer as an 'enemy of the people' that endangered social order by wrecking individual bodies. This stood in marked contrast to the rhetorical and narrative strategies pursued in East German public health films. And it had little to do with contemporaneous oncological research. But the film was not really about communicating scientific knowledge. Rather, it sought to instil in viewers' minds an image of cancer that would justify early, invasive therapy as well as the call for them to remain 'alert'.

The film depicted taking up the 'fight' against this 'enemy of the people' as a matter of individual responsibility towards oneself and one's family. At the same time, it paralleled the GDR film from 1956 discussed above by framing the fight as part of a collective effort. As an appeal to the viewer at the end of the film pointedly instructs: 'Everyone must help in the fight against cancer.' The filmmakers illustrated the steps they wanted viewers to take through a narrative about a woman who makes the 'right' decision and goes to the doctor. Apparently, the image of women harboured by German health policy had changed since the 1920s and 1930s, when films generally homed in on the 'foolish' woman who failed to go to the doctor in time. By the 1950s, men were considered to be the real 'problem children' of preventive care.

The film contrasts the actions of the female protagonist with those of three men who all avoid early detection exams. By splitting up the 'foolish' role among three different characters, the film shuttles between fearmongering and optimism, with

[137] Author's transcription of *Krebs ist heilbar*.

the latter coming out on top at the end. The first male character—the woman's neighbour—dies before viewers ever see him, his story symbolizing the tragic consequences of procrastination. One intense scene shows the man's family sitting in the hospital corridor. The doctor approaches them and, still standing, turns towards the man's wife to ask her: 'Dear Mrs Peters: Why did your husband wait so long? He should have come to us much earlier. I don't think that we can help him now. His cancer is too advanced.' This harsh criticism from the doctor standing over her has a powerful effect: the camera zooms in on the silent, stunned face of the patient's daughter as she turns away in shame and grief.

After this unmistakable, visually disturbing ascription of blame, the film only deals with death one more time. When the second male character ignores his wife's repeated reminders to get his car inspected in order to avoid having to drive her to a lecture on cancer, she relates to him how this type of behaviour had robbed many children of a parent. Her thoughts are illustrated in a short family scene in which the youngest child's question 'Where's mom?' is answered with oppressive silence. Otherwise, the film follows the protagonist, who gets examined by her doctor and learns that everything is fine. All the while, she tirelessly presses her husband to make an appointment with a radiologist, but he always finds an excuse. Whether he ever goes remains open at the film's end. A brief third plotline sketches in a few emblematic images the story of a man who rolls the dice with his own life by seeking the advice of a 'healer'.

Interspersed throughout are short sequences that depict operations and radiotherapy as safe, promising, painless treatments. The film touts both as absolutely controllable, routine procedures performed with state-of-the-art technology. Though this ignored the clinical realities of the 1950s, the film's representation of therapy as an almost guaranteed success makes the men's actions appear driven by a misguided fear. Amplifying this impression are the actions of the woman, who goes to the doctor out of sheer cautiousness and is reassured that she is healthy. Avoiding a check-up thus appears irrational, irresponsible, and 'immature', and the medical professor condemns it with a paternalistic tone and raised index finger (Fig. 14).

The wagging index finger would remain the symbol of public health campaigns in West Germany, as in the front page of a pamphlet that was printed by the Bundeszentrale für gesundheitliche Aufklärung (Federal Centre for Health Education) in 1967 and distributed up into the 1970s.[138]

Paternalistic moralizing stood in stark contrast to East Germany's strategies, which portrayed early detection exams as part of a lifelong practice of solidarity and 'love of life'. West Germany's health officials consciously rejected concepts of

[138] BArch B 142/4093, 209. The pamphlet featured the iconic image of Uncle Sam pointing his index finger at the viewer, known throughout the world from the famous recruitment poster of the US Army during the First World War.

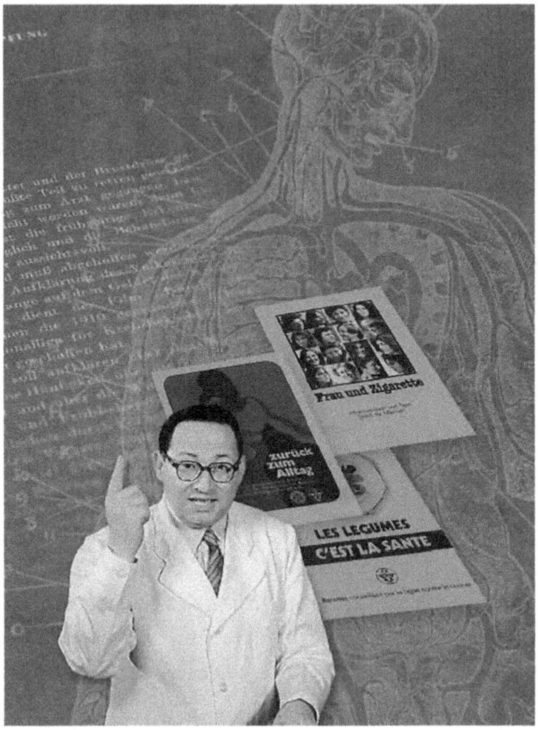

Fig. 14 Advertisement for the film *Kampf dem Krebs/Krebs ist heilbar* (*Fight Cancer/ Cancer Is Curable*, 1945/53).

social medicine developed during the Weimar Republic, while the GDR, heavily influenced by the Soviet Union, adopted them. Instead, the Federal Republic of Germany defined public health and illness prevention as the responsibility of non-governmental actors, with the state assuming the role of educating people and appealing for particular behaviours. Thus, the administration of and decision-making about actual preventive care was, for the most part, placed in the hands of doctors, a policy approach largely shaped by the representatives of doctors' associations.[139]

In the run of the 1960s, the public discussion on regular check-ups for seemingly healthy people grew. Contributing to this was increasing awareness about heart and circulatory issues such as hypertension. Labelled as 'managers' diseases' in the 1950s, they were perceived as afflicting the standard bearers of the *Wirtschaftswunder*, which had given the young Federal Republic of Germany new confidence and every citizen a standard of life that only a few years earlier would have been considered unattainable. Public discourse pointed at this

[139] Madarász, 'Prävention chronischer Herz-Kreislauf-Krankheiten', 313.

relationship to put a positive spin on coronary diseases, framing them as illnesses of successful people who unflaggingly 'toiled' for the prosperity and economic stability of their country. At the same time, epidemiological research like the aforementioned Framingham Heart Study delivered 'hard' facts to support the hypothesis that quantifiable data about the body could help predict risk of future illness. With that, the concept of risk factors was born.[140]

The concept ushered in a shift in ideas about preventive care, which moved towards health promotion through lifestyle changes. Moreover, the concept of risk factors gave added weight to preventive care as a whole and opened people's eyes to the fact that one might have an illness without showing any symptoms.

Television, too, took up health-related topics. In January 1964, West Germany's publicly funded network Zweites Deutsches Fernsehen (Channel Two) began broadcasting the show *Gesundheitsmagazin Praxis* (*Health Praxis*) once a month. Its forty-five-minute episodes informed viewers about illnesses and health risks. The first episode on cancer ran in October 1964. In contrast to its cinematic predecessors, it dispensed with narrative, instead opting for a journalistic style that placed the mic in the hands of 'real' doctors and health experts. For example, Karl Heinrich Bauer, president of the University of Heidelberg, discussed the state of cancer research in front of the construction site of the oncology research centre. The show also asked 'everyday men on the street' their opinions (women were allowed to speak neither as experts nor as laypeople).

The episode focused on the early diagnosis of cancers of the female reproductive organs and on the early detection of lung cancer, which was a secondary part of the x-ray exams for tuberculosis that were still mandatory in a few of Germany's federal states. During the interviews, doctors emphasized the necessity of such screenings, while the producers chose not to illustrate the point with images of tumours. The male passers-by, in turn, stated that they only went to the doctor when they felt something was wrong and that they wanted to avoid having to constantly mistrust their own bodies, an attitude encapsulated in one's assertion: 'I'm only going to live once and I want to live my life how I feel is right.'[141] The episode proceeded to debunk as irrational this fixation on the 'right feeling'.

Such rhetorical finger-wagging came under fire only a few years later. Criticism was primarily spurred on from the 'outside', by the marketing departments that health officials were more frequently hiring as consultants and producers of their campaigns. A vivid example is the debate over a half-hour film commissioned by the Federal Centre for Health Education. Titled *Symphonie in G-Dur* (*Symphony in G Major*, 'G' standing for 'Gesundheit', i.e. 'health') and released in 1967, it was supposed to inform young people about the principles of a healthy lifestyle.

[140] Timmermann, 'Risikofaktoren'.

[141] 'Krebs ist heilbar wenn...', episode of the series *Gesundheitsmagazin Praxis* (ZDF), premiered on 2 October 1964.

The head of the registered association Landesausschuss für gesundheitliche Volksbelehrung Baden-Württemberg e. V. (State Commission for Health Education Baden-Württemberg) railed against the film because he believed it did not contain enough facts, which he thought sufficient grounds for not showing it in schools. The production company Leonaris Films countered that they wanted to avoid communicating knowledge with a raised index finger and thus opted against lectures by experts.[142]

Happiness, Health, and the Power of Good Feelings

Health education thus shifted towards speaking to people as equals and away from paternalistic gestures, a shift that political initiatives in the 1970s and 1980s had been demanding from their government more generally. In the 1980s, a broad movement started to demand that doctors treat patients like mature people capable of making decisions for themselves.[143] This did not mark a departure from the impetus to educate, since campaigners still wanted to incite people to go in for early detection screenings. However, in the run of the 1970s, preventive care and early detection were gradually advertised as something that the medical 'market' provided to informed 'consumers'. The concrete illness that was supposed to be prevented or detected faded into the background, a development that had multiple expressions and multiple causes.

Films, television shows, posters, presentations, and other visual media almost entirely ceased showing cancerous tumours. The painful images had become superfluous, since doctors were now able to diagnose many externally visible cancers much earlier. Consequently, fewer people with such advanced tumours were coming to the doctor for the first time. As the array of diagnostic tools expanded, first with the colposcopy, Pap smear, and endoscopy, and later with mammograms and PSA (prostate-specific antigen) tests, public health campaigns focused less on 'warning signs'. Instead, they encouraged people to get into the habit of regularly getting check-ups even if they had no symptoms, and particularly if they belonged to certain 'risk groups'.

However, this did not mean that images of cancer disappeared from public view. Beginning in the late 1960s, cancer was discussed with increasing frequency in magazines, which were seeing higher print runs and greater circulation. In contrast to the informative literature distributed by cancer awareness campaigns, magazines tended to publish the stories of people who had cancer. Even when

[142] Letter from Dr Schmidt, head of the state commission for health education Baden-Württemberg, to Director Hammer, Landesbildstelle, Baden, 3 November 1967, BArch B 310/18.

[143] Axel Schildt and Detlef Siegfried, *Deutsche Kulturgeschichte. Die Bundesrepublik—1945 bis zur Gegenwart* (Munich: Carl Hanser, 2009), 277–302.

magazines ran multi-part series on early detection measures, they foregrounded the experiences of those who had been through it. The magazines' illustrated stories also dispensed with images of tumours, replacing them with pictures of cancer patients that showed the side effects of therapy. Magazine features played a role in turning the hair loss caused by chemotherapy—which was becoming a more common form of treatment in the 1970s—into a symbol of cancer. Later on, the scars left behind by surgery, and in particular the markedly visible loss of a breast through mastectomy, fuelled criticisms of 'radical operations' that had been gaining volume since the 1970s. In 1993, this trend reached a highpoint when a self-portrait of photographer and model Matuschka (Joanne Motichka) appeared on the cover of *New York Times Magazine*. Titled 'Beauty Out of Damage', it showed her in a white dress that only covered one side of her torso. The other side revealed the scar left behind by her mastectomy. The photo attracted considerable attention in the Western world. It at once broke with taboos about what could be shown and discussed while denouncing a male-dominated medical system that, in Matuschka's eyes, was all too ready to maim women's bodies and then abandon them with the grief caused by the dismemberment. Later examinations convinced her that her mastectomy had been unnecessary and she sued her doctors for medical malpractice.[144] This shift in how cancer was depicted in public forums turned the effects of therapy into the real, openly visible 'symptom' of cancer, while unspoken rules in the world of publishing and public health campaigns gradually made printing images of tumours unacceptable.

These changes in publishing are indicative of a deeper caesura that brought together two connected developments. Health policy and theory moved its focus away from *illness prevention* and towards *health production*. At the same time, social norms and sociological discourse moved away from prioritizing increased productivity and began rallying around the new concept of 'quality of life'. The optimization of individual happiness implied a healthy body as well as personal and occupational success.[145] These trends converged in the notion that health and happiness do not just happen, but must be *produced* through individual effort guided by expert knowledge.

The most pronounced, long-lasting expression of this idea was salutogenesis, a concept coined in the late 1970s by Aaron Antonovsky, an Israeli-American sociologist of medicine. In the 1980s, it gradually gained acceptance in Germany, first in the West, then in the East. Antonovsky deduced the concept from a study that inquired into how some concentration camp prisoners had been

[144] Lerner, *The Breast Cancer Wars*, 271.

[145] Heiko Stoff, 'Franz Klose, Kiel: "Auch Glück ist kein Ersatz für Arbeit!" Das Projekt der Gesundheitsvorsorge als Pflicht zur Selbstoptimierung, 1930–1970', in *Rehabilitation und Prävention in Sport- und Medizingeschichte*, ed. Christine Wolters and Christian Becker (Münster: LIT, 2004), 186–8; Stefanie Duttweiler, *Sein Glück machen. Arbeit am Glück als neoliberale Regierungstechnologie* (Konstanz: UVK, 2007), 11–12.

able to retain their physical and mental health both during and after their captivity. He concluded that the deciding factors for remaining healthy were the individual's inner sense of coherence, the conviction that events are comprehensible and can be influenced by one's own actions, and the belief that one's own life has meaning.[146]

Since the 1970s, signs of the turn towards health, well-being, happiness, and quality of life had been popping up in different places. West Germany's efforts to motivate people to go to the doctor's office for cancer screenings followed this trend, even though they were, of course, about detecting a potentially fatal illness and not about actively bringing forth health. The decision to make Pap smears available to all women free of cost certainly contributed to the shift, because it was administered regardless of the presence of symptoms, which is to say, when women felt healthy. Moreover, advances in medicine made it easier to remove the pre-cancerous cells detected during a Pap smear without surgery, thus nipping cancer in the bud. With that, the line between early detection and preventive care in the strict sense began to blur.[147] As the number of women who suffered manifest forms of cervical cancer dropped starkly around the same time, the Pap test became considered evidence of the efficacy of early detection and was celebrated as a model of success in campaigns. However, the Pap smear only has limited value as a model, because almost all other methods of early detection necessitated more invasive treatments with more potential side effects when they uncovered cancerous cells. Moreover, the rates of cases of cervical cancer fell drastically because advances in medicine had made it possible to remove pre-cancerous cells; this was not true of most other types of cancer.[148]

But this divergence in case rates between different types of cancer was not yet perceptible when legislators changed West Germany's public health insurance in law—in existence since 1911—by creating a federal programme for the early detection of cancer. In July 1971, public health insurance began covering the costs of screenings for cervical cancer and breast cancer for women, prostate cancer for men, and skin and colon cancer for both.

For the first time in West Germany, public health officials tapped pollsters and advertisers to help design campaigns and evaluate their effectiveness. Awareness campaigns in the United States had been doing this since the end of the Second World War, when Mary Lasker started engaging for the American Society for the Control of Cancer, which until then had been run exclusively by doctors. Her husband was Albert Lasker, an advertising executive who had raked in riches with

[146] Aaron Antonovsky, *Salutogenese. Zur Entmystifizierung der Gesundheit* (Tübingen: DGVT, 1997).

[147] Löwy, *A Woman's Disease*, 90–1.

[148] The extent to which the lowered rate of illness was caused by the increased availability of Pap smears and the early detection programme remains a point of contention today. See Nikolaus Becker, 'Epidemiological Aspects of Cancer Screening in Germany', *Journal of Cancer Research and Clinical Oncology* 129, no. 12 (2003): 691–702, 695–6, https://doi.org/10.1007/s00432-003-0494-y.

his campaigns for Lucky Strike cigarettes in the 1930s and 1940s. Together, the couple helped restructure the organization, now called the American Cancer Society, and transformed its campaigns with modern advertising methods.[149] Doctors and health officials in West Germany initially viewed the American Cancer Society's campaigns as too aggressive and drastic to function in their country.[150] But West German society had, over time, become more liberal, more democratic, and more open to discussion. Opinion polling institutes like the Institut für Demoskopie Allensbach (founded in 1947) acquired more influence, because citizens had won a louder voice in political debates and, as patients and consumers of 'health', their preferences were taken more seriously.

When the federal government commissioned the public health insurers to collect data on participation rates in the early detection programme, though, they were troubled that demand fell well short of their great expectations. Men's participation was particularly disappointing. Less than 20 per cent of men over 45 took advantage of the free yearly screening for prostate, stomach, and colon cancer. The television show *Gesundheitsmagazin Praxis* even dedicated an episode to the question as to why men—and not, as was thought thirty years previously, women—were particularly disinclined to go in for a check-up. The episode featured the Federal Minister for Labour and Social Affairs, Walter Arendt, discussing the findings of a study that had been conducted by the television network itself.[151]

At the University of Heidelberg's department of occupational and social medicine, which played an important role in the previous chapter, researchers studied why men were less likely to submit to routine cancer screenings. Rolf Verres, a psychologist and medical doctor based at the university, concluded that fear made men into the 'problem children' of preventive care.[152] A series of surveys supported this finding by providing evidence that this trend had been caused by campaigns' use of 'real-life images' of cancer that invoked fear and stirred up anxiety. Accordingly, the advertising agencies hired as consultants by cancer awareness campaigns recommended that they wholly dispense with informing people about treatment, since it could remind people of such images.[153] While they wrote that fear should not necessarily be silenced, they advised that

[149] Lerner, *The Breast Cancer Wars*, 49–50.

[150] Circular 5/52 of the German Central Committee for Researching and Fighting Cancer, Braunschweig, 2 July 1952, BArch B 142/412, 148.

[151] 'Männer: Sorgenkinder der Vorsorge', episode of *Gesundheitsmagazin Praxis*, screened on 12 March 1973; Letter from the ZDF to Dr Hillebrand, Federal Ministry for Labor and Social Affairs, Mainz, 19 February 1973, BArch B 149/13375, 351–7.

[152] Rolf Verres, *Psychosoziale Faktoren der mangelnden Inanspruchnahme von Krebsfrüherkennungsuntersuchungen. Eine Interviewstudie mit 115 männlichen Patienten einer allgemeinärztlichen Praxis* (Frankfurt: Peter Lang, 1977).

[153] Cancer: Education, Early Detection, Prophylaxis. Foundations for the Development of a Pamphlet. Study conducted by Item, Institute for Market, Motive, and Advertising Research, commissioned by the Federal Centre for Health Education, sent on 29 August 1975, BArch B 310/764.

campaigns should not use fear to motivate people to act. Instead, they counselled campaigns to highlight that overcoming the illness was within reach, advice that was translated into the new slogan 'Klarheit für dich' (Clarity for you).[154]

Campaigns began printing images of familial happiness to confront the frightening images they assumed people harboured in their imaginations (Fig. 15). Pamphlets suggested that such happiness could only be attained when a person's feeling of health was validated by a doctor. Thus, campaigns redefined early detection screenings as a technique to produce happiness, not just to protect already existing happiness. Though the danger of illness did, of course, continue to loom, the campaigns sought to push into the background the connection between the screenings they were promoting and the possibility that those screenings might end up detecting a fatal disease.

Anti-smoking campaigns also turned away from fear and shocking images. In the late 1960s, they started becoming more prominent in East Germany, West Germany, and a plethora of other countries in both Eastern and Western Europe. Drawing people's attention to the carcinogenic properties of cigarette smoke had developed into a key priority of preventive health policy.[155]

With a particular focus on keeping young people from smoking, West Germany's anti-tobacco campaigns initially wielded frightening stories and imagery as their tools of preference. An especially drastic example of this device was the 1967 film *Der Tod gibt eine Party* (*Death Throws a Party*), commissioned by the Federal Ministry of Health. Nominally set in youth culture with a soundtrack comprised of popular music, the film does not spare on images of weakened limbs, withered skin, and tumours. East German campaigns also employed explicit images and sometimes even went all out in framing them as 'dares' for smokers. For instance, the narrator of the film *Rauch, der uns nicht kaltläßt* (*Smoke That Makes a Difference*) ominously warns: 'If you have tough nerves, then take a look at some of the consequences.' The camera then shows close-up shots of a smoker's leg being amputated—a procedure necessitated by tissue death caused by peripheral artery disease.

But anti-smoking and anti-substance abuse campaigns, too, started questioning the effectiveness of the strategy of evoking fear and 'finger wagging'. The leaders of the Dresden Hygiene Museum beat their West German counterparts to the chase in insisting that films and exhibitions on substance abuse have a 'positive' tone. An internal paper from 1975 on an anti-smoking programme in the works maintained: 'The exclusive focus on negative consequences, and above all fomenting fear with serious illnesses, has proven ineffective. It would be better to foreground positive motivators like athletic ability, strength, and mental toughness, the

[154] Informative material of the health insurers on early detection and prophylaxis for cancer and children, gathered by the Ministry for Labor and Social Affairs, 1973, BArch B 149/13376, 49–114.

[155] Roeßiger, 'Krebskampagnen', 29.

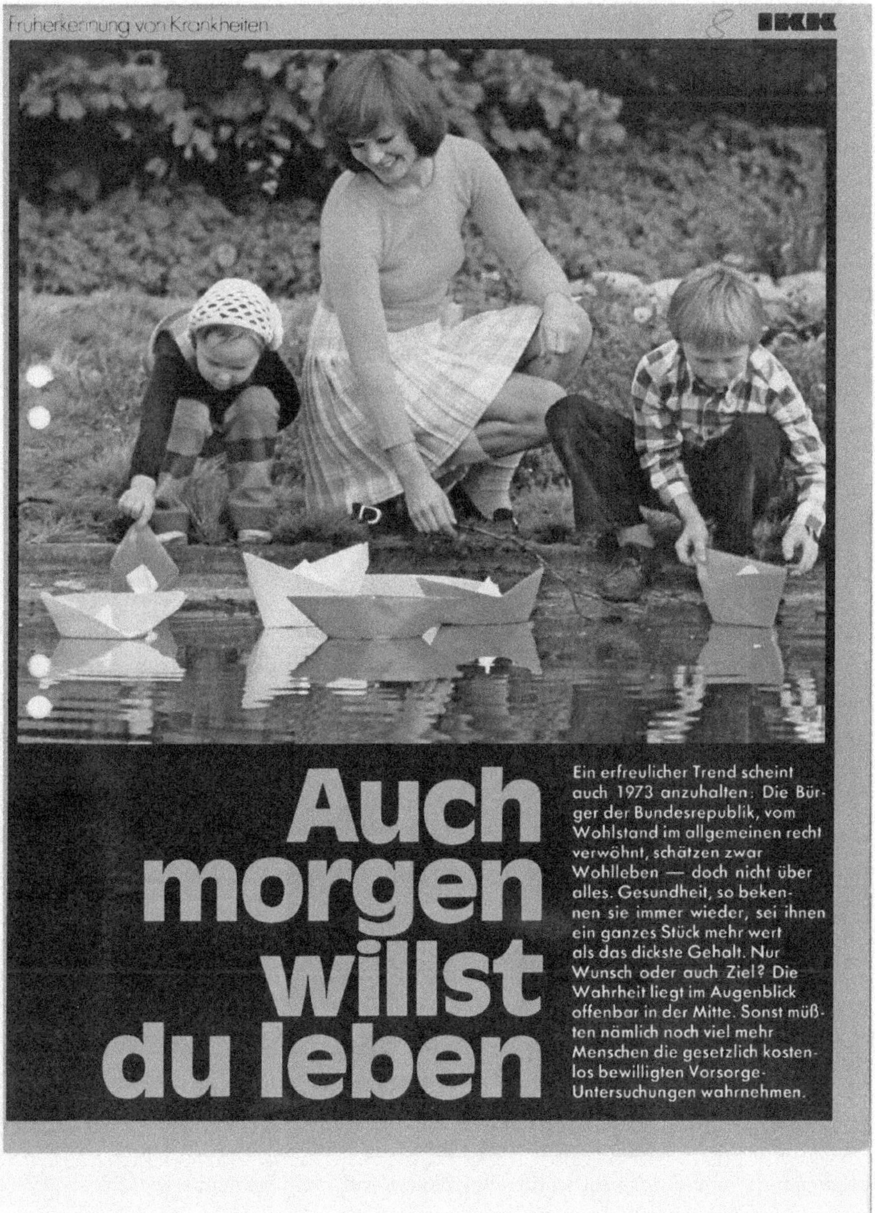
Früherkennung von Krankheiten
IKK
Auch morgen willst du leben
Ein erfreulicher Trend scheint auch 1973 anzuhalten: Die Bürger der Bundesrepublik, vom Wohlstand im allgemeinen recht verwöhnt, schätzen zwar Wohlleben — doch nicht über alles. Gesundheit, so bekennen sie immer wieder, sei ihnen ein ganzes Stück mehr wert als das dickste Gehalt. Nur Wunsch oder auch Ziel? Die Wahrheit liegt im Augenblick offenbar in der Mitte. Sonst müßten nämlich noch viel mehr Menschen die gesetzlich kostenlos bewilligten Vorsorge-Untersuchungen wahrnehmen.

Fig. 15 Illustration from *Auch morgen willst Du leben* (*You'll Still Want to Live Tomorrow*), pamphlet published by the IKK, one of Federal Republic of Germany's public health insurance corporations.

preservation of a youthful, fresh complexion, increased financial freedom by the money saved, etc., thus using for a positive purpose young people's need to conform.'[156] Discussions about a new episode of the East German cartoon series *Kundi*—named after its main character, who also served as the Dresden health museum's mascot—would make clear the degree to which those involved in public health wanted to stop showing the physical effects of smoking and abandon the old strategy of fear.

The 1985 synopsis of the episode—planned, but never produced—described an adaptation of *Little Red Riding Hood* in which the wolf is a smoker. Kundi has to coax the wolf to smoke in order to get rid of him. The film was then supposed to show how the wolf gets hooked and is so enamoured with smoking that he forgets to eat. His coat becomes grizzly and shabby and he becomes so weak that when he tries to pounce at Kundi, he misses and smashes into a tree, which kills him.[157]

The film *Der Siebente* (*The Seventh*) took a different tack. An adaptation of *Snow White and the Seven Dwarves*, the film revolves around the smallest dwarf; a clumsy fellow who does everything wrong and is distrusted by the other dwarves. In his struggle for recognition, he falls prey to the wiles of the evil stepmother, who convinces him to start smoking in order to appear older. But the plan fails. When danger comes, though, he sees through the stepmother, overcomes his fears, and rescues Snow White, winning the long-sought recognition from the others. Satisfied, he pitches the now superfluous pack of cigarettes.[158]

The strategy of using positive images and qualities to sell a product was derived from psychological research on advertising. Anti-smoking campaigns in both Germanys seized on it, marketing their product—a smoke-free lifestyle—as the choice made by mature, courageous people. They hired celebrities, and in particular athletes, whose rejection of smoking was brought into association with their mastery of their sport.[159]

They made not smoking and getting screened for signs of cancer seem like another station on the fitness trails that the West German Sportbund (Sport Federation) had constructed around the country in the 1970s. Though most of the trails had fallen into disrepair by the 1980s, fitness became ever trendier. Proponents tied fitness to wellness and exercise to endorphin-driven happiness. Cancer awareness campaigns, too, now adopted for themselves the notion that one should care for one's own body almost as if it had its own subjectivity. For example, in the late 1990s, the Berufsverband der Frauenärzte (Professional Association of Gynaecologists) together with the women's tabloid *Brigitte*, the

[156] Drafts for a five-minute film on the topic 'youth and tobacco abuse', 30 June 1975, HSTA D 13658, FV, vol. 2, no. 23, 362.

[157] Exposé for a film commissioned by the German Hygiene Museum (Kundi, the Nonsmoker) with the working title: 'Das Märchen vom rauchenden Wolf' (The Fairy Tale of the Smoking Wolf), 15 March 1985, HSTA D 13658, F VIII, no. 14.

[158] Film *Der Siebente*, 13 minutes, DHMD 2001/1669.

[159] Roeßiger, 'Bildappell', 103 and 95.

Deutsche Krebshilfe (German Cancer Aid), and the Deutscher Ärztinnenbund (German Association of Women Doctors) published a booklet intended to motivate women to examine their breasts every month. Rather than shock readers with death and tumours, it elaborated:

> The breasts play a decisive role in a woman's self-image. A woman who likes her breasts shows them more loving attention than a woman who dislikes her breasts for whatever reason. And thus, the early detection of breast cancer has to do with the emotion that a woman feels towards her body.... You should consciously feel for changes in the breast. And get used to enjoying touching your breasts: in the shower or in the bath, when applying lotion.[160]

Whether this kind of self-screening routine really produced a positive body image over the long term was, however, publicly called into question early on. The main point of contention was less the concern about the potential psychological damage it could cause and more the lingering doubts about its medical usefulness.

Towards the end of the 1970s, criticisms of West Germany's 'finger-wagging' approach piled on. They were aimed not so much at the paternalistic moralism represented by it, but at the raised index finger as a symbol of a particular type of early detection. After the above discussed 1971 law provided free annual prostate exams for all men over 45, the West German association of urologists turned the raised index finger into the symbol of their campaigns. As professor of urology Carl-Erich Alken stated, the doctor's index finger, a two-cent rubber glove, and three minutes were all that were needed to detect a potential carcinoma in a man's prostate. He described the organ as a 'ticking time bomb' for men over 50.[161] But if a urologist found a lump, a biopsy could determine whether it was cancer and, in case it was, whether it could be operated on or irradiated at an early stage, thus drastically increasing the chances of cure.

Yet despite this optimistic outlook, the number of men who went in for prostate exams remained low. Only 12 per cent of eligible men went to their urologist in 1971 and, in 1972, it was only 11 per cent.[162] While psychologists like the aforementioned Rolf Verres placed the blame on men's repression of deep-seated fears of cancer, a guest on the 21 September 1978 episode of the talk show *III nach neun* (*III after Nine*) posited, perhaps to the surprise of many, that the men who refused the exam

[160] Professional association of gynaecologists in cooperation with *Brigitte*, German Cancer Aid, and the German Association of Female Doctors, 'Aus der Praxis' 15, *Brustkrebs-Früherkennung*, DHMD 2001/1598.

[161] 'Neue Richtung', *Der Spiegel* 9 (1978): 206–10.

[162] Batelle-Institut, *Krankheitsfrüherkennung Krebs. Frauen und Männer. Aufbereitung und Interpretation der Untersuchungsergebnisse aus den gesetzlichen Früherkennungsmaßnahmen 1972. Bericht des Batelle-Instituts e.V., Frankfurt, Leiter des Vorhabens: Eckart Herwig, für das Zentralinstitut für die kassenärztliche Versorgung in der Bundesrepublik Deutschland* (Cologne: Batelle-Institut, 1975), 20.

were doing the right thing. On live television, Dr Julius Hackethal advised his 'fellow men': 'When you see a urologist, run away as fast as you can!'

Moderator Dr Marianne Koch, a long-time actor who had just completed her medical studies, was speechless. But the guest's controversial views were not unknown to her when she invited him onto the show. In the years before the show, Hackethal had gained media attention with his attacks on academic medicine, Germany's health insurance system, and conventional surgical practices; he had tried to take a few surgeons to court and lambasted medical doctors as arrogant and inhumane. An experienced orthopaedist and surgeon and former head doctor of the hospital in Lauenburg, Hackethal drew an audience because he knew the 'system' from the inside and presented himself as a person knowledgeable of American research. He proved his earnestness in 1974, when he quit his job as head doctor and renounced his licence to accept payments from Germany's public health insurers in order to be able to treat patients in his private practice as he saw fit.

Hackethal's statements on the talk show were the first salvo in his ensuing offensive against early detection screenings, which found exceptional resonance in the media. Nearly all daily newspapers reported on it, and *Der Spiegel* published a four-part series with selections from Hackethal's bestseller *Keine Angst vor Krebs* (*Don't Be Afraid of Cancer*). Hackethal's critique had three components. First, he doubted that the available early detection methods could provide a reliable diagnosis. Second, he believed that they could contribute to or even cause metastasis. Third, he railed against the serious side effects and complications that often followed out of cancer treatment, which he found all the more egregious because of his belief that the illness could not be diagnosed with certainty.

The choice of prostate cancer to exemplify his issues with early detection exams in general was not a coincidence. Scepticism towards prostate exams was more widely shared among doctors than, say, towards Pap smears. Moreover, treating prostate cancer almost always ended in impotence. In a time when sexuality was increasingly being discussed in public, this side effect grabbed people's attention.

In his 1978 book, Hackethal implored his readers to have no fear of cancer, because most cases of cancer were harmless 'house pet cancers', as he put it, that did not interrupt daily life and rarely developed into 'predator cancers'. He supported the claim with epidemiologists' findings of large discrepancies between case numbers and death rates for prostate cancer. Hackethal's star witness was Willet F. Whitmore, head urologist at the renowned Memorial Sloan Kettering Cancer Centre in New York. In 1963, Whitmore had asserted that 'many more individuals . . . die with prostatic cancer than of it'.[163] Hackethal continued that a

[163] Willet F. Whitmore, Jr, 'The Rationale and Results of Ablative Surgery for Prostatic Cancer', *Cancer* 16, no. 9: 1119–32. Hackethal quoted Whitmore in the fourth instalment of the *Spiegel* series, though he gave the wrong page number (119 instead of 1119); see Julius Hackethal, '"Keine Angst vor Krebs". Gefahren der Vorsorgeuntersuchung—Modellfall Prostata (IV)', *Der Spiegel* 44 (1978): 206–17, 216.

pathologist or histologist looking through a microscope could not distinguish cells afflicted by 'house pet cancer' from those afflicted by 'predator cancer'. And, he remonstrated, equating cancer cells in a biopsy with cancer itself was a highly questionable undertaking. The pinnacle of his argument flipped the logic of early detection and risk factor analysis on its head: 'A person with a cancerous tumour is not sick with cancer so long as he feels healthy. Further, he may only be counted among those at risk of becoming sick if it can be proven with correct scientific methods that his quality of life or duration of life will, with high probability, be negatively affected in the foreseeable future.'[164] The fact that a degree of uncertainty was involved in diagnosing cancer was something that had never before been communicated to a general audience, even though medical experts had been discussing the issue ever since histopathological early detection methods had been in use, as was touched on in the above discussion of the Pap smear.

Because less invasive forms of treatment were available for cervical cancer, gynaecologists were generally willing to accept a degree of diagnostic uncertainty. But Hackethal was not the only one who thought that deciding to treat prostate cancer warranted more discretion, because whether it was operated on or irradiated, treatment caused many men to lose their potency, and incontinence was another by no means uncommon side effect. Hormone therapy and the surgical removal or irradiation of the testicles often led to feminization, which was sometimes countered with further radiation or risky, potentially carcinogenic hormone supplements. These side effects were well known, and doctors informed patients about them before proceeding, but they generally tried to justify the risks with the argument that prostate cancer, beyond being especially aggressive and possibly fatal, could lead to an extraordinarily painful death because it often metastasized to the bones.

Hackethal did not dispute that dying of prostate cancer could be very painful, and he thought that hormone therapy was an acceptable form of pain management for advanced cases of prostate cancer. But he criticized the use of these therapies when the carcinoma could only be detected through histopathology, because he believed that such cases would rarely develop into deadly forms of prostate cancer. What bothered doctors most of all, however, was his claim that early detection methods and early treatments could make cancer 'go wild' and thus harboured significant risks in itself. He created his own graphics on how biopsies worked in order to convince his readers that they 'loosened up' the cellular structure of the carcinoma, allowing cancer cells to flow into the blood stream and lymphatic vessels, thus opening the flood gates to metastases elsewhere.

As evidence, he referenced a statistical fact that was, indeed, hard for epidemiologists to explain. Since cost-free prostate exams had been made available by the

[164] Hackethal, '"Keine Angst vor Krebs" ... (IV)', 215–16.

1971 law, the death rate for prostate cancer had climbed slowly, yet steadily. Hackethal interpreted this as a clear sign that it was the exam itself that caused cases of harmless 'house pet cancer' to mutate into 'predator cancer'.[165]

All of Hackethal's arguments were officially rejected by the Federal Chamber of Medical Doctors and the guidelines for early detection were not changed.[166] Some urologists and other doctors condemned him as incompetent, because as an 'expert of surgery of the musculoskeletal system and the spine', he had no clue about the treatment of the prostate and cancer. Professor of urology Herbert Klosterhalfen maligned him as a 'psychopath', and Hackethal returned the favour.[167] But public discussion of the potential shortcomings of early detection exams was now out of the barn. All over the country, surgeons and urologists were interviewed for their opinions. Even more astonishing was that Hackethal's criticisms occasioned Manfred Steinbach, the undersecretary at the Federal Ministry of Health responsible for early detection, to request that the non-governmental Bundesärztekammer (Federal Chamber of Medical Doctors) state their position on the matter. The chamber's scientific committee obliged: at a press conference, they publicly denounced Hackethal's claims.[168] Thus, the early detection programme remained unchanged. However, it was the first time that a medical doctor had publicly raised doubts about the utility of early detection exams in a language comprehensible by all. And a closer look at the affair reveals that a number of less belligerent doctors expressed agreement with some of Hackethal's points.

For instance, Ernst Krokowski, head of the x-ray institute and radiotherapy clinic at Kassel's city hospital, gave a talk at the 1977 Deutscher Röntgenkongress (German Radiology Convention) on his doubts about early diagnosis and treatment of prostate cancer. In an interview with *Der Spiegel*, he criticized the Federal Chamber of Medical Doctors' denunciation of Hackethal's talk-show statements, arguing that the scientific committee's claim that prostate exams were clearly

[165] Julius Hackethal, '"Keine Angst vor Krebs". Gefahren der Vorsorgeuntersuchung—Modellfall Prostata (III)', *Der Spiegel* 43 (1978): 204–18, 214. The most recent calculations show that the death rate for prostate cancer climbed after 1970, but as before, conjectures about the causes diverge. Since the 1990s, the death rate has slowly fallen, while incidence rates have continued to climb. The incidence and mortality rates of breast cancer have undergone a similar development. See Jörg Haberland and Ute Wolf, 'Trendanalysen zur Inzidenz und Mortalität an Krebs in Deutschland seit 1970', *GMS Medizinische Informatik, Biometrie und Epidemiologie* 11, no. 1 (2015): 1–10, 3–4, https://doi.org/10.3205/mibe000159. Accordingly, recent studies have concluded that early detection through digital rectal examination has not reduced the prostate cancer mortality rate. See Becker, 'Epidemiological Aspects', 693.

[166] Bundesärztekammer, 'Stellungnahme des Wissenschaftlichen Beirates der Bundesärztekammer, Das Prostatakarzinom. Vorsorge—Früherkennung—Diagnose—Therapie', *Deutsches Ärzteblatt* 75, no. 42 (1978): 2413–16.

[167] '"Schuster, bleib bei deinem Leisten" (Gespräch mit dem amerikanischen Urologen Willard Goodwin)', *Der Stern* 48 (1978): 266–9; Herbert Klosterhalfen, '"Hackethal ist ein leichtfertiger Schwätzer". Der Hamburger Urologie-Professor Herbert Klosterhalfen zur Kontroverse um Professor Hackethal', *Der Spiegel* 44 (1978): 220–3.

[168] See Bundesärztekammer, 'Stellungnahme'.

effective partially contradicted the findings of their own research.[169] In contrast, Hans-Georg Wolters, undersecretary of the Federal Ministry for Youth, Family, and Health, lambasted Hackethal's ideas as 'unserious' in January 1979 on a ZDF (public television) programme called *Vorsicht Arzt—Hackethal und die Folgen* (*Be Cautious of the Doctor—The Hackethal Controversy and Its Consequences*). Hackethal sued the federal government to prohibit all federal employees from making such claims and won the case. The government appealed, but the court of appeals in Düsseldorf refused to hear it on the grounds that while Hackethal's criticisms did not harmonize with medical consensus, he had supported his claims with a sufficient number of scientific findings.[170] This 'judgement like a punch in the face', as the tabloid *Die Bunte* put it, bolstered scepticism towards early detection exams over the long term and the press began running more critical reports on them.[171]

But most people distinguished between different types of early detection measures and drew their own conclusions about their pros and cons. While the number of eligible men who went in for a prostate exam continued to hover around 15 per cent even into the late 1980s, 55 per cent of the considerably greater number of eligible women visited their gynaecologist for a Pap test at least once every two years.[172] Data on colonoscopies demonstrate that this gap was not just a matter of women being more 'cautious' than men. In the early 1980s, more women took advantage of the free exam—25 per cent of women and only 15 per cent of men—but the discrepancy was not nearly as major.[173] Moreover, the number of women who underwent early detection exams at the gynaecologist's office climbed considerably after 1971, while the number of men who got prostate exams hardly went up. In the 1990s, after German Reunification, the numbers did not change much.

Many factors might help explain all this, among them the fact that visiting the gynaecologist became routine for many women after the invention of the pill, while men lacked a comparable experience of becoming 'habituated' to going to the urologist. Certainly, another contributing factor were the ongoing debates over the utility and dangers of prostate exams, while Pap smears are generally accepted as effective and safe.[174]

169 Ernst Krokowski, '"Mit zweierlei Maß gemessen". Professor Ernst Krokowski über den Streit um die SPIEGEL-Serie zur Krebsvorsorge', *Der Spiegel* 46 (1978): 271–73.

170 OLG Düsseldorf, 'Rechtsweg gegen ehrverletzende Äußerungen eines Behördenvertreters', *Archiv für Presserecht* 17, no. 1 (1980): 46–9.

171 Peter Schmidsberger, 'Ein Urteil wie ein Paukenschlag', *Die Bunte* 3 (1980): 84–5.

172 Becker, 'Epidemiological Aspects', 693, 696, and 698. 173 Ibid., 697.

174 Lennarth Nyström, Ingvar Andersson, Nils Bjurstam, Jan Frisell, Bo Nordenskjöld, and Lars Erik Rutqvist, 'Long-Term Effects of Mammography Screening: Updated Overview of the Swedish Randomised Trials', *Lancet* 359, no. 9310 (2002): 909–19, https://doi.org/10.1016/S0140-6736(02)08020%960; Odette Wegwarth, 'Medizinische Risikokommunikation: Nutzen und Schaden transparent kommunizieren', *Forum: Das Offizielle Magazin der Deutschen Krebsgesellschaft e. V.* 30,

At the end of the nineteenth century, cervical cancer threw Theodor Storm's fictional doctor into such despair that he thought he had no other option but to end his wife's life. Over a century later, cervical cancer has become much rarer in Germany (and in other Western European countries and North America) and the chances of curing it much greater.[175] This development doubtless played a role in the broadscale embrace of the logic of early detection and routine check-ups not only among doctors and policymakers, but also among laypeople. A long history led up to the perception that 'preventive' doctors' visits meant taking responsibility for one's own health and happiness, while the concern that they might end in being diagnosed with cancer faded into the background. The efforts of doctors, policymakers, and health insurers to promote a positive image of early detection exams did their part, as did the success of Pap smears in enabling doctors to remove 'pre-cancerous cells' with minimally invasive measures. The result of this century-long historical process is that health is no longer understood as subjectively 'feeling good'. At the same time, since the late 1970s, discussions in West Germany—and, after 1990, unified Germany—have explored the deficiencies of certain early detection screenings. Undisputed is that early detection has altered the general perception of cancer and risk factors.

Universal provision of prostate exams triggered the discussion because the available treatments—in contrast to those available for early-stage cervical cancer—were associated with detrimental side effects. In particular, the risk of causing impotence generated an emotionally charged reaction to the issue. Overdiagnosis and overtreatment continue to be topics of study and debate in Germany today. Sometimes, Hackethal's coinage 'house pet cancer' is even used without quotation marks to describe clinically inconspicuous forms of 'cancer' that grow so slowly that they rarely become fatal.[176] They often precede suspected cases of prostate or thyroid cancer, and medical practice has now switched towards 'watchful waiting', similar to the general approach to 'abnormal' Pap smears. The consequence is that the patient has to go in regularly to have their prostate, thyroid, or cervix examined, in some cases for the rest of their lives. However, the question that arises out of the entire early detection debate is: What does being healthy feel like?

no. 3 (2015): 208–13, https://doi.org/10.1007/s12312-015-1303-7; Hal R. Arkes and Wolfgang Gaissmaier, 'Psychological Research and the Prostate Cancer Screening Controversy', *Psychological Science* 23, no. 6 (2012): 547–53, https://doi.org/10.1177/0956797612437428.

[175] Sixty-nine per cent of women in Germany diagnosed with invasive cervical cancer survive for five years after the diagnosis. In absolute terms, that means that roughly 1,600 women die of the illness annually. See Robert-Koch-Institut, 'Gebärmutterhalskrebs (Zervixkarzinom)', Zentrum für Krebsregisterdaten, http://www.krebsdaten.de/Krebs/DE/Content/Krebsarten/Gebaermutterhalskrebs/gebaermutterhalskrebs_node.html. In many countries in Africa, Asia, and Latin America, however, high numbers of women continue to die of cervical cancer. See Löwy, *A Woman's Disease*, 155–75.

[176] Hartmut Wewetzer, 'Schilddrüsenkrebs. Die Ultraschall-Epidemie', *Der Tagesspiegel*, 24 February 2016, http://www.tagesspiegel.de/wissen/schilddruesenkrebs-die-ultraschall-epidemie/13006716.html.

4
Talking about Cancer

> Illness is the night-side of life, a more onerous citizenship. Everyone who is born holds dual citizenship, in the kingdom of the well and in the kingdom of the sick. Although we all prefer to use only the good passport, sooner or later each of us is obliged, at least for a spell, to identify ourselves as citizens of that other place.[1]

Monday, March 6. Franziska has an appointment with one of the clinic's oncologists in the late afternoon.... She seems very composed, very strong. I am without a doubt much more distressed and panicked than she is.

There are many reasons for Franziska's calm.... The situation is not totally foreign to her. She already experienced all of this eighteen years ago. Of course, she knows that her current situation is much worse. But she also knows what to expect; it is not like everything is dissolving into a kind of nebulous horror before her very eyes....

The oncologist who Franziska meets with alone on March 6—she didn't want any family members with her—tells her bluntly that there is no hope, none, 'not with this condition'. She would have to begin a combination of chemotherapy and radiotherapy immediately. Then, the doctor said, the tumour in her colon would have to be removed surgically, which would do nothing more than briefly delay the inevitable. The metastases on her lung were inoperable, making survival for any longer than a short period impossible anyways, because the only way to prolong her life for any time worth mentioning would have been to operate on the metastases. Thus, chemotherapy was the only option, but it, too, would only be effective for a very limited period of time. Then her life would be over. Probably before the end of the year. And the months leading up to it would be horrible.

My sister is, as she later recounted, totally numbed. She falls into a state of shock. It is not just what the doctor said, but how she says it. She shoots out the bad news with the hammering staccato of a machine gun and seems totally unaffected. My sister is just an item on her to-do list that has to be crossed off. Nothing more.

Franziska feels as if she is sitting not in a doctor's office, but in front of a firing squad. When she is able to speak again, she says: 'I have children. My daughter is only two years old.'

'That doesn't change anything', the doctor says.

[1] Susan Sontag, *Illness as Metaphor*, 3.

> *... Franziska gets up, says thanks. She has already begun staying at the clinic because they have planned to do the chemotherapy there. She returns to her room, calls home. Her mother picks up—and she begins to scream. Without saying anything. She just screamed.*

Author Charlotte Link was describing the moment when her sister Franziska learned the details about her diagnosis with 'metastasized colon cancer'.[2]

On the morning before the appointment, Link recalls, her sister was still a calm and collected woman, resolved to not give up the fight against her illness. In the evening after, her sister was in the grips of fear of death, panicked, even after nurses rushed in to sedate her with lorazepam. The shock induced by the doctor telling her the naked 'truth' was no temporary state. Although the oncologist's predictions did not come true and she did not die a painful death a few months later, she had to take anti-anxiety medication for the rest of her life. She died six years later, not of cancer, but of pulmonary fibrosis caused by radiotherapy that she had undergone as a young woman to treat Hodgkin's lymphoma.[3] In Charlotte Link's eyes, the doctor's brusque communication of diagnosis and prognosis destroyed not only her sister's hope at that moment, but also her *ability* to hope at all. This, Link asserted, irreparably shattered her sister's inner constitution.

In 2016, around 492,000 people were diagnosed with cancer in Germany.[4] Almost all learned about their diagnosis from their doctor. Many of these talks had an atmosphere totally different from the coolness that defined Franziska's experience. Not all doctors tell their patients about their chances of survival with such mechanical matter-of-factness. Many people diagnosed with cancer do not die from it. After completing treatment, they live for years without symptoms and die from something unrelated. But Franziska's experience is not unique, either. It is an instance of the 'detached' style of communicating diagnoses that has been criticized for years by medical ethicists, patients, and their loved ones. In 2001, journalist Peter Tautfest of the German newspaper *taz* described his recent diagnosis with non-small-cell lung carcinoma, which, statistically speaking, has a particularly low survival rate. His doctor, too, spoke unsparingly: 'Four months [of survival] are a lot with this disease.' Looking back at the talk, Tautfest wrote: 'Dr Krajewski belongs to a new generation of doctors who have learned not to hide the truth from their patients. He speaks dispassionately, directly, pitilessly, and without circumlocution; indeed, even a bit brashly.'[5]

[2] Charlotte Link, *Sechs Jahre. Der Abschied von meiner Schwester* (Munich: Blanvalet, 2014), 47–51.

[3] Ibid., 48. Lorazepam, a benzodiazepine, is highly addictive both mentally and physically. Franziska Link thus might have become dependent on Tavor after taking it to quell her anxiety over a long period of time.

[4] https://www.krebsinformationsdienst.de/tumorarten/grundlagen/krebsstatistiken.php.

[5] Peter Tautfest, 'Ich habe Krebs', *taz* 6461, 2 June 2001, 1001–2, http://www.taz.de/1/archiv/?dig=2001/06/02/a0274.

Werner Bartens, journalist with the *Süddeutsche Zeitung*, thinks this trend oversteps a boundary. When a doctor curtly executes his duty to inform his patient without any attempt to empathize, Bartens asserts, the hard-fought ideal of the autonomous patient devolves into a caricature of freedom.[6] Medical ethicist Giovanni Maio followed a similar line of argumentation in 2009: 'It is not ethically responsible to view people with severe illness as solo bearers of freedom, because if one exclusively insists on preserving autonomy, one would leave seriously ill people in particular all alone with their freedom. In such cases, the exclusive emphasis on freedom without caring engagement is a disguised form of indifference that disregards the central importance of understanding and helping.'[7] Maio situates this in the broader context of the economization of medicine, in which the healthcare system treats patients as freely choosing consumers of medical services. This economistic understanding of freedom, he elucidates, has usurped older concepts of autonomy, personal responsibility, and truthfulness, which had different meanings in medicine in the past.

The story of American intellectual Susan Sontag demonstrates this shift with poignancy. In 1978, her book *Illness as Metaphor* gained canonical status in the movement to name cancer for what it is and dispense with metaphors. As she argued, metaphors sugar-coat or conceal the gravity of the illness and surreptitiously burden the patient with a moral stigma that compounds their pain. Sontag's essay drew on her personal experience. In 1975, she had been diagnosed with breast cancer. The treatment lasted three years. Thirty years later, she died of leukaemia. When her doctor told her about this new cancer in 2004, he used the kind of direct language she had called for in her essay. But, as Sontag's son David Rieff would explain, he expressed no empathy with her. He expounded on the illness and her prognosis as if he were holding a lecture on the topic. Neither Sontag nor her son interrupted him, even though they found his comportment and word choice jarring.[8] Perhaps Sontag felt helpless not just because she was personally affected, but because she had—allegedly—provided some legitimation for the doctor's behaviour. Her intentions in her essay were different, and her ideas about what it meant to be transparent, open, and truthful when talking about cancer diverged wholly from the doctor's.

This thread in Susan Sontag's biography suggests that, since the late 1970s, support for speaking about cancer has converged with concepts of autonomy and truthfulness and has thus become something like a morally unquestionable

[6] Werner Bartens, 'Grenzen der Aufklärung. Die Illusion vom mündigen Patienten: Warum das Arzt-Patienten-Gespräch über eine Krebs-Diagnose oft misslingt', *Süddeutsche Zeitung* 67, no. 255, 5/6 November 2011, 24.

[7] Giovanni Maio, 'Und wo bleibt die Zuwendung? Zur Entpersonalisierung der Arzt-Patient-Beziehung in der modernen Medizin', *Der Onkologe* 15, no. 10 (2009): 972–9, 976, https://doi.org/10.1007/s00761-009-1693-1.

[8] David Rieff, *Swimming in a Sea of Death: A Son's Memoir*, 2nd edn (New York: Simon and Schuster, 2009), 6–11.

principle. Every critic of how some doctors speak about cancer is seemingly obliged to emphasize that, of course, nobody wants to return to 'the paternalism of doctors who make decisions without consulting the patient', which made cancer 'taboo among those afflicted'.[9]

This refusal to look back is informed by a specific interpretation of history, which holds that, well into the 1970s, doctors generally withheld cancer diagnoses from patients. Without their knowledge or consent, this reading goes, they were just acted upon. Consequently, they had to live their final years entangled in a web of deception and lies, often spun with the participation of relatives aware of their diagnosis. As the taboo was arduously dismantled bit by bit, the story goes, cancer patients were finally able to speak openly and honestly with their loved ones about their potentially fatal illness. They won the right to decide, as informed patients, what kind of treatment they were willing to undergo and how active a role they wanted to take in trying to beat their cancer. The unambiguous knowledge of having cancer enabled all patients to look at their life at the edge of death, so that being diagnosed with cancer could sometimes be grasped as a chance at a new beginning and a better life.

I do not want to question the basic outlines of this story. However, current developments make clear that the history of 'being diagnosed with cancer' should not be told as a straightforward story of liberation from the conventions of paternalistic dishonesty. This chapter will show that the break with silence did not occur as radically and suddenly as many in the 1980s thought they were witnessing. Because withholding information was not universal before then, and openly discussing was not universal after. Most importantly, the justifications for and logic behind remaining silent or speaking openly shifted in the run of the twentieth century.

Emotions played a crucial part in discussions on 'truthfulness with the patient', a fact that has often been overlooked because of the longstanding focus on paternalism and autonomy. What hope is, what it means, and what it depends on; whether and why it is necessary—all these questions were of enormous significance for the shift towards the general tendency to inform patients of their diagnosis. But other emotions that might run counter to, supplement, or take the place of hope also shaped the debate. What remains without hope? Just hopelessness and despair? Or does the rejection of hope open the way for courage and the assertion of self-worth? Who can handle the truth? Who must confront the truth? Everybody? Or only the brave or the faithful; the clever or perhaps just the simpler minds; men or women; people in positions of responsibility or authority? Were doctors' emotions significant? And which ones? How did the

[9] Bartens, 'Grenzen der Aufklärung'; Christa Wolf, 'Cancer and Society', in *Parting from Phantoms: Selected Writings, 1990–1994*, trans. Jan van Heurck (Chicago: Chicago University Press, 1997), 89–108, 93.

decision for or against 'truthfulness' influence the emotional relationship between doctors, nurses, patients, and their loved ones, and how did it impact trust?

These questions demonstrate that what is at stake here is not just theoretical—not just a matter of medical ethics, theology, philosophy, or law. The decision to tell a patient that they have cancer, how and what to tell them, or to conceal it from them altogether, is a decision with consequences that resonate far beyond the face-to-face meeting with the doctor. After all, if doctors cannot use the word 'cancer', then what to call clinics where cancer patients are treated? How should patients be convinced to undergo dangerous treatments associated with grave side effects and complications? How to employ methods well-known as treatments for cancer without arousing suspicions? And how to talk about emotions when the decisive matter has to be swept under the rug? All of this gives rise to a complicated historiographical question: How can a historian learn something about the emotions of a cancer patient if speaking or writing about the diagnosis was proscribed during their lifetime? How can a historian tell if the person sick with cancer might perhaps have had a notion about what they were suffering from—a notion about which they, too, may not have spoken, just as they may have remained silent about the emotions they felt about their situation?

Cancer, Taboo, and the Death of a Kaiser

Many history books for German schools mention cancer at least once: in 1888, Friedrich III, the '99-day Kaiser', died of laryngeal cancer. His brief rule made him an insignificant emperor, a sort of interregnum between the reigns of two Kaisers whose time in power fundamentally shaped the history of the German Empire. Before him, his father Wilhelm I ascended the throne to become the king of Prussia in 1858 and, in 1871, the first emperor of the German Empire. After him, his son Wilhelm II assumed the role of emperor, remaining in office until his abdication in 1918. Many historians discuss Friedrich III in connection with the hopes that liberals placed in him, hopes that were abruptly dashed by his cancer. In the years before being crowned emperor, he had shown an affinity for liberal politicians, arousing expectations that his reign as Kaiser might mark a turn away from the conservative policies of his elderly father.[10]

Because he was perceived as the harbinger of a new political era and his father's life was clearly coming to an end, his health problems attracted immediate public attention when they became known in the spring of 1887. Thus, Friedrich III's 'health report' developed into the first case of cancer covered extensively by the German media. Debates on the potential political consequences of his diagnosis

[10] Frank Lorenz Müller, *Der 99-Tage-Kaiser: Friedrich III. von Preußen—Prinz, Monarch, Mythos* (Munich: Siedler Verlag, 2013).

stood in the foreground, which structured the narrative of Friedrich's 'case' with a specific logic that did not apply to others.

Similar to other, less public cases, the opinions of his doctors and family members played a significant role in Friedrich's. But in contrast to the case histories of less prominent patients, many of those engaged with Friedrich's illness wrote down their thoughts, emotions, and reactions, even if it was often with the intention of defending themselves against accusations or supporting their criticisms of others. Public reporting on Friedrich's health during the last year of his life revealed details about an individual case of cancer in a manner previously unknown to open, public discussion. The elaborate chronicling did not end with his death. It devolved into a bitter controversy—shot through with nationalist sentiments—about whether the diagnosis was correct and the treatment he received adequate. Thus, this section tackles the first widely publicized case of cancer in Germany, that of the man who ascended the throne as Friedrich III, German Emperor, on 9 March 1888.[11]

Since January 1887, Crown Prince Friedrich had been suffering from serious hoarseness. In March 1887, Dr Carl Gerhardt, an internist and professor at the University of Berlin, examined him and discovered a lump on his left vocal cord, which he initially believed was a benign polyp. Thus, he burned it away fourteen times in succession with a hot wire, enough to make it disappear for a while.[12] By mid-May 1887, though, it had already grown back, now larger than it was before. This confirmed Gerhardt's secret fear that it might be cancer. Other doctors, including surgeon Ernst von Bergmann, were consulted. They also opined that it was cancer and recommended the surgical removal of parts of the larynx.[13] But they did not want to embark on this risky path before hearing the opinion of an internationally recognized authority. August Wegner, Friedrich's house doctor, recommended renowned Scottish laryngologist Morell Mackenzie, and Friedrich's wife Victoria, daughter of British Queen Victoria, agreed with the choice.[14]

On 20 May 1887, Mackenzie examined the crown prince in Berlin, but a clear determination of what was wrong eluded him. He thus performed a biopsy and

[11] The most recent account of Friedrich III's illness is in Müller, *Der 99-Tage-Kaiser*, 258–309. Two older books go into more detail: Michael Freund, *Das Drama der 99 Tage. Krankheit und Tod Friedrichs III.* (Cologne: Kiepenheuer and Witsch, 1966) and Hans-Joachim Wolf, *Die Krankheit Friedrichs III. und ihre Wirkung auf die deutsche und englische Öffentlichkeit* (Berlin: Berliner Medizinische Verlagsanstalt, 1958).

[12] C. Gerhardt, 'Bericht des Dr. C. Gerhardt, Königlichen Universitäts-Professors und Geheimen Medizinalrathes in Berlin', in *Die Krankheit Kaiser Friedrichs des Dritten. Dargestellt nach amtlichen Quellen und den im königl. Hausministerium niedergelegten Berichten der Aerzte* (Berlin: Kaiserliche Reichdruckerei, 1888), 1–17, 2–3.

[13] It is not entirely clear which kind of operation Bergmann recommended. In a later writing justifying his actions, he claims he recommended splitting the larynx. However, it is very likely that this was a retroactive attempt to defend himself, since contemporaneous medical knowledge held that the only advisable operation was the much riskier extirpation of the larynx. See Wolf, *Die Krankheit Friedrichs III*, 3–7.

[14] Müller, *Der 99-Tage-Kaiser*, 261–2.

commissioned Rudolf Virchow, at the time the world's most famous expert of pathology, to analyse the sample. Virchow found no evidence of cancer and thus joined Mackenzie in opining that Friedrich's illness was not cancer. Nevertheless, Virchow qualified his opinion with a 'probably', because a tissue sample free of cancer cells was not sufficient to rule out cancer with certainty. But Mackenzie assured the crown prince that he did not have cancer, and Friedrich thus declined to undergo the operation recommended by Bergmann and Gerhardt.

He continued to carry out his official duties and took to the waters a few times, as Mackenzie had recommended. When Friedrich's complaints worsened in early November 1887, Mackenzie examined him again at his vacation home in San Remo on 6 November 1887. This time, he suspected that it might be laryngeal cancer. Viennese laryngologist Leopold von Schrötter was called in for a second opinion, and he agreed with the Scotsman's assessment. But by this point, Friedrich's health had declined so drastically that the doctors would not risk taking a tissue sample, thus making it impossible to confirm the diagnosis with certainty.

Friedrich was informed of the diagnosis. He again opted against an operation, which was now much riskier than it would have been just a few months earlier in the summer. On 12 November, a report in the *Deutscher Reichs-Anzeiger* informed the public that the crown prince's illness was 'of cancerous nature'. On 15 November, an official dispatch verified that: 'the suffering [of the crown prince] is caused by the presence of a malignant tumour, which is primarily located beneath the left vocal cord and on the back of the vocal box; small growths also appear on the right side.'[15]

But a whole seven weeks later, on 7 January 1888, Mackenzie cast doubt on his own diagnosis. In an article published in the *British Medical Journal*, he ambiguously wrote: 'There is now good ground for hoping that the disease may be of the comparatively favourable character here indicated [chronic inflammation].'[16] In late January, Virchow conducted another pathological analysis of a chunk of tissue that Friedrich had coughed up. The report did not use the word 'cancer' once, nor did it say anything about a 'malignant tumour'. Ernst von Bergmann's team of doctors, however, read the total lack of nuance in its description of the tissue's cell structure as a coded cancer diagnosis.[17]

But Virchow's unclear report could be read both ways. With the backing of Mackenzie's 'authority', Friedrich and his wife decided to interpret it as saying 'not cancer' and communicated this version to the public. Official accounts now only

[15] *Deutscher Reichs-Anzeiger und Königlich Preußischer Staats-Anzeiger* 266, 12 November 1887, and 268, 15 November 1887, 1.

[16] 'The Illness of the Crown Prince', *British Medical Journal* 1410, no. 1 (7 January 1888): 31.

[17] See Rudolf Virchow, 'XII. Gutachten über ein aus dem Kehlkopfe Sr. K. K. Hoheit des Kronprinzen entleertes Gewebsstück', *Deutsches Medicinisches Wochenblatt* 14, no. 8 (23 February 1888): 159.

spoke of the crown prince's 'catarrhal' inflammation.[18] At Friedrich's request, Mackenzie wrote letters to a number of British and German medical journals in which he explained: 'at this moment medical science does not permit me to affirm that any other disease is present than chronic interstitial inflammation of the larynx combined with perichondritis.'[19] Until his death on 15 June 1888, the official story remained that perichondritis was causing 'wild flesh' to pullulate in his throat. Since 3 March 1888, though, all of Friedrich's doctors, including Mackenzie, had known for sure that he had cancer, because anatomist Heinrich Wilhelm Waldeyer had analysed another tissue sample on that day and discovered cells that were undeniably cancerous. But they never shared the finding with Friedrich and the public never heard anything about it until after his death. As late as 9 June 1888, Mackenzie told the *British Medical Journal* that the emperor's health had improved and 'that the physicians... are no longer sure about the diagnosis.... This uncertainty of course is in itself an immense improvement on the terrible diagnosis which was arrived at in November.'[20]

On 15 June 1888, Friedrich III passed away. The first reports of his death spoke only of a 'treacherous illness', saying nothing about cancer.[21] His son Wilhelm ordered an autopsy in order to be certain about the final diagnosis. The autopsy confirmed that he died of cancer.

On 11 July 1888, an official statement on 'the illness of Kaiser Friedrich III' was published. It drew exclusively on the assessments and notes of German doctors and levelled grave allegations against Mackenzie, blaming him for not recognizing the 'cancerous nature of the sickness' or only recognizing it after it was already too late. Mackenzie defended himself against the reproach by publishing his own version of the *Fatal Illness of Frederick the Noble* that same year.[22] He did not dispute that the Kaiser died of cancer. But he expounded on why he had held on to his doubt for so long, despite the fact that he, too, thought that there was considerable evidence that made cancer a plausible diagnosis. Two primary factors that influenced his indecision were his concerns about how he should speak about cancer with his patient, the 'person' Friedrich, and his estimation of the (im) probability that an operation would be successful.

Even though the official statement and Mackenzie's text both clearly try to justify decisions made and place blame on others, they offer insights into how and why doctors at the end of the nineteenth century spoke with their patients about

[18] *Deutscher Reichs-Anzeiger und Königlich Preußischer Staats-Anzeiger* 7, 1 September 1888, evening edition, 1.

[19] See Morell Mackenzie, 'The Case of His Imperial Highness the Crown Prince of Germany', *The Lancet* 131, 3364 (18 February 1888): 339–40, https://doi.org/10.1016/S0140-6736(02)28032-0.

[20] 'From Our Own Correspondent, Health of the Emperor', *British Medical Journal* 1, 1432 (9 June 1888): 1245.

[21] 'Der Tod des Kaisers Friedrich', *Illustrirte Zeitung* 2347 (1888): 652.

[22] Morell Mackenzie, *The Fatal Illness of Frederick the Noble* (London: S. Low, Marston, Searle and Rivington, 1888).

their cancer diagnosis, because Friedrich's doctors repeatedly took recourse to common-sense assumptions about what a medical professional should and should not say.

If one believes Mackenzie's retrospective account, an embarrassing mistake was what tipped off Friedrich about his doctors' initial suspicion that he may have had cancer. Carl Gerhardt, the doctor who burned away the tumour multiple times in 1887, dispatched Friedrich—who knew nothing of the cancer fears—to take the waters at Bad Ems.[23] Gerhardt's indiscretion had sent news of the doctors' worries down the grapevine. An acquaintance of the crown prince heard about it and, assuming that Friedrich was in the know, asked him about his cancer while he was at the resort. Mackenzie claims that Friedrich told him the story in May 1887, sending him into a rage about Gerhardt's carelessness: 'Although, for the sake of his family, he [Friedrich] manfully assumed a cheerful demeanour, the horrible idea that he was the subject of cancer must have frequently occurred to him.'[24]

Mackenzie's narrative was undoubtedly intended to question Gerhardt's loyalty and, at the same time, to intimate that Friedrich had a notion about the truth of the matter early on. Despite its likely having a calculated aim, the story seems fairly plausible. That Gerhardt may have said nothing to Friedrich about his yet foggy premonition that cancer might be afoot would have meshed well with nineteenth-century doctors' paternalistic understanding of doctor-patient relations.[25] And that a doctor slipped up would be unsurprising, as indiscretions permeate Friedrich's story. The remarkable part of Mackenzie's version is the acquaintance's assumption that Friedrich was aware of his situation. This suggests that not all doctors would have always concealed cancer diagnoses from their patients.

A look at the next time a diagnosis of cancer was up for discussion substantiates this hypothesis. When Friedrich underwent another examination after returning from Bad Ems in May 1887, Gerhardt and Bergmann concluded that the lump was certainly cancer and recommended that it be operated on at once. On 18 May, four doctors performed another exam. All agreed that cancer was the correct diagnosis and surgery the necessary treatment. They scheduled it for 21 May 1887.

Reports penned during these eventful days in May 1887 only permit a single conclusion: nobody told Friedrich that his doctors were nearly certain he had cancer. Letters written in this period by Victoria, Princess Royal, to her mother, Queen Victoria of England, explicitly confirm this conclusion. They reveal that the

[23] Winfried Baumgart, ed., *Kaiser Friedrich III. Tagebücher 1866–1888* (Paderborn: Schöningh, 2012), 526–34.

[24] Mackenzie, *The Fatal Illness of Frederick the Noble*, 19–20.

[25] Karen Nolte, *Todkrank. Sterbebegleitung im 19. Jahrhundert: Medizin, Krankenpflege und Religion* (Göttingen: Wallstein, 2016), 114; Barbara Elkeles, 'Die schweigsame Welt von Arzt und Patient. Einwilligung und Aufklärung in der Arzt-Patienten-Beziehung des 19. und 20. Jahrhunderts', *Medizin, Gesellschaft und Geschichte* 8 (1989): 63–91.

doctors spoke with Victoria without her husband being present, though she, too, was never informed of the 'true' diagnosis. Instead, in their conversations with her, the doctors referred to the tumour as an 'epithelioma', a rather ambiguous term.[26] She wrote of this pacifying revelation: 'I am not so frightened about danger to Fritz's life; thank God, I do not apprehend that, nor that this swelling is of a cancerous kind, nor does Bergmann, who says when once it is taken away, he does not think it will return.'[27]

Considering the fact that Victoria disputed the diagnosis with others even after she knew of her husband's cancer, it cannot be ruled out that she knew better when she claimed in her 19 May 1887 letter to her mother that Bergmann had not discovered cancer.[28] It does, however, seem likely that Bergmann proceeded as she recounted it: on the one hand, he reassured her that it was not (yet) cancer, while on the other, he hinted that it might become cancer if it was not operated on. Thus, he would have played one fear (of cancer) against the other (of surgery) in order to overcome Victoria's doubts about the risky operation scheduled for two days after the letter was written. This strategy worked at first, because she assented to the operation under the condition that Mackenzie, who had been summoned via telegram, also deemed it necessary.

Friedrich remained in the dark the entire time. Both Victoria's recollections in the 19 May letter as well as Otto von Bismarck's recollections in his memoirs corroborate one another on the fact that the doctors planned to operate on Friedrich without ever informing him of this intention.[29]

At the time, this was not so uncommon. Before the advent of anaesthesia, operating without a patient's consent was, of course, impossible. But after the advent of anaesthesia, doctors could partially or wholly dispense with obtaining consent to perform surgery. Doctors often took advantage of this new option by choosing not to discuss with their patient just how invasive an operation might get in the worst-case scenario. In a few cases, patients were chloroformed against their will and then operated on without consent or even against their express wishes. Doctors justified this practice with the paternalistic claim that only a doctor could decide what was best for the patient. But they also reasoned that the patient's fear might negatively influence the operation or drive him or her to end his or her own life.[30]

[26] Frederick Ponsonby, ed., *Letters of the Empress Frederick*, Letter from 17 May 1887 (London: MacMillan, 1928), 257–8.

[27] Ponsonby, *Letters of the Empress Frederick*, 231.

[28] Wolf, *Die Krankheit Friedrichs III*, 90–5.

[29] Ponsonby, *Letters of the Empress Frederick*, Letter from 19 May 1887, 306.

[30] Karen Nolte, 'Zeitalter des ärztlichen Paternalismus: Überlegungen zu Aufklärung und Einwilligung von Patienten im 19. Jahrhundert', *Medizin, Gesellschaft und Geschichte* 25 (2006): 59–89; Thorsten Noack, *Eingriffe in das Selbstbestimmungsrecht des Patienten. Juristische Entscheidungen, Politik und ärztliche Positionen 1890–1960* (Frankfurt am Main: Mabuse-Verlag,

Victoria clearly accepted these arguments and betrayed nothing of the planned operation to her husband, even though she found it 'so difficult to appear unconcerned when one's heart is so torn, and it is so important he should eat and sleep and feel well'.[31] In the end, Friedrich learned about the planned operation and was asked for his consent, but it was not on account of Victoria's initiative. It was Bismarck who intervened, presumably because he rejected its necessity and wanted to prevent it from taking place.[32] He argued that the heir apparent to the throne could not be operated on without the consent of the emperor. It is not clear if he demanded that the crown prince also be involved in the decision; he claimed that he did in his memoirs, which were published in 1898. But in her letter to her mother from 20 May 1887, Victoria claimed that Bismarck said to her: 'They are obliged to ask the Emperor's permission and to tell him the whole, as they cannot tell Fritz.'[33] Thus, Bismarck may have altered his account of his intervention in retrospect because the 'truth' about Friedrich's cancer had become a bone of political contention. Another reason for this likely alteration may have been a decision issued by the Reichsgericht (Imperial Court of Justice) in 1894 that classified operations without the patient's consent as bodily harm and thus made them punishable under law.[34]

In short, Bismarck demonstrably informed Kaiser Wilhelm I, who insisted that Friedrich consent before being operated on. Records are insufficient to say whether the doctors told him what they thought he was suffering from when they asked for his consent. However, considering the constant consultations with doctors, the enlistment of a doctor from Scotland, and the plan to operate that was, in the end, communicated with him, it seems unlikely that he would never have thought that it might be cancer. Indeed, in her letters to her mother, Victoria wrote that Friedrich voiced concerns that his 90-year-old father might outlive him.[35] The discussion between Friedrich and Mackenzie about Gerhardt's indiscretion thus might have been Friedrich's attempt to talk with a doctor about the possibility that he might have cancer. But Mackenzie's report does not say whether he indeed talked about it.

A few days later, however, Friedrich learned that the doctors had, at least for a time, suspected that he had cancer. Shortly after Mackenzie expressed disagreement with the German doctors' diagnosis, English newspapers reported that the previous supposition that the crown prince had cancer had now been ruled out. It

2004), 17–19; Karen Nolte (2008) '"Telling the Painful Truth"—Nurses and Physicians in the Nineteenth Century', *Nursing History Review* 16, no. 1 (2008): 115–34, 102, https://doi.org/10.1891/1062%968061.16.115.

[31] Ponsonby, *Letters of the Empress Frederick*, Letter from 19 May 1887, 263.

[32] Wolf, *Die Krankheit Friedrichs III*, 99.

[33] Ponsonby, *Letters of the Empress Frederick*, 232.

[34] Noack, *Eingriffe*, 26–43; Andreas-Holger Maehle, 'Assault and Battery, or Legitimate Treatment? German Legal Debates on the Status of Medical Interventions without Consent, c. 1890–1914', *Gesnerus* 57, nos. 3/4 (2000): 206–21, 213–14.

[35] Ponsonby, *Letters of the Empress Frederick*, Letter from 17 May 1887, 258.

is highly unlikely that Mackenzie would have given this information to the press if he was not certain that Friedrich already knew about the suspicions.

Why exactly Mackenzie disputed the diagnosis of cancer, however, has been debated ever since without reaching a satisfying conclusion. While the court's official report castigated him as incompetent, rumours circulated that he believed treating the prominent patient—a task ultimately entrusted to him—promised personal gain and a boost in reputation. Political opponents of Friedrich and Victoria asserted that Mackenzie was supposed to prevent the potentially fatal operation so that Friedrich, even if deadly sick, could still ascend the throne and thus at least defer for a while the emperorship of their son, which both feared.[36]

Mackenzie himself had a different explanation for his hesitation, and, at least when applied to the situation in May 1887, it seems fairly convincing.[37] He stated that he did not want to treat the illness as cancer without definitive evidence that it was. In his 1888 account of the case, he grounded his doubts about the cancer diagnosis in his disagreement with the planned operation:

> I did not say that it was not cancer; I only said that that opinion was 'not proven'; and in the absence of positive proof I refused to sanction surgical procedures which at present are at the best more or less of the nature of experiments, which are always dangerous to life, nearly always destructive to the voice, and which, even when 'successful', too often leave the patient unfit for the business of life, or even sometimes in a condition worse than death itself.[38]

But consideration of Mackenzie's medical writings published before 1887 suggests that he might have rejected the operation as too risky not only because he doubted that the diagnosis was correct. In part, Mackenzie had his 1880 book on diseases of the nose and throat to thank for his status as one of the world's leading laryngologists. He dedicated an entire chapter to diagnosing and treating laryngeal cancer. Drawing on his own experiences and research, he wrote that in no case of laryngeal cancer known to him had surgery cured the disease or led to a significant prolongation of the patient's life in comparison to merely treating the symptoms. He called the results of these operations 'extremely unsatisfactory', an assessment aggravated by the fact that many patients died during or immediately after the procedure.[39] Given this context, it seems plausible that Mackenzie had already recognized in May 1887 that Friedrich's tumour was cancer, but that he expressed doubts about the diagnosis in order to stop what he saw as an ineffective, risky, debilitating operation.[40] This would help explain why Mackenzie persisted in his

[36] Freund, *Das Drama der 99 Tage*, 69–70.
[37] A similar assessment can be found in Müller, *Der 99-Tage-Kaiser*, 264–5.
[38] Mackenzie, *The Fatal Illness of Frederick the Noble*, 29–30.
[39] Morell Mackenzie, *A Manual of Diseases of the Throat and Nose* (New York, 1880).
[40] Müller, *Der 99-Tage-Kaiser*, 265; Wolf, *Die Krankheit Friedrichs III*, 53–9.

scepticism about Friedrich's diagnosis all the way until November 1887—a blindness that remains confounding, considering that Mackenzie was undoubtedly a competent doctor. Because if his aim was to prevent the operation, he would have had to stick to his guns either until the diagnosis was so apparent that it could no longer be doubted, or until the surgeon Dr Bergmann judged the operation to be too risky. Both conditions held in November 1887. The examination's findings were so clear-cut that even wanting to wait for the results of the pathological analysis of Friedrich's tissue sample could only be seen as weak grounds for hesitation. And because the tumour had in the meantime grown so large that the entire vocal box would had to have been excised and Friedrich was in miserable health, Mackenzie could, despite his patient now definitively being diagnosed with cancer, refuse to carry out the operation without confronting too much resistance from his colleagues. If this thesis holds true, then Mackenzie remained silent about the diagnosis during the first phase in order to prevent the operation. In contrast, the other doctors tried to get Friedrich's family's consent to operate by warning them of the danger that the lump might develop into cancer, while encouraging them to conceal the diagnosis from him for his own good.

It is telling how the doctors comported themselves towards Friedrich, his family, and the general public after the window for operating seemed to have passed. In his self-defence, Mackenzie described a key event in the story—his examination of Friedrich on 6 November 1887:

> Without raising from my chair I informed His Imperial Highness that a very unfavourable change had taken place in his throat. He said, 'Is it cancer?' to which I replied, 'I am sorry to say, Sir, it looks very much like it, but it is impossible to be certain.' I felt that evasive answers, which for the patient's own sake medical men are often compelled to give under similar circumstances, would in the present instance have been out of place.[41]

This description of the situation doubtlessly served two ends. On the one hand, Mackenzie wanted to underscore that Friedrich was, by this point, not totally clueless about his health, thus invalidating the accusation that he, Mackenzie, had shamelessly lied to the crown prince and inflated his hopes. On the other, the passage, like so many others in the book, depicts Friedrich as a dignified, strong, courageous man. The image contrasts with his political opponents' calumnious attacks on him as a puppet of his domineering British wife. But since Mackenzie's report of the meeting does not contradict the only other account of it—that contained in Friedrich's diary—it can be safely assumed that his version is close

[41] Mackenzie, *The Fatal Illness of Frederick the Noble*, 66–7.

to the truth. The only discrepancy between the two sources concerns a not unimportant detail: while Mackenzie claims that Friedrich directly asked him if it might be cancer, the crown prince himself only noted Mackenzie's opinion that the 'potential for cancer cannot be ruled out'.[42] In the end, the source material does not resolve whether Mackenzie mistakenly or perhaps intentionally put a question in Friedrich's mouth that the latter definitively asked the physician Leopold von Schrötter five days later, or whether Friedrich asked the question to both doctors in order to gain a better sense of what he was going through. Certain, however, is that Mackenzie held his own approach to the situation as the right one, because otherwise he would not have delved into it in such detail. Read as a statement on medical ethics, the description of the scene implies an adherence to the rule that the doctor should avoid using the word 'cancer' while at the same time not denying that it might be the diagnosis if the patient explicitly asks. And he sowed hope by leaving the door open for doubt: 'but it is impossible to be certain.'

A few days later, the other doctors took a similar tack when they, after conferring with one another, told Friedrich about their findings. Their 'speaker', Professor Schrötter, avoided the word 'cancer' and evaded Friedrich's question about it, thus leaving room for doubt and, with it, for hope. But despite this strategy, the doctors felt fairly certain that Friedrich clearly understood that he had cancer.[43] Friedrich's diary entry from 11 November 1887 records his belief that his death was near, thus confirming their suspicion.[44]

Moreover, all of the doctors agreed that the diagnosis should not be communicated to the public.[45] In their report to the emperor, Friedrich's father Wilhelm I, they did not beat around the bush, clearly calling the growth a 'malignant tumour'. When Mackenzie learned a few days later that Wilhelm I had the unmodified medical report printed in the *Deutscher Reichs-Anzeiger*, he was fuming—not necessarily because the public now knew that the crown prince had cancer, but because Friedrich would hear the diagnosis 'without any disguise or palliation'.[46] The remark reiterates that the doctors' circumlocution was part of a finely tuned strategy to manage the crown prince's emotions, which demanded striking a delicate balance. On the one hand, the doctors wanted to unequivocally bring Friedrich to recognize that he would, in all likelihood, die in the near future.

[42] Baumgart, *Kaiser Friedrich III. Tagebücher*, 554.

[43] Mackenzie, *The Fatal Illness of Frederick the Noble*, 72; Baumgart, *Kaiser Friedrich III. Tagebücher*, 555 and 'Bericht des Professor Schrötter', in *Die Krankheit Kaiser Friedrichs des Dritten. Dargestellt nach amtlichen Quellen und den im königl. Hausministerium niedergelegten Berichten der Aerzte* (Berlin, 1888), 43.

[44] The entry states: 'Thus I will surely have to get my house in order.' Baumgart, *Kaiser Friedrich III. Tagebücher*, 555.

[45] Mackenzie, *The Fatal Illness of Frederick the Noble*, 73; 'Bericht des Professor Schrötter', in *Die Krankheit Kaiser Friedrichs des Dritten*, 44.

[46] Mackenzie, *The Fatal Illness of Frederick the Noble*, 73.

Indeed, in the run of 1888, Mackenzie repeatedly hinted to Friedrich that his death was approaching; he justified the tactic on the grounds that he wanted to allow him ample time to bring his official and familial affairs in order.[47] On the other hand, the message was supposed to be expressed in terms vague enough to sustain hope, not so much about the possibility that his death might not be imminent, but about the process of dying itself. The doctors wanted to distract from the cancer diagnosis because, as Mackenzie wrote, it 'was something much worse than a mere sentence of death'. It would have meant 'that he [Friedrich] was doomed only too surely to a lingering agony worse than death'.[48]

This assessment was informed by Mackenzie's knowledge that he did not really have any way to soften his patient's death from cancer. At the end of the nineteenth century, some surgeons were able to perform tracheotomies. However, they used breathing tubes made of aluminium or silver, and their lack of flexibility often led to complications. Thus, after Friedrich got a tracheotomy in February 1888, hardly a day went by that he did not suffer from bleeding, pus, or mucus build-ups in the tubes or around the hole. Regularly changing the tubes must have been extraordinarily uncomfortable and painful; the press reported on it in rather dry language.[49] Morphine and opium could be used to fight the pain caused by the tumour. In his aforementioned book, Mackenzie recommended that doctors apply a powder solution mixed with morphine to the vocal box once or twice a day,[50] and it is likely that Friedrich had been receiving this treatment since May 1887.[51] But morphine was not always sufficient to manage the pain, and medical experts and theologians had been arguing for years over whether and to what extent its use was ethically defensible. Some were concerned about the fact that numbing cancer pain often demanded high doses that rendered the patient unconscious or only partially conscious, while others feared that their patients would become addicted.[52] Both outcomes would have prohibited the crown prince from performing his future duties as emperor, placing serious limits on the degree to which his doctors could rely on painkillers. Thus, every medical professional could foresee that his last months would be defined by agonizing pain, constant complications, and increasing weakness. And the writings of everyone who met him in person during this period confirm beyond a shadow of a doubt that his final weeks were indeed wretched.[53]

[47] Ibid., 158 and 172. There is evidence that Friedrich understood the implied message even though he did not explicitly speak about his own death with Mackenzie. For instance, in May and June 1888, he and his wife Victoria shipped confidential documents to her mother in England, where she had already brought three chests filled with papers during a trip there in July 1887. See Müller, *Der 99-Tage-Kaiser*, 312.

[48] Mackenzie, *The Fatal Illness of Frederick the Noble*, 66.

[49] 'Hofnachrichten', *Illustrirte Zeitung* 2346, 10 June 1888, 616.

[50] Mackenzie, *A Manual of Diseases*, 250.

[51] Gerhardt, 'Bericht des Dr. C. Gerhardt', 11; Baumgart, *Kaiser Friedrich III. Tagebücher*, 542–52 and 562.

[52] Bourke, *The Story of Pain*, 285–7.

[53] Freund, *Das Drama der 99 Tage*, 291–393.

With their roundabout discussion of the diagnosis, Mackenzie and the other doctors wanted to ward off thoughts of such a miserable death for as long as possible. This helps explain Mackenzie's actions in the spring of 1888. By calling the disease perichondritis, he intimated to Friedrich that death was on the horizon, as this infection of the vocal box was almost always fatal. But the downgrade offered him an alternative to the cancer diagnosis from November 1887. While the new pseudo-diagnosis could plausibly explain Friedrich's ailments, it was not associated with the burden of facing a drawn-out, painful death. The same reasons probably motivated the ambiguous style of Virchow's analysis from January 1888.[54] The sources that have been preserved make it impossible to say whether Friedrich really believed Mackenzie's alternative diagnosis or whether he perhaps just accepted it for political reasons or out of 'consideration' for his family and doctor. Friedrich's wife Victoria definitely knew the facts, though, because Mackenzie had informed her about the pathologist's report that Waldeyer had completed on 3 March 1888.[55] It is unclear if she told Friedrich about its findings. Mackenzie wrote that after he had told Friedrich he was suffering from perichondritis, his patient no longer asked him about the nature of his illness and only inquired into his symptoms and how they might be lessened. The Scottish doctor interpreted this as a sort of silent mutual agreement to no longer speak about cancer, even though he surmised that the true diagnosis of cancer had found its way to Friedrich's ear through the imprudent talkativeness of others:

> What the Emperor's own inmost thoughts were as to his condition and prospects I am quite unable to say.... It may be that he hoped against hope, but he never spoke either of his hopes or fears to me. It must be remembered too that the Emperor had had far greater opportunities of hearing the truth—or what was supposed to be the truth—about his condition than fall to the lot of ordinary patients.[56]

In Mackenzie's representation, Friedrich's choice to remain silent about his hopes and fears lent him an aura of august masculinity, an image that served Mackenzie's secondary mission of defending the crown prince and Kaiser. At issue were not just masculine norms, though. Mackenzie was also dissecting which behaviours and attitudes he and other doctors thought were helpful in such situations. One of the few available resources was 'hope against all hope', an emotion that doctors counted on and did not want to undermine. Such hope

[54] Looking back, Mackenzie commented on Virchow's second analysis from 9 June 1887: 'It must be borne in mind that Virchow, knowing that his report would come under the eyes of the patient, was naturally anxious to make it as favourable as he could consistently with truth.' Mackenzie, *The Fatal Illness of Frederick the Noble*, 34.

[55] Wolf, *Die Krankheit Friedrichs III*, 33–4.

[56] Mackenzie, *The Fatal Illness of Frederick the Noble*, 185–6.

was only possible in the kind of space opened up by Mackenzie's ambivalence about the diagnosis, even if that space required Friedrich to not speak to his doctor about some of his feelings. It is possible that Friedrich experienced this as a form of emotional isolation that had been forced upon him, but that he did not want to disturb in order to fulfil others' expectations. But it is also possible that he was authentically convinced of the necessity of 'stabilizing' his own emotions. He might have embraced not speaking about his hopes and fears as a conscious way to disengage from the existential question facing him, instead opting only to ask his doctor to palliate the symptoms and concentrate on his duties as crown prince and emperor.

Friedrich's diary contains numerous complaints about his father Wilhelm treating him dismissively and many recollections about medical procedures he underwent. But it only contains one brief note on his feelings about his illness and death. On 4 November 1887, after a summer and autumn full of hopes that he might recover, he learned that his doctor had telegraphed for Mackenzie. His diary entry from that day reads: 'Therefore, I am at the same place as I was at the end of May.... I am very dispirited, especially since only 8 days ago everybody found that my voice had very much gained in strength—which, however, I myself never perceived.'[57]

When he learned a few days later that all of his doctors believed his illness was cancer or 'something related', he described the situation in his diary in some detail, but he dispensed with writing about his own emotions, focusing on his wife's reaction instead: 'Wife admirable as ever, in her constitution and in her courage.'[58] These curt words fit with the memories and letters of observers and people close to the couple at the time, who generally wrote that Friedrich and Victoria reassured both others and themselves that there was still hope, while emphasizing anything that might suggest that a cure could still be found.[59] Even though Victoria knew it was cancer by March 1888 at the latest, her letters to her mother all the way up until a few days before Friedrich's death insist that he was suffering from perichondritis, not cancer.[60] Many observers conjectured that she believed in her own hopeful messaging, and like her, they were convinced that one could decide to remain composed, hopeful, and courageous until one's own resolve turned into 'real' inner emotions.[61]

[57] Baumgart, *Kaiser Friedrich III. Tagebücher*, 554.

[58] Ibid., 555 (entry from 11 November 1887).

[59] Anton von Werner, *Erlebnisse und Eindrücke 1870–1890* (Berlin: Mittler, 1913), 502; Ernst Curtius, *Ein Lebensbild in Briefen*, ed. Friedrich Curtius (Berlin: Springer, 1903), 675–6; Margaretha von Poschinger, *Kaiser Friedrich. In neuer quellenmäßiger Darstellung*, vol. 3 (Berlin: Schröder, 1899), 432–3.

[60] Wolf, *Die Krankheit Friedrichs III*, 94.

[61] Werner, *Erlebnisse und Eindrücke*, 526; Anna von Helmholtz, *Ein Lebensbild in Briefen*, ed. Ellen von Siemens-Helmholtz, vol. 1 (Berlin: Verlag für Kulturpolitik, 1929), 310.

Many of these details did not surface in public, at least not at first. But some did. The disagreement among Friedrich's doctors about his diagnosis; the official, public description of the illness as a 'malignant tumour' in November 1887; the re-evaluation of the diagnosis in January 1888 as a 'chronic infection and perichondritis'—all these things provided fodder for the German newspapers for weeks.[62] Friedrich's case underscored with unsettling clarity how a group of renowned medical specialists could remain at odds for months on end over whether an illness was cancer.

While Friedrich was still alive, questions about the 'truthfulness' of cancer diagnoses entered into public discussion, too. Friedrich's political opponents in particular were convinced that Mackenzie and Victoria had devised a coverup to keep him in the dark about his health and thus prevent the German doctors from taking the necessary steps.[63] Though this imputed deception was instrumentalized for political purposes, the case sparked heated public debate on whether doctors should tell a patient that he or she has cancer. Many doctors reported that the crown prince's illness had stirred up broader interest in cancer. Educational associations organized events where doctors explicated the anatomy of the vocal box and surveyed available forms of treating cancer. Some doctors claimed that patients latched onto Friedrich's experience as an argument against heeding their doctors' recommendations to operate.[64]

Accounts published after Friedrich's death deepened these conversations. While they were likely only read by educated middle- and upper-class people, media coverage distributed the debate among all social classes in the German Empire. Two issues stood front and centre: the (un)certainty of medical knowledge and the ethical issue of whether and what doctors should tell cancer patients. Some newspapers, such as the national-liberal *Heidelberger Zeitung*, defended Mackenzie's approach with the argument that not knowing he had cancer enabled Friedrich to retain hope. Its editors thus read Mackenzie's not telling him—whether it was an act of consciously misleading him or just an error, they did not yet know—as a good deed.[65]

The story of Friedrich's illness uncovers the complex machinery of late nineteenth-century strategies of how to talk about cancer. It involved circumlocution, unspoken, yet implied understanding, euphemisms, and plain suppression. These tactics served diverse ends. All of the crown prince's doctors avoided definitively stating that the diagnosis was cancer. Even when it came to deciding

[62] Wolf, *Die Krankheit Friedrichs III*, 104–15.

[63] 'Die neuesten Nachrichten über den Zustand des deutschen Kronprinzen', *Schwäbischer Merkur* 268, 12 November 1887, 1961–2.

[64] Wolf, *Die Krankheit Friedrichs III*, 116–17; Max Schaeffer, 'Larynxcarcinom', *Deutsche Medicinische Wochenschrift* 16, no. 28 (1890): 608–10, https://doi.org/10.1055/s-0029%961207315; Bernhard Fraenkel, 'Die intralaryngeale Behandlung des Kehlkopfkrebses', *Archiv für Laryngologie und Rhinologie* 6 (1897): 361–74, 364.

[65] 'Zu Kaiser Friedrichs Heimgang', *Heidelberger Zeitung* 140, 18 June 1888, 1.

how to treat the illness, they did not tell their patient what precise illness was being treated. After all, the doctors held obtaining the patient's consent before operating to be superfluous; indeed, they believed doing so might even be harmful. Not everybody was prepared to accept the doctors' paternalistic attitude, however. While Victoria tended to accept it, Bismarck and Kaiser Wilhelm I opposed it on the grounds that Friedrich had political—and, one might say, occupational—responsibilities to fulfil. Normative expectations about stoic masculinity in the face of death probably also played a role in their rejection of surgery without consent.

The doctors did inform family members about what was going on, for the most part without allowing gender to determine what they said. By warning them that the lump might develop into cancer, the doctors evoked fears of cancer in order to win the family over to the treatment that they had already decided upon. But in order to protect their patient, they used ambiguous terms, and not 'cancer', when speaking with the family. They pursued similar rhetorical strategies when the patient himself asked whether or not he had cancer. Without directly denying that he did, they evaded the question or emphasized that the course the illness might take was unforeseeable, despite the fact that they knew better. Uttering words like 'cancer' and more technical synonyms like 'malignant tumour' remained taboo. But out of this taboo unfolded a paradoxical communicative structure. Though they never said the words, the doctors were convinced that their patient understood that he had cancer. By refusing to call the disease by its name, the doctors aimed to disaffirm it the status of an indisputable fact. The strategy was informed by the belief that humans' need for hope in life was so great that they would want to maintain it despite knowing that things were grim, so long as they lacked absolute certainty that the situation was irredeemable. Out of this followed the belief that hope could amplify the significance of a minor doubt into a major one. The consensus opinion among medical professionals was that abiding in this paradoxical structure of tiptoeing around the taboo would enable the patient to speak about their emotions with doctors and family members. Many doctors sternly resisted calls to depart from this model of circumlocutory communication, because they feared something that their colleague Carl Haberlin would articulate clearly thirty years later: 'He [the doctor] can kill if he kills hope.'[66]

But Friedrich's case paved the way for a shift. After all, a pillar of this communicative structure's efficacy was patients' ignorance of the strategy itself. But as details about it found their way out of the exclusive domain of medical and theological discourse and into the discourse of the 'lay' public after Friedrich's death, this pillar was, at least in principle, undercut. Now, tacit agreements made in silence would be much harder to maintain.

[66] Carl Haeberlin, *Vom Beruf des Arztes*, 2nd edn (Munich: Verlag der Ärtzlichen Rundschau Gmelin, 1925), 108.

Fear and Hope at the Turn of the Twentieth Century: The Patient's Consent and Discussing Diagnoses

It might seem a bit astonishing that, for the time being, nothing initially changed after all this. But as Friedrich's case pointedly illustrates, an integral component of maintaining the unspoken rule against talking about cancer was the patient's knowledge that their doctor would use coded language and their ability to decipher it. Thus, the public discussion about concealing the diagnosis from the patient did not necessarily impact its communicative structure.

However, the strategy was called into doubt by a different debate, one that had also played an important role in Friedrich's story: should a doctor have to obtain a patient's consent before conducting medical procedures that he viewed as necessary? As the nineteenth century drew to a close, courts grappled with the question in an ever-increasing number of cases. Under discussion were two different situations. First, judges, doctors, ethicists, and others discussed if and when a doctor could operate on a patient without that patient having given explicit consent or having been informed of the potential invasiveness of the procedure, an issue that confronted the doctors in Friedrich's case. Second, they inquired into whether patients could be 'used' for medical experiments without their consent, which might serve the progress of medical science and thus be beneficial for others, but not the patient themselves.

In the second half of the nineteenth century, doctors often carried forth in both types of cases without their patients' knowledge or consent, which rarely garnered protest from colleagues. In a sense, both practices were associated with the accomplishments of 'modern' medicine. As discussed in the previous section, operations without consent had only become possible with the advent of general anaesthesia with ether or chloroform. In contrast, human experiments without therapeutic value for the individual patient were often employed to test bacteriological hypotheses about if and how certain diseases were transmitted and if their transmission could be halted with vaccines. Moreover, such experiments usually took place in hospitals, which had significantly grown in number since the 1870s.

Doctors believed they were making their decisions in the name of health: the patient's in the former instance, humanity's in the latter. Implied was that the two practices were not on equal footing, since doctors performing human experiments clearly valued what they thought was the general good over the welfare of their patients (often women), thus turning the person into a sort of experimental 'thing'.[67] It was no accident that the decision regularly affected people whose

[67] Katja Sabisch, *Das Weib als Versuchsperson: medizinische Menschenexperimente im 19. Jahrhundert am Beispiel der Syphilisforschung* (Bielefeld: Transcript Verlag, 2007); Barbara Elkeles, *Der moralische Diskurs über das medizinische Menschenexperiment im 19. Jahrhundert* (Stuttgart: Fischer, 1996); Barbara Elkeles, 'Wissenschaft, Medizinethik und gesellschaftliches Umfeld: Die

chances of recovery were seen as slim or whose occupation or lifestyle were deemed 'immoral'. Thus, experiments were almost exclusively conducted on prostitutes, underclass women with 'dubious' reputations, orphans, or 'incurable' persons and terminally ill patients.

Around 1890, operations and human experiments without consent gained prominence as topics of medical law and medical ethics. Despite the differences between the two issues, both involved a common point of contention: Should doctors, on account of their specialized knowledge and training, decide for themselves what happens to their patients' bodies, whether it be in the service of what they believed to be the patient's best interest or that of the general good? Should they be allowed to make such decisions? And if so, did this permit them to conceal from the patient information about their illness and the invasiveness and risks of the medical procedure they planned to perform? How people answered these questions depended not least on the significance they attributed to fear and hope.

It seems to have been a coincidence that the discussion picked up after Friedrich III's death, because it tied together a series of older developments of which Friedrich's case was more symptom than cause. Among them were the aforementioned advances in therapeutic techniques; the pathbreaking success of bacteriology, which augmented doctors' self-confidence and their standing as specialists; and institutional changes like the professionalization of doctors, the construction of new hospitals and the expansion of old ones, and the implementation of a public health insurance system in the 1880s. These developments bolstered many doctors' already paternalistic attitude. They also helped reduce the frequency of previously standard negotiations between doctor and patient, especially as the newly built hospitals were receiving a growing number of publicly insured patients from the underclasses, whom doctors did not believe had even the most minimal understanding of medical matters.[68]

But another development in the medical world also factored in here. In the late eighteenth and early nineteenth century, doctors argued that the power of emotions justified not telling patients about their illness, an upcoming operation, or their approaching death. For instance, in 1836/7, Christoph Wilhelm Hufeland, a renowned practitioner of natural medicine and, for a time, house doctor of the family of Prussian king Friedrich Wilhelm III, wrote in his guide for doctors about concealing things from the patient:

Diskussion um den Heilversuch um 1900', in *Medizingeschichte und Medizinethik. Kontroversen und Begründungsansätze 1900–1950*, ed. Andreas Frewer and Josef N. Neumann (Frankfurt: Campus Verlag, 2001), 21–43.

[68] Noack, *Eingriffe*, 19–20.

> Is it not well-established that fear—especially fear of death—anxiety, and terror are the most dangerous poisons and that they immediately paralyze a person's vitality; but that hope and courage are the greatest vitalizers, which often are more powerful than any medicine, yes, without which the best medicines lose their efficacy? Thus, the doctor must above all seek to retain the patient's hope and courage—better to play the matter down, conceal all danger.... Announcing death is the same as giving death, and that cannot ever be the business of he who is only there to spread life.[69]

Vitalists like Hufeland believed that all human existence was propelled by a special life force. But they were not the only ones who were convinced that emotions like fear and hope had a direct corporeal effect and could thus literally kill a person. For some, this conviction provided a strong argument against revealing the 'truth' to a patient, which led to a series of conflicts between doctors on the one hand and nurses and ministers on the other. As nurses were almost always employed by religious organizations, they insisted on telling terminally ill patients about their impending death in order to prepare them for their last rites.[70] However, cellular pathology and bacteriology rejected this conviction and many 'modern' doctors did, too.[71] After all, if cells and bacteria—the 'agents' of disease—could be studied under a microscope, where human emotions were wholly absent, then the latter's effect on bodily afflictions could only be negligible. The paradigm shift swept the rug from beneath an important argument for 'benign deception', and indeed, some doctors drew conclusions from this turn. For example, Scottish gynaecologist James Matthews Duncan, member of London's College of Physicians, told his colleagues: 'It had been said that a knowledge of the truth will accelerate the progress of a cancer of the liver. I do not believe it.... I am among those who believe that the truth communicated to an inquiring doubting patient has a decidedly beneficial therapeutic effect, at least in the majority of cases.'[72] While many doctors had believed that doubt was the shepherd of hope, and that deception was thus justified, Duncan ripped into this belief as more dangerous than the destruction of hope through knowledge of the truth could ever be. Initially, such forceful criticism of hopeful doubt and such support for clear-cut communication of the facts were the exception, not just in Great Britain, but also in the German Empire, where no written statement of comparable clarity was to be found.

[69] Christoph Wilhelm Hufeland, *Enchiridion medicum oder Anleitung zur medicinischen Praxis: Vermächtniß einer fünfzigjährigen Erfahrung* (Herisau: Litteratur-Comtoir, 1837), 502.

[70] Nolte, '"Telling the Painful Truth"', 116–28.

[71] Bettina Hitzer, 'Healing Emotions', in Frevert et al., *Emotional Lexicons*, 118–50, 124–32.

[72] J. Matthews Duncan, 'Concerning Medical Education: An Address Delivered at the Opening of the Session of the Abernethian Society, October 14th, 1886', quoted in Oswald Browne, *On the Care of the Dying: A Lecture to Nurses* (London, 1894), 23.

Medical laypersons, and above all jurists, were the first to voice criticism publicly. The critique's foundation was the legal principle that citizen-subjects have inviolable rights over their body just as they do over their property.[73] This argument has a connection to Friedrich's story. When discussing the case in his published memoirs, Bismarck wrote that he had asserted that Friedrich must himself decide whether to undergo an operation. Though he supported his position with arguments about political and domestic responsibility, and not with claims about the autonomy of the subject, the end result of both positions overlapped, since such responsibilities might necessitate that an ill person make decisions on the basis of duty alone, not on the basis of feelings that needed protecting.

But there is another, subtler connection between this juridical critique and Friedrich's case. In 1891, criminal defence lawyer Lassa Oppenheim presented the first German-language casuistic analysis of the issue of consent at his inaugural lecture at the University of Basel.[74] His motivation stemmed from his outrage over a case that had recently become public. Interestingly, the case involved two central characters in Friedrich's story: Berlin-based surgeons Eugen von Hahn and Ernst von Bergmann. In an open letter to the *Nationalzeitung*, a government official named Dr Leidig accused the two men of transplanting parts of patients' cancerous tumours onto healthy skin in order to discover whether the cancerous cells would live and grow.[75] Since the press had extensively reported on similar 'surgical crimes' in France, many were shocked to learn such acts were possible in the German Empire.[76] Berlin's magistrate reacted quickly, first summoning Eugen von Hahn to testify and then, after Prussia's culture ministry intervened, Ernst von Bergmann.[77]

In his affidavit from 14 July 1891, Bergmann wrote that he had conducted the experiments in the early 1870s at the surgical clinic in Dorpat (today, Tartu, Estonia), where he had been a professor of medicine.[78] If Bergmann had not presented the findings of these decade-old experiments at the Kongress der deutschen Chirurgen (Conference of German Surgeons) in April 1889, Eugen von Hahn would have probably been the sole target of critique in the 1891 letter. But Bergmann had good reason to publicly discuss his results at precisely this time. He had been trying to undermine all doubts about his position in the case of king and Kaiser Friedrich III. As his studies sought to show, if cancer began as a

[73] Noack, *Eingriffe*, 21.

[74] Lassa Francis Lawrence Oppenheim, *Das ärztliche Recht zu körperlichen Eingriffen an Kranken und Gesunden* (Basel: Schwabe Verlagsbuchhandlung, 1892).

[75] Eugen Leidig, 'Brief von Dr. Eugen Leidig an die Redaktion', *Nationalzeitung*, 5 July 1891, GStA PK I. HA Rep. 76 VIII B, no. 3846, 16.

[76] 'Ein chirurgisches Verbrechen', *Nationalzeitung*, 1 July 1891; 'Medizinisches Verbrechen', *Das Rhein-Journal*, 6 July 1891, GStA PK I. HA Rep. 76 VIII B, no. 3846, 3–4.

[77] Letter from the Magistrate of the Royal Capital and Residence to the Minister of Education and Medical Affairs, 13 July 1891, GStA PK I. HA Rep. 76 VIII B, no. 3846, 17.

[78] GStA PK I. HA Rep. 76 VIII B, no. 3846, 18–29.

local disease, then the only correct way to treat it was early operation. But if, as some critics countered, cancer began as a disease that encompassed the entire body, after which a tumour developed in a certain spot, then operating did not make any medical sense and might even be harmful. Bergmann's experiments found that a surgically removed tumour would grow and expand if transplanted to another, 'healthy' part of the body. He believed this provided clear evidence that cancer started with the primary tumour.

Against the accusation that his experiments had transgressed 'the limits of the medical profession and the doctor's authority over patients', Bergmann defended himself with a series of arguments.[79] First, he explained that all of the test subjects were already suffering from metastases and thus would soon die of cancer. Therefore, he claimed, the additional tumours did not shorten their lives. Moreover, he asserted that the procedure was painless, because he had removed tumours that were especially painful on account of their location in places like the armpit and transplanted them to less sensitive places, like the thigh. In short, he claimed, the experiments had reduced the patients' pain, not caused more of it. He depicted them as an 'act of humanity' crowned by the fact that the terminally ill patient had contributed to science and thus helped future patients' chances of being cured. For this reason, many patients had 'gladly' consented to participate in the experiments.[80] However, Bergmann believed that the issue of consent was irrelevant anyways: 'The patients' consent to be part of the experiment was not lacking, although I do not attribute any weight to it, because the doctor who cares for such patients, who does them the good deed of treating their pain, who gives them a bed, and who treats them with all means available at our time, need not fear their objection about whatever procedure he chooses.'[81] This passage offers a poignant look at the relationship between a professor of medicine and his mostly poor patients in a late nineteenth-century hospital. The doctor's power, knowledge, reputation, benevolent occupation, and access to medical instruments and financial support stood against the patient's dependency on the doctor, lower status, and physical weakness. Bergmann's contempt towards the patient's consent was thus an expression of an almost cynically realistic perspective on the situation, which afforded no space for the patient's autonomous choice. His statement reveals his intent to use his power as he saw fit. It was precisely this intention that the official at the ministry of culture took issue with, notating it—and not any other passage in the twelve-page letter—with a big question mark.

Professor Lassa Oppenheim did not know of Bergmann's affidavit, because it was never published. He learned about Bergmann and Hahn's experiments through newspaper reporting in 1891. This spurred him to engage with the

[79] Leidig, Letter, GStA PK I. HA Rep. 76, VIII B, no. 3846, 16.

[80] GStA PK I. HA Rep. 76 VIII B, no. 3846, 23 RS.

[81] GStA PK I. HA Rep. 76 VIII B, no. 3846, 24 VS.

question of how medical procedures should be legally defined and regulated.[82] He ultimately arrived at the conclusion that medical procedures performed without the patient's explicit consent were, with a few exceptions, a form of coercion.[83]

In 1894, the Reichsgericht adopted this position in its first case dealing with a complaint against a surgeon who had performed a procedure against the express will of the patient. In this case, it was the patient's legal guardian, her father, who did not consent to her foot being amputated in order to cure her osseous tuberculosis (which was ultimately successful). The decision, later nicknamed the 'Hamburg decision' after the city in which the events in the suit took place, created the general legal framework for questions of consent that lasted well into Weimar Republic. However, few doctors were ever convicted on these grounds. This was true in the 'Hamburg case' itself. After the high court sent the case back to the Hamburg district court, the judges acquitted the doctor on the grounds that the amputation was an emergency operation and that the doctor was thus justified in performing it without consent and even against the expressed will of the patient's father. The majority of doctors disagreed with the Reichsgericht's decision, since it qualified a doctor's actions as bodily harm, the punishability of which was simply suspended when certain conditions maintained, such as medical necessity and the patient's consent. But jurisprudential thinkers also remained divided on the decision. A particular point of dispute was whether the patient's entry into a clinic or practice did not itself constitute consent to all measures deemed necessary by the doctor, thus making their explicit consent superfluous.[84]

Consent and informing the patient about the measures to be taken were not necessarily treated as an indivisible unit in these debates. Some people held that explicit consent was necessary while at the same time believing that it was legitimate for doctors to give the patient only a rough sketch of the planned operation without informing them about its potential risks or invasiveness. As a 1912 court decision explained:

> The doctor providing the patient with comprehensive information about all potentially negative effects of the operation would not seldom even be acting incorrectly, whether it be because it might frighten the patient from undergoing the operation although it might be necessary or helpful, or whether it be because the thought of the risks associated with the operation might place the patient in a state of fear and excitement and thus jeopardize the favourable outcome of the operation and recovery.[85]

[82] Noack, *Eingriffe*, 23. [83] Oppenheim, *Das ärztliche Recht*, 21.

[84] Noack, *Eingriffe*, 17–147; Elkeles, 'Die schweigsame Welt'.

[85] 3rd Civil Law Panel, Decision from 1 March 1912, III. 231/11, 1. Ist der Arzt verpflichtet, den Kranken auf die nachteiligen Folgen aufmerksam zu machen, die möglicherweise bei einer beabsichtigten Operation entstehen können? 2. Zur Frage der Beweislast beim Eintritte schädlicher Folgen einer Operation, in *Entscheidungen des Reichsgerichtes in Zivilsachen* 78 (1912): 432–6, 434.

The decision applied similar reasoning to informing patients about their diagnosis, because in the judges' minds, the issue was not whether the doctor's plans were medically purposeful, but whether the patient was prepared to live with the effects of the operation.

But the discussion on consent put pressure on proponents of 'benign deception' to justify the practice. The legal notion that patients have a right to decide for themselves whether they undergo a certain medical treatment put a fissure in the often 'silent world of doctor and patient'.[86] The fracture was not just a matter of legal theory or medical ethics. It had real consequences: asking for a patient's consent gave them an opportunity to ask why the treatment was necessary, and the answer could factor into their decision for or against going forward. Moreover, the concept of explicit consent relativized the assumption that *every* suggestion of future health risks should be suppressed in order to avoid evoking fear or hopelessness and their potentially harmful effects. Though this assumption had long been relegated to the margins of medical research, it retained validity in medical practice and law, as the quoted decision from 1912 shows.

Hope against Hope: Facets of an Emotion

Shortly after the turn of the twentieth century, one of the most extensive analyses of 'benign deception' in the Germanophone world appeared in the form of the 650-page book *Ärztliche Ethik* (*Medical Ethics*). Published in 1902, it was authored by Albert Moll (1862–1939), a doctor, psychiatrist, and sexologist based in Berlin.[87] Outrage over experiments conducted on non-consenting patients had also occasioned him to reconsider the ethics that determined 'the duties of the doctor in all aspects of his work', as the book's subtitle read. Moll believed that doctors and researchers had allowed their moral standards to slip under the auspices of 'modern', scientific medicine.

He reconceived the doctor-patient relationship as a contractual relation, which he understood not in the sense of an actual paper contract, but in the sense of a general ethical framework. He wanted the patient to be treated as a client who entered into a relationship with the doctor for a distinct purpose, and he thought that the doctor's duties and latitude to act were in turn delimited by this

[86] Jay Katz, *The Silent World of Doctor and Patient* (Baltimore: Free Press, 1984); and, relativizing Katz's claims, Nolte, 'Zeitalter des ärztlichen Paternalismus', 82–4.

[87] Albert Moll, *Ärztliche Ethik. Die Pflichten des Arztes in allen Beziehungen seiner Thätigkeit* (Stuttgart: Enke Verlag, 1902); Andreas-Holger Maehle, '"God's Ethicist": Albert Moll and His Medical Ethics in Theory and Practice', *Medical History* 56, no. 2 (2012): 217–36, https://doi.org/10.1017/mdh.2011.34; and Andreas-Holger Maehle, 'Zwischen medizinischem Paternalismus und Patientenautonomie: Albert Molls "Ärztliche Ethik" (1902) im historischen Kontext', in *Medizingeschichte und Medizinethik. Kontroversen und Begründungsansätze 1900–1950*, ed. Andreas Frewer and Josef N. Neumann (Frankfurt am Main: Campus, 2001), 44–56.

contractual bond.[88] In this schema, the doctor could fill three roles: medical expert, treating physician, and family doctor/general practitioner. The contractual relationship's defined purpose was supposed to immediately make clear whether and to what extent the 'relatively immoral means' of deception were permitted.[89] In Moll's ethical theory, if the client-patient commissioned the doctor's 'expert opinion on their state of health', then the doctor was obliged to truthfully and candidly offer his assessment, even if it was 'an exceptionally painful [feeling] when he has to tell his patient that they are suffering from a fatal illness'.[90] To help the patient retain a 'shimmer of hope', Moll recommended communicating the diagnosis in a 'gentle manner' and to qualify it by reminding them 'that all knowledge and prediction only have conditional validity'.[91] Another technique was not to tell the diagnosis directly to the patient, but to a third party such as a family member, who would have to be advised on how to truthfully relay the information to the patient. He reasoned this would help the patient hold onto hope because learning about the impossibility of recovery 'from the mouth of the doctor must have a much more serious influence on the spirit than from the mouth of a layperson'.[92] Only when the doctor had strong reasons to believe that the patient would end their own life after learning about their condition was the doctor justified to deceive them, Moll wrote. But he explicitly framed this scenario as an exceptional one and elaborated that the reason could not just be the incurability or terminal nature of the illness, but must be rooted either in a particularly dreadful diagnosis (his example was progressive 'encephalomalacia') or in the patient's mental state.[93]

Moll's plea that deception only be deployed in the most extreme cases was informed by his moral convictions and his belief that, for the most part, people had a robust disposition to keep hope afloat. He went so far as to state: 'In general, one need not take the "last hope" so seriously. After the "last attempt" [to defeat their disease], patients usually make many more very last attempts, as everyday experience shows.'[94]

However, if the client-patient contracted the doctor to treat them, Moll believed there was more room for deception. Again, the power of hope played a decisive role in his reasoning, while he was less concerned about the potentially fatal force of hopelessness that had bothered 'older' doctors like Hufeland. As a psychiatrist specializing in hypnosis, Moll felt certain that the patient's conviction that their condition was curable could in itself help rid them of their illness or, if they had an incurable disease, at least improve their symptoms. Thus, he thought that generating hope through deception was permissible so long as it was in the 'interest of the patient's health'.[95] But he explained that doctors should only rely on hope as a

[88] Moll, *Ärztliche Ethik*, 33–183.
[89] Ibid., 219.
[90] Ibid., 121, 123, and 213.
[91] Ibid., 212–13.
[92] Ibid., 125.
[93] Ibid., 214.
[94] Ibid., 216.
[95] Ibid., 217–19.

therapeutic means after careful consideration. If the treating physician could foresee that it would only hold for a short period of time, then it would do more harm than good, because as soon as the patient realized the doctor had deceived them, they would lose trust in him. Moreover, the patient might have expended time and money to undergo such therapy through hope. If it only had temporary efficacy, the patient would suffer. Thus, Moll placed strict limits on how he thought doctors should try to produce hope through deception.

Finally, Moll thought that family doctors and general practitioners could only legitimately deceive in a few exceptional cases. He asserted that because the family doctor was working in the interest of the entire family, not just in the interest of the individual patient, the doctor was obliged to inform them of their loved one's incurable state or approaching death so that they could wrap up that person's familial and occupational affairs. But he rejected solely informing family members out of concern that they would then 'tell the client about his state in [the doctor's] absence, whether intentionally in words, or unintentionally in being unable to suppress their restlessness and fear'.[96] His book applied to this situation rules of communication similar to those it outlined for the medical expert providing a diagnosis.

Moll's *Ärztliche Ethik* thus did not argue that doctors had an unconditional duty to tell their patients the truth about their diagnosis. Still, it criticized many doctors' default choice of suppressing the truth out of their belief that knowledge of it would result in devastating hopelessness. Moll countered that human hope was essentially indestructible. Additionally, he maintained that truthful communication was necessary before a patient made important medical decisions. He declared that patients had an absolute right to make such decisions because they immediately affected them as human beings. This led him to expound on other forms of hope alongside that of survival, which was often the exclusive focus of his fellow doctors. They included the hope of some form of salvation, though not necessarily in the Christian sense, or the consolation won by knowing that one had ordered one's affairs and said goodbye to family before passing away.

In a newspaper article published in the *Berliner Tageblatt* on 28 May 1916, Moll took his nuanced analysis of hope to its logical conclusion. The text made clear that his conception of medical ethics placed normative expectations on the patient. Titled 'The Right of the Sick to Truth', the article implied that patients should bear the knowledge of their inevitable death and derive hope and solace from the fact that they were part of something greater that transcended their individual existence. This argument marked a consequential shift away from placing primacy on the notion that patients *could* 'survive' knowing they had a potentially fatal disease like cancer and towards the assertion that patients *should*

[96] Ibid., 122–3 and 217.

have the fortitude to bear the burden of this knowledge and maintain hope. The moment at which Moll chose to publish this position was no matter of coincidence. In May 1916, the Battle of Verdun—the most horrific, deadliest fight of the First World War—had been raging for months. Moll thought it necessary to make people recognize the omnipresence of death around them and act accordingly. In the article's final passage, he wrote:

> One should educate people such that they look at death as serenely as possible. There can be no doubt that education can accomplish very much in that respect, but here a type of education is necessary that teaches the individual to reach for something higher. It is certain that the previously dominant purely materialistic worldview, which only viewed the soul as a function of the body, was not conducive to this type of education. And a worldview that sees the comfort of the individual as the highest good will not contribute either. Only [the individual's] dissolution into the whole, whether it be of the people, of humanity, of the entire world, can lay the foundation for such an education. Only then can the individual learn to perceive themselves as a small part of the whole, and the resulting state of mind will help them overcome the fear of death that dominates their microcosm.[97]

Moll left open what this 'greater good' could or should be. One was certainly religious faith, which he had already touched on in his book. But in 1916, Moll, who saw himself as a conservative patriot, placed the '*Volk*', the 'people', on equal footing with humanity and the world.

His criticism of individualism and his holistic orientation placed him in the camp of conservative cultural criticism, of which the critique of medicine was one component. However, this led him to support 'truthfulness' in the doctor-patient relationship, which most of his colleagues, including those who would have subscribed to his other positions, rejected. A prominent counter-voice on this question was Albert Krecke—a surgeon, head of a private clinic in Munich, and co-editor of the *Münchener Medizinischen Wochenschrift* (*Munich Medical Weekly*). Krecke categorically rejected telling patients or their family members that they had been diagnosed with cancer and offered as an alternative a list of euphemisms: colon cancer was an 'appendix infection', rectal and stomach cancer were 'benign ulcers', breast cancer an 'innocent breast tumour'.[98] Krecke justified his position with the argument that the knowledge of having cancer would cause a 'heavy psychic shock' that would enduringly shatter the patient's mental stability. He continued that 'from then on, [the patient loses] their joy in life

[97] Albert Moll, 'Das Recht des Kranken auf Wahrheit', *Berliner Tageblatt und Handels-Zeitung* 45, no. 272, 28 May 1916, 2nd supplement.

[98] Albert Krecke, *Vom Arzt und seinen Kranken* (Munich: Lehmanns, 1932), 108.

and their work.... The wife of the cancer patient also loses all confidence and hope the moment that she learns of the nature of the illness; but she absolutely needs them in order to give her husband consolation and stability in the difficult period that is to come.'[99] This claim documents an important shift in psychosomatic thought, away from the 'old' notion that fear and hopelessness directly affected the body, and towards the concept of shock as an event that could cause long-term psychological harm. Military psychologists had formulated the concept of shock during the First World War, as an unprecedented number of soldiers from all armies on all fronts left its battlefields with mental illnesses. German psychiatrists in particular blamed personality traits like a 'weak constitution' for why the experience of war left psychological scars on certain soldiers. Nevertheless, it was now a matter of consensus that the sudden traumatic experience—and not longstanding fear—caused mental illness.[100]

Implicit in the assumption that learning about a cancer diagnosis would constitute such a shock event was the belief that 'cancer' was itself a traumatic experience that radically, inescapably threatened a person's life. Because only then did it make sense to think that the mere application of the word to an individual could afflict their psyche so severely. Even though Krecke himself had had cancer patients who lived for years with cancer or after recovering from cancer, he observed this belief in public discourse.[101]

Some oncologists wanted to push back against this image of cancer as an incurable, unspeakably dreadful illness. The early detection campaigns discussed in the previous chapter were one component of this movement. Another was the establishment of special institutes that offered state-of-the-art treatment and conducted cutting-edge research to improve patients' chances of recovery, particularly for cancer patients who had long been cast away as 'inoperable'.

The taboo proved a considerable hurdle and constantly entangled early oncologists in contradictions. The difficulties began with what they should call their planned institutes. Vinzenz Czerny, who piloted the founding of the Heidelberger Institut für experimentelle Krebsforschung (Heidelberg Institute for Experimental Oncological Research) in 1906, engaged in tiresome negotiations with the state's health ministry, the university's medical faculty, funders, and the grand duke and duchess over the name of the institute's forty-seven-bed clinic. They ultimately agreed on a name that would not wear the 'stigma of incurability on its forehead': 'Samariterhaus (Heil- und Pflegeanstalt für Geschwülste und Geschwüre)'

[99] Ibid., 65 and 57.

[100] Susanne Michl (2014), 'Erster Weltkrieg 1914–1918: Gefühlswelten—Konzepte von Angst in der Kriegspsychiatrie', *Deutsches Ärzteblatt* 111 (2014): 3–34, A1414–A1416; Susanne Michl and Jan Plamper, 'Soldatische Angst im Ersten Weltkrieg. Die Karriere eines Gefühls in der Kriegspsychiatrie Deutschlands, Frankreichs und Russlands', *Geschichte und Gesellschaft* 35, no. 2 (2009): 209–48, https://doi.org/10.13109/gege.2009.35.2.209.

[101] Krecke, *Vom Arzt*, 58 and 108.

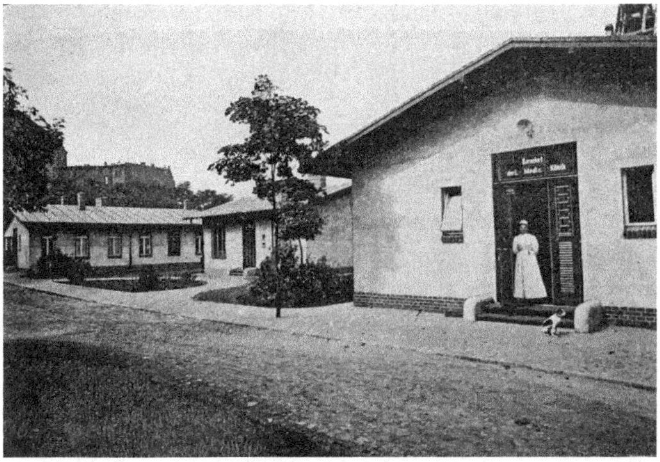

Fig. 16 View of sick bay 1 of the division for cancer research at Berlin's 1st Medical Clinic (1904).

(Samaritan House (Cure and Care Institute for Tumours and Ulcers)).[102] The Institut für Krebsforschung (Institute for Cancer Research) at Berlin's Charité hospital, founded in 1902/3, also had a sick bay with ten beds for women and ten beds for men.[103] Even though newspaper reports on the institute's opening ceremony clearly called them wards for cancer patients, the signs above the doors simply read: 'Pavilion I [or II] of the 1st Medical Clinic' (Fig. 16).[104]

But staff and doctors were supposed to call it 'Ca.-Pavilion' when talking to patients and their family on the assumption that laypersons would not be able to decipher what 'Ca.' stood for. That the institute's leadership invested considerable significance in this innocuous label is revealed by a complaint filed by Georg Klemperer, who took the reins of the cancer wards in 1910. In a letter to the Charité's directors, he remonstrated that when patients and visitors asked the reception about the Ca.-Pavilion, they were told: 'Oh yeah, you mean the cancer wards', whereby they were 'most unsettled'. The directors took the complaint seriously and ordered the receptionists to only use the name 'Ca.-Pavilion'. All employees had to sign an agreement certifying they would adhere to the order.[105]

But the longer specialized cancer institutes existed, the less their doctors were bothered by calling cancer clinics what they were. The tendency began during the First World War, a good ten years after the establishment of the two clinics. For

[102] Vinzenz Czerny, ed., *Das Heidelberger Institut für experimentelle Krebsforschung*, part 1 (Tübingen: Laupp, 1912), 2–4.

[103] Voswinckel, *Erinnerungsort Krebsbaracke*, 9–10.

[104] Dr M., 'Eröffnung des Laboratoriums für Krebsforschung', *Berliner Lokalanzeiger*, 8 June 1903, evening edition, 1.

[105] Copy of a Letter from Prof. Dr Klemperer to the Royal Board of the Charité, Berlin, 21 August 1911, HU Archiv, Charité-Direktion, 949, 293.

instance, in 1915, Ferdinand Blumenthal, who had just assumed leadership of the Charité hospital's Institute for Cancer Research, coordinated with Berlin's poor relief to set up 'consultation for cancer patients, tumour patients, and suspected cancer patients'. Held three times a week, it offered indigent persons with 'suspicious' symptoms the chance to be examined. The consultation sessions' 'circumlocutory' name was indeed supposed to enable the doctors to play down the fear of cancer. But Blumenthal clearly no longer thought it necessary to avoid the word 'cancer' altogether.[106] His reasoning drew on his past experience as an assistant to the institute's first director, Ernst von Leyden. He realized that 'not a small number' of patients came to the institute precisely because they knew it specialized in treating cancer and offered therapies not available elsewhere. In his experience, the name 'Institute for Cancer Research' evoked more trust and hope in these patients than the attempted deception ever could have.[107]

Czerny said similar things about his experiences as head of Heidelberg's oncology institute. Initially, all parties involved feared the clinic would never reach capacity either because other doctors would refuse to send their patients there despite its 'innocuous' name or because patients themselves would avoid it. Indeed, in the clinic's first years, many beds, particularly in the third-class section, remained empty, even though private philanthropic donations had made some free of charge. In order to shake its reputation as a home for the dying, the Samaritan House's administration decided in 1907 to receive not only inoperable cancer patients, but also patients with benign tumours and potential but unconfirmed cases of cancer. However, in Czerny's estimation, it was the clinic's specialized 'modern' cancer treatment that helped people overcome their initial reservations, because it gave them new hope of 'finding help after [their] hopes had elsewhere so often been disappointed'.[108] He maintained this despite the fact that doctors at the clinic themselves admitted that they only successfully cured a fraction of their cancer patients. Still, Czerny thought that the Samaritan House might offer a nugget of hope because it was expressly dedicated to cancer patients considered inoperable and because it used all means available at the time to try to help them:

> But we almost always succeed in reviving the hope of these hopelessly ill people and in palliating their suffering and improving their state of being. They feel benefitted that they are visited daily by a doctor who they trust, treated by talented, good-hearted, young colleagues, and cared for by self-sacrificing, well-trained nurses; they feel good that something new is always at hand when

[106] Ferdinand Blumenthal, Letter to the Royal Board of the Charité, Berlin, den 5. Mai 1915. HU Archiv, Charité-Direktion, 950, 135–6.

[107] Ferdinand Blumenthal, Report on the Institute for Cancer Research for the Minister of Education and Medicine, Berlin, 21 June 1915, HU Archiv, Charité-Direktion, 950, 152.

[108] Czerny, *Das Heidelberger Institut für experimentelle Krebsforschung*, 11.

> another means fails, which strengthens their courage and makes the painful suffering more bearable. And when inexorable—yet, in many of these painful cases, salvific—death claims its victim, the patient dies with the conviction that everything in man's power has been done to palliate and ease his suffering if curing it was impossible.[109]

The hope of the clinic's 'hopelessly ill' patients thus derived from their perception that nobody knew more about cancer than the doctors working there. A good bit of Czerny's account is dedicated to why he thought patients at the Samaritan House never lost their will to fight: because personnel never gave up on them and always tried new means of pain management; because doctors and nurses continued to care for them even though a cure was out of the question.

The Samaritan House and the Berlin cancer clinic were exceptions. Most doctors and policymakers insisted on keeping cancer diagnoses secret from patients. As late as 1935, Berlin's mayor ordered borough mayors to compel doctors in the city-run hospitals to never give patients discharge papers marked with the diagnosis 'Ca.' His reasoning was that: 'Patients today generally know what "Ca" means and such communication might negatively affect them psychologically.'[110] The order was occasioned by a complaint from Karl Frik, who had been running the Werner-Siemens-Institut für Röntgenforschung (Werner Siemens Institute for Radiological Research) since 1924. Frik wrote that, in April 1935, another hospital had sent him two female patients to undergo radiotherapy. They learned of their diagnosis from the unsealed referral note marked with their diagnoses, 'Ovarial-Ca.' and 'Portio-Ca.', respectively.

The effort invested in hiding a cancer diagnosis from a patient sometimes went to extreme lengths. In a few cases, doctors opted against radiotherapy even though they found it medically expedient because they or the patient's family feared that it would tip the patient off to the truth about their condition. After all, everyone had by then seen enough early detection campaigns to know that radiation was the therapy of choice for cervical and ovarian cancer.[111] Evidently, some doctors and family members feared triggering despair in the patient to such a degree that they risked foregoing the chance to hinder—or at least delay—that person's death. Perhaps, too, they wanted to avoid having to witness that despair themselves. At the time, doctors' emotions were rarely thematized in public. An exception was an article published in 1938 by Austrian psychoanalyst Anton Mißriegler in the journal *Hippokrates*:

[109] Ibid., 11–12.

[110] Letter of the Mayor of Berlin to the Borough Mayors of Districts 2, 3, 5–9, 11, 14, 16–20, Berlin, 2 May 1935, LAB A Rep. 003-04-03, no. 143.

[111] Ferdinand Blumenthal, 'Die Bekämpfung des Krebses', *Krankenpflegezeitschrift* 2 (1930): 13–16.

> In cases of cancer, fear makes us [doctors] put our heads in the sand. Even while checking which possible diagnosis is correct, it is always the last diagnosis considered (not just in the textbooks). In unclear cases, do we immediately recommend the patient undergo a serology test for cancer like we do with a Wassermann test [test for syphilis]? . . . It is our own fear that makes us cowardly in the face of cancer and that holds us back from dispelling the patient's fear. We cannot dispel it by ignoring the danger; we dispel it by looking them honestly in the eyes, 'calling the child by its name', and beginning procedures in a timely manner.[112]

The practice of 'benign deception' complicated things for doctors because it prohibited them from informing patients about their diagnosis. But what if the patient sought a second opinion and the other doctor told them they had cancer? In an advice guide for doctors published in 1932, Albert Krecke assessed this as a realistic scenario. This was just one more crack in the shroud of silence cloaking the doctor-patient relationship, which was beginning to peel away despite many doctors publicly clutching on to 'humanitarian' deception.

Krecke maintained that withholding cancer diagnoses from patients was absolutely necessary. Indeed, he was so committed to this position that he disregarded his own fear that doctors might harm their professional reputation if they did not tell a patient that they had cancer and that patient then proceeded to learn the correct diagnosis when seeking a second opinion from another doctor. At the most, he stated, a doctor should only reveal the diagnosis to a friend or extended family member of the patient in order to have a 'witness' for his own diagnostic competence. He thought telling close relatives was out of the question. On the one hand, he thought the knowledge would, on account of their emotional connection to the patient, throw them into despair, crippling their ability to give the patient hope and confidence. On the other, he feared that an unloving relative might write the patient off while they were still living, stop caring for them, or tell them their diagnosis out of sheer malice.[113]

In doctors' offices, though, it seems to have been normal for doctors to tell close relatives that the patient had cancer.[114] The few preserved documents from the period between the 1920s and 1940s in which patients' family members either wrote about or were quoted on their experiences attest to this fact.[115]

[112] Anton Mißriegler, 'Die Krebsangst', *Hippokrates* 18 (1938): 469–71, 470–1.

[113] Krecke, *Vom Arzt*, 60, 109, and 129–30; Gustav Schulte, 'Erfahrungen bei der ambulanten und stationären Krebsbehandlung', *Strahlentherapie* 60 (1937): 323–9, 327. Published by the renowned Thieme Verlag publishing house, five new editions of Krecke's manual were printed between 1932 and 1946.

[114] Carly Seyfarth, *Der 'Ärzte-Knigge'. Über den Umgang mit Kranken und über Pflichten, Kunst und Dienst der Krankenhausärzte* (Leipzig: Thieme Verlag, 1935), 61.

[115] Letter from Luise B., Altona, to the President of the Imperial Health Department Dr Reiter, Altona, 3 January 1934, BArch R 86/4136, 96–8, 96 RS.

A particularly impressive example stems from the archives of Heidelberg's university clinic during the period when it was led by Karl Heinrich Bauer. In April/May 1944, retired 60-year-old Major Anton K. was treated there. Complaining of stomach pains and weight loss, he first went to a doctor friend in Saarbrücken, who referred him to get x-rays at the city's hospital. The radiologist concluded that it was, with 'overwhelming probability', stomach cancer, which is why he sent K. to Heidelberg to be operated on. In his referral letter, he described the patient as a 'very life-affirming and active, joyful man and a caring father... [of] four daughters' and stated that he had told him he was going to have an operation on a benign stomach ulcer. But he did communicate his fears that it might be cancer to Anton K.'s wife, reasoning that: 'I know his wife to be a very brave woman, she wanted to know unconditionally and wants to try everything to keep her husband alive.'[116] Performed on 17 April 1944, the operation revealed that the cancer had already spread throughout the entire digestive tract, making it impossible to surgically remove the tumour. Thus, the operation did not proceed: the surgeons ultimately just took a tissue sample before stitching the abdomen back together.

In Heidelberg, too, doctors adhered to the strategy that the radiologist and friend of Anton K. had pursued. Dr Bauer, the hospital's head doctor, told the patient's wife that the surgery had confirmed the diagnosis and entrusted her with his assessment that her husband only had a few months to live. As expected, she supported the doctors' efforts to keep the truth a secret and deceived her husband into believing that he was suffering from a 'serious infection of the stomach lining', which would 'disappear with rest'.[117] After releasing him in early May 1944, the head doctor in Heidelberg praised Anton K.'s wife in a letter to the doctor in Saarbrücken, who would continue to treat the major: 'Thanks to the especially intelligent disposition of his wife, he [Anton K.] took the quick recovery from the immediate post-surgical reaction as a good sign of his recovery, so that he could be sent to A. on Starnberger Lake [his place of residence] in a sick car of the Reichsbahn [train] without knowing anything about his true state.'[118]

A while after her husband's discharge from the hospital, Anton K.'s wife Lotte wrote a letter to the head doctor in Heidelberg. She thanked him for treating her husband and described the deterioration of his health:

> But now to his physical condition, I have the impression that gradually the worst is coming. —For a few days now, the patient suffers nausea almost every time he eats and otherwise has serious difficulties. —I now only give him fluid food and

[116] Letter from Prof. Dr H. Erbsen, MD, to Prof. Dr Bauer, MD, Saarbrücken, 11 April 1944, UAH, provisional signature: Acc. 11/02 (Chirurgische Klinik), inventory 2, 1944, 95.

[117] UAH, provisional signature: Acc. 11/02 (Chirurgische Klinik), inventory 2, 1944, 95.

[118] Letter from K. H. Bauer, Heidelberg, to Prof. Dr Noetzel, Saarbrücken, 5 May 1944, UAH, provisional signature: Acc. 11/02 (Chirurgische Klinik), inventory 2, 1944, 95.

> 2–3 pantopon injections.[119] But I think that I must now switch to morphine. His body is very hard, and circulatory problems are noticeable. His feet swell up to his ankles and his face is already very yellow, even his eyeballs are discoloured. Otherwise, my husband is still very interested in everything, goes into the garden every day, and believes firmly that he will recover.... [I] only hope that I can uphold the illusion until the end, that he gets a little better each day, though it's often bitterly hard.[120]

This letter is the last document about the death of Anton K. contained in his Heidelberg patient file. The file does not hold the notice of death that house doctors regularly sent to the Heidelberg clinic, sometimes at the clinic's request. But based on Lotte K.'s narration, it is likely that her husband died in 1944.

In this case, too, the preserved documents do not go to the core of the taboo; they do not reveal if Anton K. truly 'firmly believed in his recovery' or whether he remained ignorant about his cancer. On the one hand, this is not very surprising, since the taboo was all about silence: like the eye of a storm, stillness predominates in the centre of the space artificially created by not telling the truth. This silence gives the lie its stability. On the other hand, if almost all patients knew that they had cancer and 'just' conformed with expectations—at the cost of their own emotional isolation—then it seems remarkable that there exist hardly any documents of patients breaking the silence. What does it mean that, up into the 1950s, there are no (or perhaps very few) preserved sources that reveal patients' attempts to break through the silence and talk about their feelings of isolation and loneliness with family members, doctors, nurses, or hospital pastors?

The exchange between Lotte K. and the head doctor at Heidelberg's clinic might offer some clues. The letters contained in Anton K.'s patient file show that an unquestioned hierarchy dominated the relationship between Lotte K. and the doctor, despite her social status, her education, and her wealth, which would have made her the doctor's equal in any other situation. This hierarchy derived from the head doctor's medical authority. He explicitly demanded that she conceal her husband's diagnosis from him and 'bravely' support the doctors' campaign of deception. The doctors promised that in doing so, she was helping her husband stay 'cheerful', as she notes elsewhere in her letter. Both she and the doctors believed that this saved him plunging into undignified despair, which would have been especially difficult for a former officer to bear.

[119] Pantopon is an opioid preparation that was put on the market by Hoffmann-La Roche in 1909; it had fewer effects on the respiratory system than morphine. On its effects, see H. Winternitz (1912), 'Ueber morphinfreies Pantopon und die Wirkung der Nebenalkaloide des Opiums beim Menschen', *Münchener Medizinische Wochenschrift* 59, no. 16 (1912): 853–4.

[120] Letter from Lotte K. to Professor Karl Heinrich Bauer, A. am Starnberger See, undated, UAH, provisional signature: Acc. 11/02 (Chirurgische Klinik), inventory 2, 1944, 95.

By adopting the doctors' communicative strategy for herself, she became part of their team. They praised her for her contribution, and in turn, they allowed her to serve as her own husband's nurse and decide which pain medications to give him. Her letter demonstrates that she accepted this role, at least when she was talking with the head doctor. As soon as she begins describing her husband's health and the measures she is taking, she calls him 'patient', and she writes about his 'body', 'feet', and 'eyeballs' in a way that detaches them from him as a feeling subject. In doing so, she imitates the doctor's medical gaze. She only returns to her husband as a person when discussing his interests.

She only gave cursory mention to how difficult upholding this demeanour was for her, because she knew very well that complaining to the doctor was not befitting of a 'brave' wife and she seems not to have wanted to lose her role as medical assistant and caretaker. This shows that 'benign deception' could have advantages for family members who shared the underlying assumption that hope, cheerfulness, and a dignified attitude would ease the process of dying for *everyone* involved. Those who deviated from the path and told the patient about their cancer and their approaching death risked more than causing the patient to fall into despair as the doctors warned. They also risked being condemned by others for actually or allegedly robbing the patient of hope, joy, and dignity. So long as most people saw death and emotions about it like this, it is likely that only few would have wanted or been willing to undertake this risk and that the few who might have done so either concealed it or did not write about it.

But this does not entirely explain why there is little documentation of cancer patients rejecting the taboo and talking with family about their belief that they had cancer. Did this take place in private so that nobody wrote about it? Or did every attempt at speaking 'openly' fail? Doctors' manuals and medical journals do contain evidence that patients like Anton K. explicitly asked about the nature of their illness and whether they were suffering from cancer. And not all of them let themselves be satisfied by doctors' and nurses' evasive responses. They inquired again and again or tried to peek into their patient's file, which was supposed to remain out of their sight.[121]

However, most accepted—or at least acted as if they accepted—the claim that they had a benign tumour or the like without asking any further questions, perhaps because they tacitly understood its meaning. This is supported by a letter written in 1934 by Luise B. from Altona near Hamburg. Addressed to the president of the Reichsgesundheitsamt (Reich Health Office), the letter's main topic was its author's theory that roundworms and other parasites were the cause of cancer. Almost in passing, she interprets her doctor's statements as a coded cancer diagnosis:

[121] Irmgard Linde, 'Krebsfürsorge im Rahmen der Krankenhausfürsorge', *Strahlentherapie* 97 (1955): 633–42, 636.

> The doctor used the expression 'cramps' for the x-ray findings. To my question if it was cancer I received the reply that it was not yet, but could easily become cancer. This information bolstered my fears, which already tended in this direction—shortly before, namely, my father had died of cancer according to the evaluation of reputable doctors and he had very similar symptoms like those described above. It occasioned me to carefully observe the illness's progress, all symptoms, and my body's reaction to them.[122]

Did Major Anton K. surmise the same thing ten years later about his 'serious infection of the stomach lining' without needing to ask any further questions? His wife's report details the intensity of his pain and how it worsened with every passing day in the summer of 1944. Moreover, the 60-year-old Anton K. had certainly seen materials published by early detection campaigns and probably knew people who had died of cancer. It thus seems highly unlikely that he did not at least for a time doubt the truth of the 'infection of the stomach lining' diagnosis and did not at least for a time suspect that cancer was the disease that was destroying his body. That his wife did not note that he asked any more questions about his state despite his rapidly declining health makes it seem more plausible that he had already deciphered the real meaning of the diagnosis. Perhaps it is more likely that it was not his 'illusions' that had to be maintained, but those of his wife. Perhaps he rejected discussing the 'truth' because he feared that *she* would fall into despair. Without uncovering more documentation, it is impossible to know for sure, and further documentation might not exist.

Our contemporary conceptions of emotions view speaking about them as beneficial, while suppressing negative emotions like fear or despair are seen as dangerous forms of self-alienation. From this perspective, the possibility that Anton and Lotte K. did not speak about the former's cancer might have produced and perpetuated loneliness and emotional isolation. But as the second chapter showed, this understanding of emotions is itself a product of history. During the interwar years and even more in the early 1950s, another theory of emotions dominated public discourse. It held that mastering emotions like fear and despair and not speaking about them were attributes of a mature, 'dignified' person.[123] The taboo on speaking about cancer with a patient meshed well with this normative position. If one embraces the notion that emotions and perspectives

[122] Letter from Luise B., Altona, to the president of the Imperial Health Department Professor Dr Reiter, Altona, 3 January 1934, BArch R 86/4136, 96–8, 96 RS.

[123] Hitzer, 'Jim Button's Fear'; Peter N. Stearns and Timothy Haggerty, 'The Role of Fear: Transitions in American Emotional Standards for Children, 1850–1950', *American Historical Review* 96, no. 1 (1991): 63–94; Nelleke Bakker, 'The Meaning of Fear: Emotional Standards for Children in the Netherlands, 1850–1950: Was There a Western Transformation?', *Journal of Social History* 34, no. 2 (2000): 369–91; Michael Roper, 'Between Manliness and Masculinity: The "War Generation" and the Psychology of Fear in Britain, 1914–1950', *Journal of British Studies* 44, no. 2 (2005): 343–62, https://doi.org/10.1086/427130.

on them change throughout history, are culturally variable, and are to a certain extent learned, then the K.'s summer of 1944 was not necessarily one of laborious deception, lonely despair, and burdensome silence. It is possible that both knew or sensed that Anton K.'s death was near. And it is possible that they chose not to speak about it not just because of the pressure of the doctors' expectations, but because they had a sort of silent pact that they did *not* want to share their feelings of fear and despair. It is possible that they were in agreement that this would make it easier for them to keep those feelings in check and more happily spend their remaining days together. Ultimately, this cannot be anything more than speculation, because there are no (further?) traces that lead us further into the inner workings of the taboo.

Dispassionate Dying: Appeals to Courage and Truth during National Socialism

Thus, well into the 1940s (and thereafter), doctors and family members were practising 'benign deception', suppressing the truth about a patient's or loved one's cancer diagnosis. But in some places, people began to speak more openly, and sometimes, the spaces that cultivated silence were not far away from those that fostered speaking. At Heidelberg's surgery centre, where Anton K. was treated, suppression was seemingly standard. But in the same hospital's clinic for internal medicine, and particularly in its neurology division, things were different. Patients treated for cancer there were suffering either from tumours or metastases in the brain or spinal cord. As far as can be discerned from patient files, they were generally told about their diagnosis. A married, 36-year-old machinist with brain metastases, a 35-year-old deaconess with metastases in her pelvic bone, and a married, 61-year-old painter with a brain tumour—the doctors in Heidelberg spoke with all three patients about their cancer. They did not hide from the deaconess that she would soon die, nor did they leave the machinist in the dark about the fact that only a high-risk operation could save his life.[124]

Age, gender, and marital status fail to entirely explain why these patients—in contrast to those in the surgery centre—were told about their diagnosis, as the differences among them are too stark. Perhaps the deaconess's faith played a role in her case, but indices about the other two patients' religious beliefs are lacking. Moreover, there is no evidence that the doctors viewed these three patients as extraordinarily stable personalities. In fact, the doctor described the machinist in his anamnesis as a 'somewhat unreasonable, uncritical, but otherwise

[124] Patient records of Frieda Sch., single nurse from Karlsruhe; patient records Wilhelm St., machine worker from Neulußheim; patient records Eduard Th., married painter from Landau, UAH, provisional signature: Acc. 30/01 (Neuro), new: L-V, 1938, no. 917; no. 930; and no. 977.

unremarkable man'.[125] The only common link between all three patients was that they were afflicted with forms of cancer that had little chance of being cured. But the head doctor treating Anton K. had the same assessment about his illness and still did not speak openly with him. Thus, it seems justified to assume that neither the patient's disposition nor the severity of the diagnosis or prognosis were necessarily the deciding factors in whether a doctor communicated with the patient that they had cancer. Rather, who the attending doctor was determined the limits of discussion, and it seems that their primary guide was their beliefs about whether one should speak about cancer or death with a patient.

What conditions helped form these beliefs? One might have been how particular medical specializations shaped doctors' relations with patients. Did surgeons speak less with their patients about cancer and death because they were more focused on the body part to be operated on and less on the 'whole' person? Because they only had patients for long periods of time in exceptional cases? Did neurologists and internists inquire into the interrelations between body and psyche as a matter of habit? Did they pay more attention to patients' mental state because they cared for them over longer periods of time and thus had more opportunity to develop an amicable relationship with them? Though these hypotheses might seem intuitive, a look outside Heidelberg shines light on their weaknesses. While the head surgeon opted for silence in the case of Anton K., his prominent colleague, Berlin surgeon Ferdinand Sauerbruch, pleaded with doctors to inform cancer patients about their diagnosis.[126] In contrast, internist Ludolf von Krehl—who led Heidelberg's clinic for internal medicine until 1931 and, as Viktor von Weizsäcker's teacher, helped pave the way for psychosomatic medicine—categorically refused to tell his cancer patients the truth.[127] This lack of consensus among doctors suggests that the deciding factors must have lain elsewhere. Like around 1900, the debate on whether to inform patients of their diagnosis was carried out in two domains: in law, and in medical, psychological, theological, and philosophical discussions about death and the role of emotions in the success of medical treatment.

In 1932, a high court decision grappled for the first time with whether doctors were obligated to tell patients that they had been diagnosed with cancer.[128] It made waves in discussions on medical ethics and medical law. The case concerned Frau L. from the East Prussian town of Braunsberg. In 1930, she sought out a 'healer'

[125] Patient records Wilhelm St., machine worker from Neulußheim, UAH, provisional signature: Acc. 30/01 (Neuro), new: L-V, 1938, no. 930.

[126] Ferdinand Sauerbruch, *Das war mein Leben* (Bad Wörishofen: Kindeler and Schiermeyer, 1951), 123.

[127] Ludolf Krehl, *Die Behandlung innerer Krankheiten*, 2nd edn (Berlin: Vogel, 1934), 79; Ludolf Krehl, *Der Arzt* (Stuttgart: Hippokrates-Verlag, 1937).

[128] Willy Schumacher, 'Inwieweit darf der Arzt den Kranken über eine gefährliche Erkrankung wahrheitsgemäß aufklären', *Monatsschrift für Krebsbekämpfung* 3 (1933): 135–6; Gustav Schläger, 'Aufklärung und Verschwiegenheit bei Krebsverdacht', *Monatsschrift für Krebsbekämpfung* 10 (1943): 150–5, 153.

and told him about her somewhat unspecific medical concerns. By means of hypnosis, he diagnosed her with an early onset of cancer and promised to cure it. Learning this placed her in such a feverishly fearful state that another doctor diagnosed her with severe depression and psychosis and evaluated her as being at a high risk of suicide. Consequently, Frau L. was deemed 'mentally ill' and checked into a psychiatric clinic.[129] Her family accused the 'healer' of bodily harm, claiming that his openly telling Frau L. she had cancer was what caused her psychosis.

The case was first heard by a local court in Braunsberg; the appeal at the Braunsberg district court. The appeals court sided with the plaintiff and judged the defendant guilty of negligent bodily harm, because 'the defendant, through *unsparingly* informing Frau L. about her cancer, "at least contributed to causing" her mental illness'.[130] The 'healer' appealed, sending the case to the Reichsgericht in February 1932. The high court's second panel for punitive law overturned the ruling and returned the case back to the district court. Their reasoning was clear:

> Insofar as the ruling is supposed to say that it should be *regularly* concealed from the patient that they have cancer, the judges cannot agree. Even with serious illnesses like cancer, the patient has an interest and entitlement to be truthfully told about the nature of his illness by the doctor or natural healer to whom he entrusts his care. The patient can only then make a reasoned decision about whether he wants treatment and which treatment he wants. Thus, a medical professional also must tell a cancer patient about their illness—even if not necessarily about all its details and consequences—so long as specific reasons in the individual case do not lead to fear that this may impede the process of recovery.[131]

The Reichsgericht turned on its head the district court's argumentation, which had adhered to the dominant position propagated in advice manuals and medical textbooks. Their ruling asserted that concealing the diagnosis should be the exception, not the rule. It relied on the same principle that the Reichsgericht had used in past decisions requiring doctors to obtain the patient's consent before performing surgery: namely, the principle that people have a right to decide what happens to their own body and that they must be given the necessary medical facts in order to make an informed decision. But the 1932 judgement was novel in the sense that it was not just about a doctor telling the patient about the planned medical procedure and its potential complications and side effects. Rather, it

[129] 2nd Criminal Law Panel [Strafsenat] (1932), Decision from 29 February 1932, II 57/32, Inwieweit ist ein Heilbehandler verpflichtet, den sich ihm anvertrauenden Kranken, auch den gefährlich Erkrankten, über sein Leiden aufzuklären?, in *Entscheidungen des Reichsgerichts in Strafsachen* 66 (1932): 181–5, 181–2.

[130] Ibid., 184 (emphasis in original).

[131] Ibid., 182–3.

concerned talking about the patient's illness itself. Moreover, the high court's ruling established a connection between 'truthfully' telling the patient about their diagnosis and that patient's trust in their doctor. By making trust a pillar of their argument, the judges followed a line of reasoning similar to Albert Moll's in his vision of the doctor-patient relationship as a contractual relation. They only considered silence legitimate when the patient was in a particularly volatile mental state. The strict limits they placed on what constituted such an exception can be gleaned from their instructions to the district court mandating that a professional investigate whether Frau L. had a mental illness before learning about her cancer diagnosis and, if so, whether this had been known to the 'healer'.

Although the judges did not explicitly write about emotions in their decision, they made a judgement about the plausibility of the notion that telling a patient they were diagnosed with cancer could completely rob them of hope and thereby set their death in motion. By placing primacy on the right to self-determination, they suggested that they did not believe this reasoning.

The Reichsgericht's third panel for civil law explicitly affirmed the principle of self-determination in a decision published on 8 March 1940.[132] The judgement concerned a surgeon's appeal against a lower court's order that he pay his patient Hedwig H. 6,000 Reichsmarks in damages. In February 1936, he had amputated her right breast in the belief that he had detected a cancerous tumour, which a biopsy later proved to be false. However, before the operation, Hedwig H. knew nothing about the doctor's concern she had cancer, assuming it was a benign tumour. Based on this assumption, she assented to a local surgical removal of the tumour. Only when her bandage was changed for the first time after the operation did she realize that the doctor had performed a mastectomy. The operation also seriously restricted her ability to move her right arm, disabling her from fully returning to work.

The appeals court in Leipzig and the district court in Dresden awarded her damages because the doctor had not conducted a biopsy to confirm his suspicion, neither before nor after the operation. The Reichsgericht upheld the grant of damages but did not follow the lower courts' reasoning. Drawing on expert opinions, they held that it was medically plausible for a doctor to decide to operate after formulating a diagnosis of breast cancer solely based on how the tumour looked and felt. The opinions explained that a biopsy was not without its own risks and that in this case, the doctor's clinical observations suggested that it was highly probable the tumour was cancer. However, the Reichsgericht denied the doctor's appeal exclusively on the grounds that he should have informed his patient about

[132] 3rd Civil Law Panel (1940), Decision from 8 March 1940, III 117/39, 1. Zur Sorgfaltspflicht des Arztes vor einem schwerwiegenden Eingriff. 2. Wie ist die Rechtslage, wenn der Arzt bewußtermaßen einen schwerwiegenden Eingriff ohne die Einwilligung des Kranken vorgenommen hat, obwohl ihm deren Einholung möglich gewesen wäre, und wenn sich der Eingriff später als nicht erforderlich herausstellt?, in *Entscheidungen des Reichsgerichtes in Zivilsachen* III 117/39 (1940).

her illness before the operation and should have obtained her consent before performing the mastectomy. The judges thus rejected the doctor's argument that this case represented precisely the sort of exception carved out by the high court's 1932 decision. He had claimed that the patient would not have been able to bear the emotional burden of the diagnosis because her mother had recently died of cancer, and obtaining consent to amputate would have been impossible without communicating the diagnosis. The Reichsgericht judges countered:

> The legal principle that . . . the individual must retain self-determination over their body, even in relation to their doctor, is of such general nature and is necessitated by such well-founded considerations . . . that it must be maintained even against such concerns as the appeal raises. Of course, a doctor will try to protect the patient from harmful fearfulness . . . . But this must give way to the necessity that the doctor must, before every operation, ensure that he has the consent of the patient, consent based on clear, accurate information about the nature and effects of the operation (even if naturally not encompassing every detail). Though the communication required to receive such consent might lower the patient's mood or general state of being, such are the unavoidable disadvantages that must be accepted.[133]

Thus, the judges placed the right to self-determination higher than concerns about the potential harm that might be caused by fear. And they characterized the emotional effects of learning one had cancer as a 'lowered mood' or 'fearfulness', which might indeed be 'disadvantageous' for the patient, but would not threaten their life or make it unbearable and might only be temporary. This re-evaluation of fear, hopelessness, and death deserves some analysis.

Decisive for this shift were medical, psychoanalytic, and theological discussions about the meaning of modernity. In the mid-1920s, some psychoanalysts criticized Freud's atheism, because they viewed 'modern' rootlessness as a primary cause of neurosis. They contemplated how they could establish bonds for their patients and wondered if religion might provide a suitable means to do so.[134] Many appealed to Alfred Adler's individual psychology, which centred on the individual's social relationships and their feeling of community. At the same time, a number of pastors, both Catholic and Protestant, began engaging

[133] Ibid., 137–8.

[134] Viennese psychiatrist Viktor Frankl remains the most influential progenitor of this approach; however, while he thought religion was likely a suitable means to forge such bonds, he thought that therapists and doctors should refrain from trying to influence patients' religion or worldview. See Victor Frankl, 'Psychotherapie und Weltanschauung. Zur grundsätzlichen Kritik ihrer Beziehungen', *Internationale Zeitschrift für Individualpsychologie* 3 (1925): 250–2.

with psychotherapy with the aim of integrating this 'technique of the soul' into pastoral theology.[135]

One result of this mutual effort was the founding of the Arbeitsgemeinschaft 'Arzt und Seelsorger' (Working Group 'Doctor and Pastor'), which had been publishing a book series of the same name since 1925 and met multiple times a year.[136] The initiative was started by Protestant theologian Carl Gunther Schweitzer, who believed such dialogue was necessary to give doctors some orientation beyond what he saw as the 'materialism' of medical science and to inform theologians working 'in our nervous time' about developments in medicine.[137]

Psychiatrists Fritz Künkel and Johannes Heinrich Schultz played a key role on the medical side of the organization. Both practiced in Berlin and both had made names for themselves among Germanophone doctors interested in psychotherapy. In 1936, both joined Matthias Göring's Deutsches Institut für psychologische Forschung und Psychotherapie (German Institute for Psychological Research and Psychotherapy), which, as discussed in Chapter 2, promoted National-Socialist Deutsche Seelenheilkunde (German Psychotherapy) as an alternative to what its representatives vilified as Freud's 'Jewish' psychoanalysis. While Schultz, who invented autogenic training, remained the institute's deputy director until 1945, Künkel did not return to Germany from a 1939 lecture tour in the United States.[138]

In the 1920s, Künkel began urging psychotherapists to open themselves to ideas from religion and philosophy. His position led him to inquire into the meaning of courage and a sense of community for mental health.[139] One part of this analysis involved promoting a more dispassionate, detached perspective on fear. Like National-Socialist writer Charlotte Köhn-Behrens, who was also close to

[135] Benjamin Ziemann, *Katholische Kirche und Sozialwissenschaften 1945–1975* (Göttingen: Vandenhoeck & Ruprecht, 2007), 266–71; Benjamin Ziemann, 'The Gospel of Psychology: Therapeutic Concepts and the Scientification of Pastoral Care in the West German Catholic Church, 1950–1980', *Central European History* 39, no. 1 (2006): 79–106, 81–2.

[136] R. Gaupp, 'Psychotherapie', *Verhandlungen der Deutschen Gesellschaft für Innere Medizin. 39. Kongress, gehalten zu Wiesbaden vom 25.–28. April 1927*, ed. A. Géronne (Berlin: Bermann-Verlag, 1927), 11–35, 29. Some sources also refer to it as the Arbeitsgemeinschaft zwischen Geistlichen und Ärzten.

[137] Ernst Jahn, 'Geschichte und Problematik der Arbeit', in *40 Jahre Berliner Arbeitsgemeinschaft Arzt und Seelsorger* (*Berliner Hefte zur Förderung der evangelischen Krankenseelsorge*, 18) (Berlin: Evangelisches Konsistorium Berlin-Brandenburg, Generalkonvent für Krankenseelsorge, 1965), 13–31, 20.

[138] Michael Gregor Kölch, 'Theorie und Praxis der Kinder- und Jugendpsychiatrie in Berlin 1920–1935. Die Diagnose "Psychopathie" im Spannungsfeld von Psychiatrie, Individualpsychologie und Politik' (PhD diss., Freie Universität Berlin, 2006), 265–73; Jürgen Brunner and Florian Steger, 'Johannes Heinrich Schultz (1884–1970). Begründer des Autogenen Trainings. Ein biographischer Rekonstruktionsversuch im Spannungsfeld von Wissenschaft und Politik', *BIOS: Zeitschrift für Biographieforschung und Oral History* 19, no. 1 (2006): 16–25.

[139] Johannes Neumann, 'Über den IV. allg. ärztlichen Kongreß für Psychotherapie in Bad Nauheim 12.–14. April', *Internationale Zeitschrift für Individualpsychologie* 7 (1929): 303–5; Kölch 'Theorie und Praxis', 268–9.

Deutsche Seelenheilkunde, Künkel thought that fear of fear itself was unwarranted, because people would generally muster up courage in the 'open' confrontation with their own fears.[140] He equated avoiding fear with cowardice and identified it as the symptom of a 'character type' lacking in courage and bravery. Such emotional strategies had earlier been propagated by the 'Mental hygiene' section of the aforementioned exhibition 'Kampf dem Krebs'.[141]

These morally charged concepts reappeared in 1937 in a series of talks organized by the Working Group 'Doctor and Pastor' on the question 'Should one tell the patient the whole truth?'.[142] Fritz Künkel himself had posed the question during a lecture he held on the 'ethics of medical treatment' in June 1937 at Berlin's Lutheran Consistory. Speaking to members of the group, he situated the doctor-patient relationship within a larger 'unitary front' of relations, which included family members and the *Volkskörper* (body of the German people). Künkel claimed that if the patient recognized their place within this extended social circle, they would be freed from their 'egoistic' disposition. This, in turn, would enable doctor and nurse to see through the 'illusory subject' along with that subject's stated wishes and uncover the patient's true essence, their 'will to health' and 'health conscience'. He asserted that this ethics would allow the doctor to treat the patient against their expressed, yet 'illusory' will.[143] Only at the end of his lecture did Künkel touch on what this meant for dying patients, spurring the group to plan another session on 'Truth at the sickbed' for 2 September 1937.

So many members of the Working Group and their guests convened on this day in the Consistory's grand Baroque building at Lindenstrasse 14 that seats ran out. Many had to stand and some were sent home, a measure of interest in the topic.[144] The discussion was introduced by professor of medicine Dr Schwarz, who offered a survey of the positions represented in the most popular books on medical ethics. He rounded it out by asserting that Albert Moll's was the only well-reasoned position that went beyond the mere 'exchange of opinions'. In contrast to Moll, though, Schwarz concluded his introduction with some reflections on the difference between truth and truthfulness:

[140] Köhn-Behrens, 'Das Kapitel von der Angst'.

[141] Bettina Hitzer, 'Körper-Sorge(n). Gesundheitspolitik mit Gefühl', in *Performing Emotions. Interdisziplinäre Perspektiven auf das Verhältnis von Politik und Emotion in der Frühen Neuzeit und in der Moderne*, ed. Claudia Jarzebowski and Anne Kwaschik (Göttingen: Vandenhoeck & Ruprecht, 2013), 43–68, 60–1.

[142] Arbeitsgemeinschaft 'Arzt und Seelsorger', January 1936–November 1942, Evangelisches Zentralarchiv [EZA] 1/2899.

[143] 'Zur Ethik der Krankenbehandlung. Bericht über einen Vortrag Dr. Künkels auf einer Tagung der Arbeitsgemeinschaft zwischen Ärzten und Geistlichen am 8. Juni 1937', LAB A Rep. 003-04-03, no. 55.

[144] 'Soll man dem Kranken die volle Wahrheit sagen? Vortrag von Professor Schwarz sowie anschließende Diskussion', Conference of the Arbeitsgemeinschaft zwischen Ärzten und Geistlichen on 2 September 1937, 1, LAB A Rep. 003-04-03, no. 55.

> So, truthfulness for the doctor! But not truth and certainly not the whole truth; who would be so arrogant as to claim to be in possession of it! Rather, truthfulness in all 'statements that one cannot avoid'—this remains the great, difficult task that we have to fulfil, and indeed have to fulfil in such a way that we do not kill or harm, but heal and promote life, whereby we have to treat people not only as bodies but above all as soul and spirit.[145]

This represented a regression to a time before the Reichsgericht's 1932 decision. Many of the theologians present argued against Schwarz, because, in the words of the Catholic pastor of the Berlin-Buch hospital, dying should be consciously experienced as a 'holy end' and 'the highpoint of life'.[146]

Künkel and Schultz took a position that went in the opposite direction of Schwarz. Schultz emphatically affirmed the 1932 high court decision and stressed that not telling patients the truth about their diagnosis must be the exception, not the rule. But in contrast to the judges' ruling, the patient's right to self-determination played no role in his argument. He was exclusively concerned with outlining the necessity for 'Germans' to adopt a new, warriorlike emotional tenor that necessitated they prove themselves in dying and death:

> Today, the courage to [say and hear] the truth is one of the most important demands of our time. The new Germany wants courageous people who also have the courage to [know] the truth. The German should not just live courageously, he should also be able to die courageously.... A living Christian will also know how to die and there is no reason to keep the truth from him.[147]

Excepted from this rule were, in his opinion, only 'unstable, internally fragile people', for whom 'doctor and pastor [must] decide... what is to be done'.[148] He thus elevated dying—be it on the battlefield or in the hospital—as the 'final' test of courage of a 'German', a test that nobody should be denied because of a lack of knowledge.

Künkel took an even more radical approach to the concept of death as a test of courage, speaking out against making the process of dying more comfortable through methods like pain management. He advocated for detachment:

145 Professor Schwarz, 'Soll man dem Kranken die volle Wahrheit sagen?', Conference of the Arbeitsgemeinschaft zwischen Ärzten und Geistlichen on 2 September 1937, 3, LAB A Rep. 003-04-03, no. 55.

146 'Soll man dem Kranken die volle Wahrheit sagen?' (discussion), Conference of the Arbeitsgemeinschaft zwischen Ärzten und Geistlichen on 2 September 1937, 1, LAB A Rep. 003-04-03, no. 55.

147 'Soll man dem Kranken die volle Wahrheit sagen?' (discussion), 3.

148 Ibid.

> One should not try to make dying for a person easier than it is. From the experience of war, where everything proceeds in a much more matter-of-fact way, we know the simplicity of dying, like we know from farmers and all people who still exist in the original we (*Urwir*), this matter-of-fact way of dying. One should refrain from 'soothsaying' the sick. The dying person's time has come. Now *he* is confronting the last big test. Will he pass the test? One can only prepare somebody for this final test and one does it uprightly by not shielding him from the truth.[149]

In Künkel's eyes, consciously experiencing dying represented the final crisis in the process of character development—the 'Werde-Leid' (becoming-suffering), as he put it.[150] He only briefly mentioned the role that community played in overcoming this suffering when describing farmers as an example of people captured in a sort of motherly 'original we'. The farmer, he seemed to claim, does not conceive of himself as a discrete individual, which enables him to take a simple, detached perspective on his own death. Soldiers, he stated, also learned this attitude in war through the everydayness of death in their units. The argument recalls Albert Moll's article 'The Right of the Sick to Truth'. Penned in the middle of the First World War, Moll upheld training people to 'dissolve into the whole' as *the* curative measure against the desperate finality of death.

Thus, there was a tight connection between, on the one hand, calls for a detached approach to death under the auspices of a new community united through war and, on the other, pleas to speak 'openly' about cancer diagnoses with patients. Some doctors invested this relationship with a clear National-Socialist stance. For instance, August Mayer, head of Tübingen University's women's clinic, wrote in an article published in a 1941 issue of the specialist journal *Strahlentherapie* (*Radiotherapy*) that he had given up his earlier reservations against cancer wards and 'cancer houses' for terminally ill cancer patients. He was swayed by his observation that more and more women sick with cancer bore 'the awareness of their suffering with remarkable and joyful stoicism'; thus, there was no need to conceal their diagnosis from them. Mayer, who had forcibly sterilized women in his clinic even before 1933, then proceeded to engage with the question as to whether the lives of terminally ill cancer patients were 'worthless' and thus should be 'exterminated', a notion that he said was 'seductive from the purely rational point of view'. But because patients clung to life and stopped wanting to die as soon as their pain was relieved, and in order to maintain people's trust in doctors, Mayer relativized this position: 'There are serious concerns

[149] Ibid., 5 (emphasis in original).

[150] Fritz Künkel, *Charakter, Krisis und Weltanschauung. Die vitale Dialektik als Grundlage der angewandten Charakterkunde*, 3rd edn (Stuttgart: Hirzel Verlag, 1976), 147 (original edition published 1935).

against the extermination of unworthy life by the doctor.'[151] It is unclear whether he was using coded language to speak out against euthanasia or simply did not want doctors to participate in it. However, his thought clearly established an inner connection between the promotion of a detached approach to death, which reached its extreme in Nazi euthanasia programmes, and the matter-of-fact approach to fatal cancer, which was supposed to make possible open, 'stoic' discussion about the 'truth'.

Hope after the War

After the end of the Second World War, August Mayer was allowed to continue leading the women's clinic at the University of Tübingen. Despite having been a member of the SA and despite having overseen forced sterilizations, a denazification tribunal declared him 'exonerated'.[152] Because of his age, the now 73-year-old Mayer was named professor emeritus in October 1949. But even in retirement, the topic 'truth at the sickbed' left him no peace. In 1951, he published a long article in the Catholic journal *Die Kirche in der Welt* (*The Church in the World*) in which he revised some of his positions from his 1941 article without, however, explicitly referring to it.[153]

His new ruminations on 'truth' were informed by a markedly different take on suffering and dying. Drawing on the work of Viktor von Weizsäcker, he concluded that physical illness was a 'means to heal the personality and mind', while society's caring for sick people, including the terminally ill, now appeared to him as a 'school of suffering' that would cultivate 'valuable ethical powers' for the 'whole of the people'.[154] He opposed constructing 'cancer houses' for the care of dying cancer patients, because he now thought doctors should only tell them and their loved ones the 'truth' 'drop by drop' so as not to exclude them from the community.[155] In 1955, psychiatrist Max Mikorey established a similar argumentative connection between communicating a diagnosis and the danger of abetting euthanasia. He characterized telling someone they had cancer as an event that made the patient dead while they were still living. This, he believed, opened up a slippery slope that, by way of the patient's wish for assisted suicide, could lead to euthanasia:

[151] August Mayer, 'Die Entwicklung unserer Therapie beim Uterus-Kollumkarzinom', *Strahlentherapie* 69 (1941): 17–28, 26–7; Thorsten Doneith, 'August Mayer—Direktor der Universitäts-Frauenklinik Tübingen 1917–1949' (PhD diss., Universität Tübingen, 2007), 72 and 100–5.

[152] Ibid., 159–64.

[153] August Mayer, 'Wahrheit am Krankenbett', *Die Kirche in der Welt* 4, no. 9 (1951): 59–66 and no. 29 (1951): 209–16. The only publication of his own that Mayer referenced was an article from 1929.

[154] Ibid., 214. [155] Ibid., 212.

> Whosoever predicts the death of a sick patient today might be asked by them tomorrow to execute this death sentence in the subjectively most comfortable form. But whosoever complies with such wishes for death can easily become entangled in state-run euthanasia programmes against sick people who are in no way ready to die so quickly.[156]

In contrast to Mayer, Mikorey's text was not informed by thoughts about suffering and its potentially humanizing effects. As a psychiatric consultant for the newly founded Bundeswehr (the army of the Federal Republic of Germany), he was more concerned with the notion that fear of death could easily turn into panic.[157]

Juridical discussions on the doctor's duty to inform their patient also returned to the perception of fear and dying as threatening emotions that had the power to consume the patient and destabilize their mental health. But at the same time, they highlighted the irrational aspects of fear. These debates began in West Germany in the mid-1950s and closely followed the American legal concept of informed consent, which had only recently been defined.[158] On the primary issue of consent, West German courts' judgements differed little from the decisions handed down by the Reichsgericht. Courts on all levels affirmed that doctors could only operate on patients with their consent and that this necessitated informing them of the nature of the treatment and its potential effects.

But on the question as to whether doctors were obligated to tell patients about their diagnosis, West German courts diverged from their National-Socialist predecessors. And in 1959, the Bundesgerichtshof (Federal Court of Justice) set their position on the matter in stone. The case concerned a woman with cervical cancer who had consented to undergo radiotherapy. She sued her doctor for informing her neither about her diagnosis nor about the possible side effects of the treatment.[159] The radiotherapy caused chronic inflammation of the bladder, which in turn shrank it and ultimately required surgery. The Federal Court of Justice decided in favour of the patient, writing that the doctor should not have performed the radiotherapy without having first informed her about possible complications. However, the judges underscored that it would have been acceptable to

[156] Max Mikorey, 'Der Arzt und die letzten Dinge', *Medizinische Klinik* 50, no. 22 (1955): 954–61, 960. On Mikorey's actions during National Socialism, see Andreas Michael Weidmann, 'Prof. Dr. med. Max Mikorey (1899–1977). Leben und Werk eines Psychiaters an der Psychiatrischen und Nervenklinik der Ludwig-Maximilians-Universität München' (PhD diss., Technical University of Munich, 2007), 89–101.

[157] Ibid., 250–8.

[158] Bettina Hitzer, 'Oncomotions. Experiences and Debates in West Germany and the United States after 1945', in Biess and Gross, *Science and Emotions after 1945*, 157–78, 164–5; Ruth R. Faden and Tom L. Beauchamp, *A History and Theory of Informed Consent* (New York: Oxford University Press, 1986).

[159] Hans Römer and Ernst Steindorff (1960), 'Zur Aufklärungspflicht des Arztes gegenüber Krebskranken', *Juristenzeitung* 15, nos. 5/6 (1960): 137–42, 138; Wilhelm Adam, 'Zum Thema: "Die barmherzige Lüge"', *Medizinische Welt* 2 (1959): 1185–9, 1185.

'sufficiently inform [the patient] about the dangers of the planned treatment without explicitly revealing the cancer diagnosis'. Still, they qualified that if the patient's consent could only be obtained by telling the patient about their diagnosis, then the doctor was obligated to do so:

> But that does not mean that [the patient] should be abruptly told 'the naked cancer diagnosis'. Rather, the doctor will delicately inquire into what the patient already knows about their condition, perhaps from statements of the doctors who treated them previously. If it then still proves necessary, the doctor will carefully inform the patient about their diagnosis and will not conceal the gravity of his serious situation, among other things in order to bolster their will to get better. Finding the right words is another one of the doctor's duties in this situation.[160]

These instructions on how to avoid directly confronting patients with the 'naked cancer diagnosis' manoeuvred away from the Reichsgericht's 1940 assessment that learning about a cancer diagnosis could at worst only 'lower' the patient's mood. Before the Federal Court of Justice's decision, Frankfurt's district court had already opined that the knowledge of being diagnosed with cancer represented, 'empirically, a serious mental shock'. And in an article surveying various positions on the doctor's duty to inform their patients, Munich-based surgeon Wolfgang Perret emphasized:

> If the patient has heard his death sentence or infers it from the doctor's all-too extensive remarks, then it is not, as the judge supposes, a 'lowering of his mood or general state of being' that follows. What results in the doctor's experience are dread, concern, horror, terror, fright, anxiety, but above all, fear. Clear deliberateness is obscured by affects of fear.[161]

Perret thus re-evaluated the question in two ways. First, he harkened back to discussions from the 1920s that equated cancer with a death sentence and that framed the fear unleashed by the expectation of death as an emotion that squelched the person's remaining life. Second, he defined fear as an irrational emotion that made arriving at a rational decision impossible. This opinion drew

[160] M., BGB §§ 276, 823 (Duty of the doctor to inform the patient in cases of cancer). In cases of cancer, the doctor is generally not permitted to omit telling the patient about the particular risks of radiotherapy. BGH, Decision from 16 January 1959—VI ZR 179/57 (Düsseldorf), *Neue Juristische Wochenschrift* 12, no. 18 (1959): 814–15, 815.

[161] Wolfgang Perret, 'Über das Ausmaß der Aufklärungspflicht des Arztes bei Krebserkrankung', *Medizinische Klinik* 4 (1959): 138–40, 139. For a similar perspective, see Adam, 'Zum Thema', 1186.

on concepts of fear that had been gaining credence in economics, the social sciences, and politics.[162]

The judges at the Federal Court of Justice shared Perret's understanding of fear, and it informed their reasons for reversing the Reichsgericht's order to tell patients about their diagnosis. Nevertheless, the so-called 'ray decision' from 1959 caused a furore, not because it deviated from the Reichsgericht's reasoning, but because it threatened, at least in some cases, to criminally punish doctors who concealed diagnoses, a practice that many doctors had again adopted as a rule with few exceptions.

In an article in the journal *Die Strahlentherapie* (*Radiotherapy*), jurist Gerald Grünwald described the defining character traits of jurists as those of a person 'who does not allow himself to be overwhelmed by outside events or internal motivations and fears, but rather whose insight and will master and steer everything that pressures him from the outside and from the deep layers of his personality'.[163] In 1962, 'Dr Fabian, MD', alias of surgeon Dr Willy Erich Josef Schneidrzik, wrote a series of columns in the popular magazine *Bunte* expounding on why these character traits were not up to the task of medical practice. He reported on an experiment in which he told a prosecutor they had cancer in the straightforward, no-holds-barred manner that the prosecutor himself had demanded of doctors.[164] When the man broke out in panic, Schneidrzik revealed to him that he did not, indeed, have cancer. After this visceral experience, the prosecutor grasped that the 'juridical character' was just an abstract theory and admitted to Schneidrzik that the patient 'loses all courage when they are told such a thing'.[165]

Both Grünwald and Schneidrzik justified their opinions on the Federal Court of Justice's judgement with the claim that hopelessness was a powerful emotion that gripped the entire person and could thus kill without any further medical issues. So, they asked, how much deadlier must hopelessness be when the person also had cancer? As their primary source for the existence of 'death from hopelessness', both authors referenced Arthur Jores (1901–82), a professor at the University of Hamburg who specialized in psychosomatics. Towards the end of the 1950s, Jores published a series of studies in which he sought to demonstrate that hopelessness was, in sickness and in health, 'the decisive factor for death'.[166] In order to prove

[162] Hitzer, 'Oncomotions'; Frank Biess, 'The Concept of Panic in Postwar Germany: Military Psychiatry and Emotional Preparation for Nuclear War in the West German Army', in Biess and Gross, *Science and Emotions after 1945*, 181–208; Biess, *German Angst?*.

[163] Gerald Grünwald, (1961), 'Die Aufklärungspflicht des Arztes (Lecture held on the invitation of the Lower Saxony X-Ray Association on the occasion of the annual conference in 1960 in Bad Pyrmont on 1 October 1960)', *Strahlentherapie* 114 (1961): 165–78.

[164] Clarissa, *Clarissas Krambude. Autoren erzählen von ihren Pseudonymen* (Neckenmarkt: Novum Publishing GmbH, 2011), 209–10.

[165] Dr Fabian, MD (W. E. J. Schneidrzik), 'Der Arzt als Messerstecher', *Die Bunte* 42 (1962): 71.

[166] Arthur Jores, 'Der Tod des Menschen in psychologischer Sicht', *Medizinische Klinik* 54, no. 7 (1959): 237–41, 239.

his claim, he analysed the experiences of concentration camp prisoners and prisoners of war, asserting that their survival depended on whether they had maintained hope that they would be able to return to their past lives.[167] Jores also supported his hypothesis with findings from a study he led together with his colleague Hans-Georg Puchta on the death rates of retired Hamburg civil servants. They concluded 'that those civil servants live longer who were able to give their life a new goal and new content'.[168] Jores thus suggested that hope cannot necessarily be reduced to hope of mere survival.

The multifaceted nature of hope developed into an important topic of discussion, especially for those who fought against concealing cancer diagnoses from patients. East German doctors also engaged in the conversation, although it was primarily carried out in Western journals. It revolved around distinguishing between two types of hope: the hope to live and survive, and a more fundamental practice of hoping cemented in what was perceived to be the indestructible core of a person, a hope that was not linked to any particular goal or desire. Many doctors saw untangling the relation between hope and hoping as the key to deciding whether doctors could safely convey to patients knowledge of their illness.

Internist Herbert Plügge was one of the first doctors in Germany to describe hope as a complex emotion. In 1949 and 1950, he received a number of mostly young patients who had non-fatally attempted suicide.[169] He observed that growing up during the war had stricken them with a sort of existential boredom, an ennui. He asserted that existential hope was its countervailing force and thought that it was the reason why the 'suicidal sick' rarely had grave physical ailments. This seeming contradiction did not mesh with the theory that people informed about their cancer diagnosis would end their own lives. Plügge sought to explain the contradiction by drawing a distinction between 'common hope', the loss of which would result in hopelessness, and 'fundamental hope', without which a person would fall into life-negating despair. His most significant insight was that only through the 'loss of common hope... can fundamental hope become recognizable and effective'.[170] In contrast to 'common hope', 'fundamental hope' was, in Plügge's mind, not directed towards concrete goals, but towards an indeterminate 'certainty that somehow, things are progressing towards a future, and that there is not an end that is just a hole, a nothingness'.[171] This imbued 'fundamental hope' with a transcendental dimension that could function as a segue to Christian hope, but did not necessarily have to. Plügge's engagement with the work of philosopher and reformist pedagogue Otto Friedrich Bollnow led him to see 'fundamental hope' as a core feature of an inner 'healthy being' that was shielded from the

[167] Ibid., 239. For a similar perspective, see Helmut Gollwitzer, *... und führen, wohin du nicht willst. Bericht einer Gefangenschaft* (Munich: Kaiser Verlag, 1951).

[168] Jores and Puchta, 'Der Pensionierungstod', 1164.

[169] Herbert Plügge, 'Über suizidale Kranke', *Psyche* 5, no. 7 (1951): 433–50.

[170] Ibid., 438.

[171] Herbert Plügge, 'Über die Hoffnung', *Situation* 1 (1954): 54–67, 60.

illness.[172] The argument turned hope into an emotion related to the present, not just to the future; an emotion that, in contradistinction to 'common hope', represented a certainty that could not be disappointed or lost.[173]

In 1954, Walter Brednow, professor of medicine at the University of Jena (East Germany), offered a different take on two distinct types of hope that drew on the work of Georges Bernanos. At a lecture convened by the school's Protestant student congregation, he called object-related hope *espoir*, describing it as a 'vital, animalistic force'. Only over the course of an illness would it become weaker and give way to *espérance*, which would make tolerable the knowledge that one was approaching death.[174] This reasoning led Brednow to conclude that so long as a person's vital hope was strong, doctors should not immediately inform patients they were diagnosed with cancer. He asserted that only when this hope dissipated in step with the weakening body should doctors speak with their patient about cancer and terminal illness—if, that is, the patient was even interested in doing so.[175]

Brednow's position aligned with those of some theologians and psychologists. Though they all had different arguments, they shared the conviction that doctors should not immediately reveal an unfavourable diagnosis. Instead, they believed that doctors should slowly lead patients to realize the truth so that the person could, in the search for the inner truth of their being, 'grow' to bear the truth of their illness.[176] The emphasis on coming to terms with the truth as a process coincided with a new conception of death as the final, most existentially significant chance to grasp the uniqueness and indestructibility of one's own being. These positions shifted away from conceiving of death as a test and towards seeing it as a deep inner experience that a person has to prepare for over time.[177]

Proponents of this reconception of death rejected the deindividualization and objectification of death in the hospital and on the battlefield. Criticizing medicine and modernity more generally, both Brednow and theologian Helmut Thielicke quoted poet Rainer Maria Rilke's distinction between the 'little' death and the 'great' death that he had first drawn in his 1910 novel *The Notebooks of Malte Laurids Brigge*:

172 Ibid., 62. 173 Ibid., 65.

174 Brednow drew on Georges Bernanos, *Journal d'un curé de campagne* (Paris: Plon, 1936), 230–1.

175 Walter Brednow, 'Der Mensch und die Hoffnung (nach einem am 5.3.53 im Rahmen der Ev. Studentengemeinde Jena gehaltenen Vortrag)', *Die Sammlung* 9 (1954): 529–39 and 596–608, 606–8.

176 Helmut Thielicke, 'Der Konflikt zwischen Wahrheit und Liebe', *Theologie als Glaubenswagnis: Festschrift zum 80. Geburtstag von Karl Heim* (Hamburg: Furche-Verlag, 1954), 137–54, 149–50.

177 Similar ideas were published in Protestant nursing journals: 'Zur Aussprache: Darf der Arzt schweigen?', *Die Evangelische Krankenpflege* 3, no. 5 (1954): 133–4; Nurse H. Goldammer (Diakonie Nursing School), 'Die Schwester in der Begegnung mit Sterbenden', *Die Diakonieschwester* 58, no. 7 (1962): 135–7 and 58, no. 8 (1962): 169–73.

> Now there are 559 beds to die in. Like a factory, of course. With production so enormous, each individual death is not made very carefully; but that isn't important. It's the quantity that counts. Who is there today who still cares about a well-finished death? No one.... the desire to have a death of one's own is becoming more and more rare. In a short time, it will be as rare as a life of one's own.... you die the death that belongs to the sickness you have (for since all sicknesses are well known, it is also known that the various fatal endings belong to the sicknesses and not to the people; and the sick person has, so to speak, nothing more to do).[178]

Brednow valued consciously experiencing one's own 'great' death and the existential hope wedded to it. But this butted up against the early GDR's socialist vision of human life, which rejected the notion that the meaning of life could be found in the individual or in something transcendent. Instead, the dominant ideology in the GDR asserted that meaning could only be produced through active participation in the realization of communist society in the present and for the future. Thus, it championed optimism as a central virtue that had significance exclusively for the living, while maintaining that death definitively ended the individual human's existence and thus that there was no reason to hope for life after death.[179] Medical law and ethics in the East Germany of the 1950s and 1960s were firmly grounded in this belief and thus valued the maintenance of health above all else.

While in the 1950s, the East German government still tolerated the public expression of opinions that deviated from the party line, by 1961, the ruling SED party enforced its Marxist-Leninist version of medical ethics with more repressive measures. Walter Brednow experienced this first hand. In 1960 and 1961, he detailed his ethics of hope in a lecture that he read at the concluding session of the Gesellschaft Deutscher Naturforscher und Ärzte (Society of German Natural Scientists and Doctors) conference in Hannover (West Germany) and at a public meeting of the Deutsche Akademie der Naturforscher (Leopoldina—German Academy of Natural Scientists) in Halle (East Germany). The lecture was even printed and recorded on vinyl as part of the 'Die Stimme des Arztes' (The Voice of the Doctor) series, thus making it available to a broad audience.[180] It occasioned the University of Jena's party leadership to undertake a campaign against Brednow. A number of regime-conforming professors countered his position

[178] Rainer Maria Rilke, *The Notebooks of Malte Laurids Brigge*, trans. Stephen Mitchell (New York: Vintage International, 1990), 8–9. This passage was also quoted by Thielicke, 'Der Konflikt', 152.

[179] Andrea Quitz, *Staat, Macht, Moral. Die medizinische Ethik in der DDR* (Berlin: Metropol, 2015), 134–5.

[180] Susanne Zimmermann and Sebastian Tomesch, 'Der Vortrag von Walter Brednow "Der Kranke und seine Krankheit" und seine Folgen', in *Hochschule im Sozialismus. Studien zur Geschichte der Friedrich-Schiller-Universität Jena*, vol. 2, ed. Uwe Hoßfeld, Tobias Kaiser, and Heinz Mestrup (Cologne: Böhlau, 2007), 1336–45, 1337.

with their concept of 'socialist humanism'. In the end, the 66-year-old Brednow retired on 1 September 1962 and was relieved of his leadership positions at the medical faculty, neurology clinic, and tuberculosis clinic on 31 January 1963.

Interpersonal Relationships: The Emotions of the Doctor and the Trust of Their Patients

After that, discussions on the significance of hope and despair in medical treatment abruptly ceased in the GDR. Now, most publications on the issue of communicating diagnoses and obtaining consent restricted themselves to discussing East Germany's laws and how to comply with them. While West Germany's civil law held fast to the principle of individual self-determination, a principle that stood at the centre of the Reichsgericht and Federal Court of Justice decisions discussed above, East Germany broke with it. The GDR's legal code considered medical treatment not as an act of bodily harm the punishability of which was simply suspended under normal operating conditions, as discussed above, but as a curative intervention that was permitted on the basis of an unspoken contract between the patient and the state-run health institutions.[181] The intent to heal was the superseding legal principle in the matter: it was deduced from Article 35 of the GDR's constitution, which guaranteed citizens a right to healthcare. The official ideology that individual and social interests coincided precluded the formulation of civil or punitive medical liability laws. Thus, doctors could only be held accountable through labour laws or disciplinary measures brought down by a supervisory authority.[182]

Just as in West Germany, doctors in the GDR were supposed to tell people about their diagnosis and prognosis and receive their consent before performing treatment. But the imperative was not rooted in the legally enforceable principle of the individual's inviolable right to self-determination. Rather, it was floated on the wager that knowledge and consent would facilitate the patient's readiness to cooperate with the doctor. In what would become a standard text on the doctor's 'legal duties' in the GDR, jurists Gerhard Hansen of Jena and Herbert Vetterlein of East Berlin explained:

[181] G. Hansen and H. Vetterlein, *Ärztliches Handeln—Rechtliche Pflichten in der Deutschen Demokratischen Republik*, 2nd rev. edn (Leipzig: Thieme, 1962), 62.

[182] These rules were initially grounded in a law regulating hospitals passed in 1954. They were specified and further developed in the licensure rules for doctors and those for dentists (both from 1977) and the 1976 civil law code of the GDR, § 331. See contemporaneous interpretations of the rules in G. Hansen and H. Vetterlein, *Ärztliches Handeln—Rechtliche Pflichten in der Deutschen Demokratischen Republik*, 1st edn (Leipzig: Thieme Verlag, 1959); G. Hansen and H. Vetterlein, *Arzt und Recht in der Deutschen Demokratischen Republik* (Leipzig: Thieme, 1959) which had multiple print runs; Günter Becker, *Arzt und Patient im sozialistischen Recht* (Berlin: Verlag Volk und Gesundheit, 1973); and Günther Becker, *Arzt und Patient im sozialistischen Recht*, 2nd edn (Berlin: Verlag Volk und Gesundheit, 1978).

> An understanding of the illness should occasion the patient to adhere to the necessary diagnostic and therapeutic measures and to actively participate in the process of recovery. From this follows that informing the patient is a duty of the doctor, a duty that is subordinated to the goal of curing.[183]

Thus, it was left up to doctors to decide if and how they would inform their patients about their sickness and the potential side effects of treatment. However, there was consensus that informing 'has its limit where it appears no longer bearable by the psyche of the patient; that is, where informing causes one to fear a worsening of the patient's state of health or a slowing of recovery'.[184] One high-ranking doctor explicitly advised his colleagues to deceive cancer patients about their illness and to only tell them about their diagnosis if they refused treatment.[185]

Though these official positions in medical ethics hardly changed until the early 1980s, sources indicate that doctors sometimes opted for their own approach. They often argued on the grounds of everyday clinical experience, not ethical principles or laws—likely a calculated attempt to avoid getting wrapped up in conflicts with the politically prescribed guidelines. For instance, in 1975, H. Schilling, gynaecologist at the Carl Gustav Carus Medical Academy in Dresden, wrote:

> Sooner or later, the patient will certainly learn about the diagnosis of the cause of their suffering, whether it be through an indiscrete remark or simply through the symbols of contemporary organized treatment of tumours, e.g. intensive radiotherapy. The code numbers for diagnoses that appear on the doctor's notes excusing patients from work and on their social insurance identification card are also known among some patients. Then there are the later rehabilitation measures, the gathering of statistics, and the care provided by the post-treatment centre for cancer patients, etc.[186]

In 1962, radiologist Dr Claus, head of the radiotherapy institute at the Bergarbeiter Hospital Erlabrunn in Saxony, employed similar reasoning when describing 'modern' cancer treatment:

[183] G. Hansen and H. Vetterlein, *Ärztliches Handeln—Rechtliche Pflichten in der Deutschen Demokratischen Republik*, 5th edn (Leipzig: Thieme Verlag, 1973), 72. The 1st and 2nd editions did not contain the phrase 'duty of the doctor to inform the patient'.

[184] Ibid., 72. The head judges of the Leipzig district court had a similar argument: Becker, *Arzt und Patient*, 2nd edn, 62.

[185] Namely, the head doctor and medical director of the second clinic of the Dresden-Friedrichsstadt District Hospital: O. Günther, 'Aufgaben und Probleme des Internisten bei der Aufklärung', in *Aufklärungs- und Schweigepflicht des Arztes und seiner Mitarbeiter. Medizinisch-juristische Grundlagen*, ed. Gerhard Burkhardt and Wolfgang Reimann (Dresden: Steinkopff Verlag, 1975), 38–42, 39. See also Becker, *Arzt und Patient*, 2nd edn, 63.

[186] H. Schilling, 'Spezielle Fragestellungen in Gynäkologie und Geburtshilfe', in *Aufklärungs- und Schweigepflicht des Arztes und seiner Mitarbeiter. Medizinisch-juristische Grundlagen*, ed. Gerhard Burkhardt and Wolfgang Reimann (Dresden: Steinkopff, 1975), 63–72, 65.

> The cancer patient totally uninformed about their illness does not really exist, at least not after the completion of intensive radiotherapy. The patient slowly comes to more or less understand that they suffer from cancer through the admission to the radiotherapy ward, the radiotherapy itself, [and] fellow patients in the same uncertain situation who gladly tell the new patient—who surmises something similar is happening to him—the 'truth' concealed from him by doctors.[187]

The observations of Dr Claus and Dr Schilling underscore two important points. First, they bear witness to how many actors in the GDR's health system continued to exert themselves, even in the 1960s and 1970s, to shield patients from the knowledge that they had cancer. Second, all doctors involved in treating a cancer patient sought to coordinate amongst themselves what they should tell the patient about symptoms and possible forms of treatment. This encompassed the patient's family practitioner, surgeon, radiologist, and internist. Nurses and caretakers, too, had to regularly answer the patient's questions in line with the strategy agreed upon by the doctors, and post-treatment centres had to be informed as well.

Similar strategies were pursued in West Germany, and they did not just involve doctors, nurses, and other clinical personnel. The success of 'benign deception' necessitated keeping health insurance providers, care associations, and the agencies running post-treatment facilities in the loop. For example, the Bundesarchiv (German Federal Archives) contains an exchange of letters from 1958 between the director of the Landschaftsverband Rheinland (Rhineland Regional Council), which was responsible for paying for the care of terminally ill patients in the place of the public health insurers, and the head of North Rhine-Westphalia's Gesellschaft zur Bekämpfung der Krebskrankheiten (Society for Fighting Cancer), which established recovery centres and other post-treatment care facilities. The heads of the two organizations agreed to avoid using the word 'cancer' in all writings accessible to patients. Moreover, they agreed that patients not be informed that the costs of care were being covered by the Landschaftsverband, because the transfer of the patients from the insurance system for working people to the retirement/disability insurance system might also have been interpreted as a sign of their 'hopeless' condition. In order to prop up the illusion, the public health insurers agreed to pay the patients' bills on paper and then recover the funds from the Landschaftsverband with a form specially designed for the purpose.[188]

But deceiving patients became increasingly difficult as cancer treatment moved away from single operations or sets of radiotherapy sessions. Arrangements between the family doctor and surgeon or radiologist were thus no longer

[187] H.-D. Claus, 'Zu einigen praktischen Fragen der Metaphylaxe nach Strahlentherapie der Geschwulstleiden', *Das Deutsche Gesundheitswesen* 17, no. 35 (1962): 1489–98, 1490.

[188] Director of the Rhineland Landschaftsverband, division III, social welfare and health, Klausa, to the director of the Gesellschaft zur Bekämpfung der Krebskrankheiten of North Rhine-Westphalia, Dr Spohr, Düsseldorf, 23 June 1958, BArch B 142/3434, 311–13.

sufficient. Doctors Claus and Schilling argued that because the facts of treatment would make the patient aware of the nature of their illness, medical ethics could no longer support the practice of concealing diagnoses. But not all doctors followed them. Many admitted that numerous patients had learned of their illness through gaps in the machinery of deception, but they insisted that patients' need for hope was so great that they were often open to being pacified and deceived anew by their doctor.[189]

Claus and Schilling sought to draw attention to what they saw as the conflicts that could result out of the tension between deception and disclosure during cancer treatment. One was the patient's loss of trust in the doctor. Claus detailed its potentially disastrous consequences:

> If one tries to deceive the patient [about the fact that they have cancer] with see-through expressions, a tense distrust and insincerity develops between doctor and patient, which might conceivably have a negative effect not only on the patient's comportment and disposition towards the doctor, nurses, other patients, and to his situation in general, but might also indirectly contribute to the weakening and detriment of the stamina of his organism. Thus is brought about the precise effect that one sought to circumvent by suppressing the facts. Moreover, such a patient often does not believe that the treatment was selected in his best interest and distrusts every medical intervention and instruction.... Such a patient feels fear. But the fear leads him to hopelessness and paralyzes his vitality.[190]

Strictly speaking, the radiologist did not depart here from the guidelines set out by the GDR's official medical ethics. He simply put them on different footing. Claus agreed that the desire to recover and the patient's consent were essential if the patient was to be expected to take an 'active' role in treatment. But by asserting that disclosure of the diagnosis was an inevitable consequence of treatment, he positioned the doctor-patient relationship as the highest principle. The integrity of that relationship, he thought, required trust. And retaining the patient's trust in the doctor necessitated that the doctor inform the patient about their diagnosis with a circumlocutory formulation that would not shock them.

The patient's trust in the doctor's honesty and the perceived correlation between that honesty and the doctor's desire to 'do what is best' for the patient had not featured much in previous debates on disclosure, deception, and the doctor-patient relationship. Doctors' manuals of the 1920s and 1930s elaborated

[189] Johannes Kretz and O. Pötzl, 'Die Psyche des Krebskranken (Wien)', *Der Krebsarzt* 1 (1946): 19–29, 23–4; Charlotte Neumann, 'Psychische Besonderheiten bei Krebs-Patientinnen', *Zeitschrift für Psycho-somatische Medizin* 5, no. 2 (1959): 91–101, 91.

[190] Claus, 'Zu einigen praktischen Fragen', 1490.

on how the doctor could get the patient to trust their medical capabilities, not them as a person. The point had been to set the doctor apart from their colleagues who might divulge 'naked' cancer diagnoses (as opposed to communicating them through third parties that the patient knew, as Krecke had done), and from 'quacks', whom some patients trusted more with cancer treatment than trained medical professionals.

There were multiple causes for why health professionals in the early 1960s began seeing a different, more robust form of trust as a necessary foundation for the doctor-patient relationship. One reason was likely that during the twentieth century, more moral significance was placed in personal trust.[191] But certainly of much greater weight were public discussions about the actions of doctors under National Socialism. About two years before Dr Claus published his article, Alexander Mitscherlich and Fred Mielke had released a new edition of their protocols of the Nuremberg Doctors' Trial. Overnight, it ignited a heated debate on the causes and consequences of 'medicine without humanity'. While the debate played out in West German media, East German doctors followed it closely.[192] The suspicion that doctors might not always act in their patients' best interests had indeed been discussed as early as 1900. But that doctors systematically destroyed life and conducted sadistic human experiments was seen as a new dimension of medical misconduct that severely damaged trust in doctors' adherence to the Hippocratic Oath.

In this context, the meaning of trust was reformulated, with the emotional quality of the doctor-patient relationship placed front and centre. Medical publications in West Germany reflected the shift. However, their writings on emotions and trust generally drew on psychoanalysis in a broad sense. Already in 1949, internist Richard Siebeck, a former student of Weizsäcker, expressed his reservations about concealing cancer diagnoses from patients. To underline the problem, he quoted a saying he claimed a psychoanalyst once told him: 'If you have a guilty conscience when you lie, then you'll do a bad job of lying!'[193]

At first glance, the remonstration seems simply to mean that a doctor's guilty conscience could get in the way of the doctor's performance. However, by calling a psychoanalyst as his star witness, it is evident that Siebeck was not just interested in the question of performance, but in the deeper psychoanalytic issue of transference and countertransference. Freud identified the phenomenon as a key aspect of the relation between analyst and analysand: while the analysand projects emotions and behavioural patterns of their childhood ego onto the psychoanalyst, the analyst reacts to the perceived projections with emotions stemming from their

[191] Frevert, *Vertrauensfragen*, 213.

[192] Freimüller, *Alexander Mitscherlich*, 100–33 and 267–71.

[193] Richard Siebeck, *Medizin in Bewegung. Klinische Erkenntnisse und ärztliche Aufgabe* (Stuttgart: Thieme, 1949), 406.

own life, which thus have more to do with the personality of the analyst than that of the analysand. Countertransference was important, because the analyst's emotions could influence the decisions they made in the therapeutic process and might be perceived by the analysand even if the analyst said nothing about them. This complex necessitated that the analyst explore her own emotions and their meaning and origins.

Michael Balint, a Hungarian psychoanalyst who emigrated to England in 1939, applied this model to the relationship between medical doctor and patient. Inspired by his experiences working at the Family Discussion Bureau of London's Tavistock Clinic, Balint initiated in 1950 a sort of supervision group by doctors for doctors. The doctors were supposed to discuss their 'cases' with others in order to analyse how the relationship between patient and doctor was being influenced by the doctor's own emotions and assumptions as well as to reflect on the extent to which the doctor themself could productively intervene in their own relation to the patient.

Balint's groups convinced doctors to think about the impact that their own inner life had on their comportment, anamnesis strategies, and therapeutic decisions. His research arrived in West Germany in 1958 in a translation of his book *The Doctor, His Patient and the Illness*. While it was initially met with a cool reception, by the end of the 1960s, it was making waves. In the early 1970s, a number of Balint groups were founded in West Germany, offering a space for doctors, psychologists, pastors, and nurses to collectively ruminate on their clinical work. In the GDR, too, Balint's theories were read and applied in so-called 'problem case' seminars. In contrast to West German Balint groups, the East German variant gave a central role to the group leader and generally excluded psychoanalysis.[194]

Balint did not discover *that* the doctor's words and emotional comportment could have an effect on treatment. His real innovation was recognizing that the doctor's *unconscious* emotions shaped the dynamics of the doctor-patient relationship. This insight had special bearing on doctors' relationships to seriously and terminally ill patients. Balint exhorted doctors to first critically examine their motivations before following their impulse to console patients, reasoning that 'reassurance is much too often administered for the benefit of the doctor, who cannot bear the burden of either not knowing enough or of being unable to help'.[195]

[194] Michael Geyer, Werner König, and Sigmar Scheerer, 'Die Arbeit der Regionalgesellschaften—Der Aufbau der Psychosomatischen Grundbetreuung und der regionalen Balint-Arbeit', *Psychotherapie in Ostdeutschland. Geschichte und Geschichten 1945–1995*, ed. Michael Geyer (Göttingen: Vandenhoeck & Ruprecht, 2011), 345–9; Hans-Joachim Maaz, 'Zur Geschichte der Psychotherapie in der DDR', *European Journal of Mental Health* 6, no. 2 (2011): 213–38, 226–7.

[195] Michael Balint, *The Doctor, His Patient and the Illness* (New York: International Universities Press, 1957), 231.

A year before the book appeared in English, the American Psychological Association, the world's most influential consortium of psychologists, convened a panel on the topic of 'death' at its annual conference for the first time. The panel was organized by 41-year-old psychologist Herman Feifel, who worked for the Los Angeles Veterans Administration Mental Hygiene Clinic. One of the panel's guests, psychologist August M. Kasper, explicitly inquired into doctors' emotions and their thoughts about death. His interviews with some doctors had led him to the conclusion that many doctors chose their occupation because they had a strong, usually unconscious fear of death that they wanted to stave off through their work.[196] This defensive disposition, he thought, would encourage them to conceal from a terminally ill or dying patient knowledge about their imminent death. Thus, the practice of 'benign deception' answered 'more to the personality of the doctor than [the] ... need of the patient', a claim similar to that made by Balint about doctors' behaviours in general in his 1957 book.[197] Feifel published the panel's lectures in 1959 in a volume titled *The Meaning of Death*. It emphatically sought to put death on the agenda of psychologists, who had until then mostly avoided the topic, making his search for a publisher difficult.[198]

Feifel's book also had a part in cultivating, in the early 1960s, American sociologists' budding interest in the process of dying. His work was the first reference in a trailblazing study published in the United States in 1965. *Awareness of Dying* by sociologists Anselm Strauss and Barney Glaser was the end result of three years of research on clinics in the San Francisco Bay Area. The book was built on the authors' own observations and interviews with doctors, patients, and others.[199] Their data led them to develop the concept of 'awareness contexts' to denote '[w]hat *each* interacting person [i.e. patient, doctor, family members, etc.] knows of the patient's defined status, along with his [the patient's] awarenesses of his own definition'. They delineated four different awareness contexts, each comprising different forms of behaviour: 'closed awareness', in which the patient does not know or surmise that she is dying; 'suspected awareness', in which the patient is told nothing, but realizes that she is dying and becomes distrustful of doctors, nurses, and family members; 'mutual pretense awareness', in which both sides know but choose to conceal this knowledge from one another; and 'open awareness', in which all involved openly speak about the patient's coming death.[200]

[196] August M. Kasper, 'The Doctor and Death', in *The Meaning of Death*, ed. Herman Feifel (New York: Blakiston Division, McGraw-Hill, 1959), 259–70, 260.

[197] Balint, *The Doctor*, 229: 'In fact, it is not so much the patient's needs but the doctor's individuality that determines the form in which the doctor administers himself.'

[198] William M. Lamers, 'Classics Revisited: Herman Feifel, The Meaning of Death', *Mortality* 17, no. 1 (2012): 64–78, https://doi.org/10.1080/13576275.2012.654709.

[199] Barney C. Glaser and Anselm L. Strauss, *Awareness of Dying* (Chicago: Aldine Publishing Company, 1965).

[200] Ibid.

By writing the study, Glaser and Strauss wanted to encourage families, doctors, and other healthcare professionals to take a more reflective, empathetic approach to patients' experience of dying.[201] Though they identified problems with each 'awareness context', they highlighted that the first three—in which others do not speak with the patient about dying—could place a significant psychological burden on care personnel in particular. The strain could manifest itself in a tension-saturated atmosphere or lead nurses or doctors to completely avoid talking with the patient and just focus on their corporeal needs. In doing so, they 'spared' themselves direct confrontation with the patient's emotions. Ultimately, Glaser and Strauss observed, this avoidance left patients to spend most of their time alone. Still, they reached no definitive conclusion as to whether patients experienced this as emotional isolation. Of 'mutual pretense awareness', they wrote:

> For the patient, the pretense context can yield a measure of dignity and considerable privacy, though it may deny him the closer relationships with staff members and family members that sometimes occur when he allows them to participate in his open acceptance of death. And if they initiate and he accepts the pretense, he may have nobody with whom to talk although he might profit greatly from talk.[202]

They conceptualized the four awareness contexts as phases that did not necessarily end up in open discussion. But they believed that the model demonstrated the benefits of openness. Moreover, they thought that the initial difficulties brought on by openness could push the patient's personal development forward. The patient might pass through depression and despair in a process that had two possible outcomes: they would either again repress the knowledge of their coming death or finally accept it.[203]

Elisabeth Kübler-Ross's 1969 *On Death and Dying* charted a similar path. But in contrast to Glaser and Strauss, the University of Chicago professor did not seek to *observe* interactions between dying patients and doctors. She wanted to *speak* with them in order to learn about their experiences and desires.[204] Her discussions led her to infer that dying persons go through five phases of grief about their own death: a phase of denial in which they reject the knowledge of their coming death and pursue strategies like 'talking it down' as a mistaken diagnosis; a phase of anger, in which they angrily and jealously react to those who will survive them; a phase of bargaining, in which they try to prolong their life by doing things like making promises to God or another higher power; a phase of depression and

[201] Ibid. [202] Ibid., 77. [203] Ibid., 123–35.

[204] Elisabeth Kübler-Ross, *On Death and Dying: What the Dying Have to Teach Doctors, Nurses, Clergy and Their Own Families* (New York: Routledge, 1969).

despair; and finally, a feeling of acceptance, which leaves open little space for other emotions. When the patient accepted their coming death, she wrote, they generally turned inward and sought peace with themselves.

Kübler-Ross thought that giving the patient hope was important in all phases. However, she specified that cultivating hope of survival or even the kind of existential hope promoted by Plügge and Brednow was unhelpful. Beneficial for the patient, she wrote, was the hope that they would not be left alone, that doctors, nurses, and loved ones would do all they could to help them and palliate their pain. This type of hope was thus less hope of something in the future and more an act of hoping in the present.

Feifel, Glaser and Strauss, and Kübler-Ross all argued in their own ways why speaking about approaching death did not necessarily induce hopelessness. But, they added, the patient could not avoid 'negative' emotions, because such emotions were just part of grappling with the situation. At the same time, they opened up new perspectives on how the inner lives of both doctor and patient could affect the doctor-patient relationship and how speaking openly about their emotions might positively impact this relationship. This created space for speaking about oneself and one's innermost emotions. Many doctors embraced openness as a powerful tool of therapy, and many patients came to perceive it as a way to maintain healthy interpersonal relationships during the process of dying. Speaking about one's emotions with a professional also became a means for patients to seek inner peace by confronting the reality of their death. Indeed, these theories revealed that speaking about emotions—and not just emotions as such—could itself serve as the primary medium of the doctor-patient relationship.

These theories about the emotions that are caused by the knowledge of dying and the effect emotions could have on the dying patient were radically different from the discussions of the 1950s, which idealized approaching death with 'masculine', silent dignity.

Speaking about Oneself

In the first half of the twentieth century, people with cancer had neither a public voice nor a public face. Photographs and wax models of real tumours were, of course, displayed in exhibitions, and the 1930 film *Krebs* showed the face of a woman with breast cancer, but she remained anonymous and without personal expression. She was reduced to being the vessel of her breast tumour. And the stories told by early detection campaigns were fictive. Actors and statistics gave the fictional protagonists a semblance of reality, but people who were really sick with cancer remained faceless and voiceless. Ever since the event of Friedrich III's death in 1888, newspapers had stopped reporting in detail on cancer cases and patients' deaths. This began to change in the 1950s, but only in West Germany. East German media did not feature any personalized reporting.

'Until Death Do Us Part' read the headline of one of the first West German newspaper articles to thematize an individual coming to terms with the recognition that they were terminally ill with cancer; it was published in 1952 in the popular magazine *Stern*.[205] The human-interest story revolved around the happiness and homesickness of a young Bavarian woman who had moved to the United States with an American soldier in 1948. 'Ever since Maria has known that she is going to die, she only has one wish: home!' read the first sentence of the article about 27-year-old Maria Stürzer, who was considered a 'hopeless case' after four operations failed to cure her cancer. She had resolved to return to her family's home to die accompanied by her American husband. The photos that illustrate the article show not despair and grief, but smiles and loving, caring gestures. The article describes the mood: 'They desperately fight for every minute of happiness that is afforded them.'

Knowledge of her coming death did not shuttle this young woman into a paralyzed state of hopelessness. Instead, it enabled her to make a decision to return to where she felt safe and secure, at home with her family. Films of the 1950s often valourized the wish to be home with family. And the fact that Maria Stürzer chose her Bavarian home over the United States was crucial for the *Stern* story, even though cancer was its broader topic. Perhaps unintentionally, the piece revealed that there could be an alternative to 'surrendering' to cancer, an alternative in which knowledge of death enabled the patient to consciously shape and intensely experience their last days.

In the run of the 1950s, masculine traits saturated this 'alternative narrative'. Two stories that garnered considerable media exposure were primarily responsible for this turn. They associated knowledge of one's own terminal illness with masculine dignity, a topic that was not entirely new, as it had partially informed 1930s discussions on 'dying courageously'—like in the above discussed story of Major Anton K. However, never before had it really influenced medical praxis. The two narratives were about the dying and death of American *Time* journalist Charles Wertenbaker and of American Secretary of State John Foster Dulles.

Charles Wertenbaker died by suicide in January 1955 after being diagnosed with advanced-stage colon cancer. Most West German readers would have been unfamiliar with him at the time, and German newspapers did not write anything about his death. This changed abruptly in the autumn of 1957 upon the publication of a German translation of his wife and fellow *Time* journalist Lael Tucker Wertenbaker's book *Death of a Man*. In it, she chronicled the last months of her husband's life. The book was heatedly discussed in the United States and was

[205] 'Bis daß der Tod uns scheidet. Maria Stürzer will in ihrer bayerischen Heimat sterben', *Der Stern* 5, no. 7 (1952): 11.

quickly translated into multiple languages, including French, Dutch, Danish, Swedish, Japanese, and Spanish. The most provocative part of the book recounted in remarkable detail how she assisted his suicide: he slit his wrists, while she injected him with morphine and remained at his side until he expired.

But the book's reputation derived not solely from its breaking taboos about suicide and death. Controversial, too, were the Wertenbakers' 'cold, masculine' openness with one another and their consciously formulated, soberly communicated demand that their doctors tell them in unornamented terms the truth about Charles Wertenbaker's diagnosis and prognosis. The media reported on this approach with a mixture of fascination and abhorrence. *Der Spiegel* summed up this ambivalent reaction to the book in their review of it:

> In this spirit of masculine dignity and self-discipline, which does not even permit a lie out of mercy, the Wertenbakers live in daily awareness of the grim certainty that 'Wert', as his wife calls him, is sentenced to death. After this point, the book primarily deals with the couple's almost arrogant attempt to elevate themselves above the weakness of their flesh, the hardness of fate, and every emotion of the heart that borders on sentimentality. Humility is a word unheard of in their discussions.[206]

Many perceived such lack of humility in the couple's insistence, against the advice of all doctors, that Charles Wertenbaker be told the whole truth about his illness. A key scene illustrated this point in stark terms. While Charles had not yet awoken from anaesthesia after an operation, the surgeon, a friend of the couple, talked with his wife. He told her that he had not completed the operation because he found metastases in the liver, which meant that the cancer was incurable. In response to her question about how long her husband would survive, the doctor, 'in his unprotected concern and affection blurted out his real guess: three months'. He then tried to revise his judgement and make it sound more hopeful, before asking:

> 'Now', said Jim [the doctor] gently, 'what shall we tell Wert?' 'Tell him the truth', I said. 'You can't', said Jim. 'You can't take away hope from a human being.' '*Is* there any hope?' I asked him. 'No', said Jim.... 'Then', I said, 'that's that.' Jim's big, benign face was very drawn and I felt pity for him. 'Have you ever seen anyone die?' he asked me. 'No', I said.... 'I have', Jim said. 'In my profession, many, many people. During the war—many courageous men who had proved their courage. Lael, I tell you, it is better if they hope. It is one thing to take a brave chance on dying and another to know that you are going to die—soon. You

[206] 'Tod eines Mannes', *Der Spiegel* 40 (1957): 57–9, 58.

> cannot take hope away from Wert.' 'I cannot lie to this man', I said. 'That would take his dignity away from him. He would rather have dignity than hope.' 'You cannot know *any* man that well', said Jim. 'I know this man that well', I told him .... 'He may change', said Jim. People change, he told me, faced with death. He might get paranoid or suicidal. He might want to find quacks to tell him they could cure him. People clung to hope from any source, Jim said. Wert might, on the other hand, become very religious, saintly, turn to God.... I had half-smiled when Jim said Wert might take to quacks and now I think I smiled wholly and made an amused gesture of dismissal.... 'Wert's faiths are his own and they are strong ones. I think he will die by them. If he needs more, something else, to die by, I hope he has time to find, finds—God. It's his life and his death, not mine or yours, and you can't judge him for all you know.'[207]

In this passage, Lael Tucker Wertenbaker juxtaposed two positions. On the one hand, there was that of the doctor, who wielded his experience to draw general conclusions about what he believed people could bear. On the other, her own position was not based on professional expertise, but on an intimate familiarity with this in her eyes unique individual whose radical subjectivity could not be reduced to generalities, and on the promise she made to not withhold the truth from him. While the doctor feared causing hopelessness above all else, she placed more weight on the ideals of dignity, honesty, and the knowledge that one could freely choose and thus retain control over one's own life. In doing so, she flipped the power relation between her and the doctor who had tried to moralizingly pressure her into concealing the truth from her husband. By proving that she could better control her own emotions than he himself, she forced him to justify his own reasoning, which she recounted in her book by describing the doctor's gestures and her own.

A few pages later, Lael Tucker Wertenbaker makes clear that she summoned the energy to remain composed from her unconditional desire to help her husband retain his masculine dignity and to hold on to her identity as his soulmate. She finds confirmation that her actions were justified when she recounts what he said to her a couple of days after the operation:

> 'If *you* had been skittish—if you had lied to me by one word, by one intonation, that morning, I'd be a sniveling paranoiac by now, suspicious of everything and everybody.... The truth is the whole truth as you know it and nothing else sounds the same. You were telling it and I knew it and so I felt fine. It would be no damn good for me if you hadn't. I'm a suspicious son of a bitch by nature and afraid of fooling myself or being fooled.'[208]

[207] Lael Tucker Wertenbaker, *Death of a Man* (New York: Random House, 1957), 54–7.
[208] Ibid., 67.

Wertenbaker thus acted on his conviction that his own dignity as a person and, above all, as a man superseded the doctor's worry that all people feared death. This was why the review accused the Wertenbakers of being 'almost arrogant'. Publicly revealing this attitude in what most considered to be private details was even seen by some as 'embarrassing'.[209]

A look at contemporaneous film underscores that, indeed, other conventions of self-representation still dominated. Whether German or Hollywood, when cancer did, in a few isolated instances, play a significant role in movies of the 1940s and 1950s, the characters involved carried themselves in dignified self-composure, while intimacy was expressed through their choice to remain silent about illness and death. In 1939, it was Bette Davis playing doctor's wife Judith Traherne; in 1944, Paula Wessely playing x-ray assistant Maximiliane Frey; in 1950, Margaret Sullivan playing young wife Mary Scott—all of these characters had cancer that they usually learned about by mistake, sometimes from the doctor himself.[210] All decided on their own free will not to tell their loved ones about it. And although their partners always found out one way or another, they still did not talk about it. Thus, while the characters did not discuss emotions, emotions stood at the forefront of the films' plots. The protagonists demonstrated dignified self-control tinged with self-sacrifice in the name of love. In all of these films, the happiness of the couples' last weeks together was depicted as deriving from their implicit agreement not to talk about cancer.

The films thus championed an ideal of heroic loneliness, a type of dignity at once self-chosen and self-sacrificial, and overwhelmingly connotated as female. This was challenged by the Wertenbakers' ideal of self-determined, masculine dignity loudly expressed to the outside world. Lael Tucker Wertenbaker publicly represented her husband as someone who, despite being terminally ill, embodied virility and insisted on remaining the master of his own body in the face of the doctor's demands to the contrary. While this collided with many social expectations, it linked up with other contemporaneous images of masculinity, such as that propagated by Ernest Hemingway, whom Charles Wertenbaker knew personally. This all makes it somewhat less surprising that, in the run of the 1950s and 1960s, West German media tended to display men as examples of an open, dignified approach to cancer. But the fact that these men were usually American or British demonstrates that this attitude still needed to be cast as something foreign to get past the enduring taboos of West German society.

West German doctors' criticisms of reporting on the death of US Secretary of State John Foster Dulles in 1959 illustrated just how strong those taboos were. For

[209] 'Tod eines Mannes', 59.

[210] The films are *Dark Victory* (1950), *Das Herz muß schweigen* (*The Heart Must Stay Silent*, 1944), and *No Sad Songs for Me* (1951). See also Susan E. Lederer, 'Dark Victory: Cancer and Popular Hollywood Film', *Bulletin of the History of Medicine* 81, no. 1 (2007): 94–115, https://doi.org/10.1353/bhm.2007.0005.

instance, *Der Spiegel* wrote about some doctors' concerns that the reports granted cancer 'an unsettling publicity' that would 'agitate cancer patients around the world'.[211] Unlike Wertenbaker, Dulles's private reflections had not been entrusted to the public and he did not end his own life. But he insisted on being open and publicly revealed that he had cancer as soon as he found out about it.[212] Dulles was diagnosed with colon cancer during surgery on 4 November 1956. The next day, the *New York Times* published an article titled: 'Dulles' Surgery Removed Cancer'.[213] Dulles initially hoped that he would defeat his cancer, and when he suffered pains again in late 1958, doctors at Walter Reed Hospital could not find anything wrong. But during an operation in January 1959, they found a relapse. Again, Dulles chose to inform the public about the discovery and his choice of treatment. On 15 April 1959, President Dwight Eisenhower accepted Dulles's resignation after metastases were discovered in his spine. Dulles remained at the hospital, where journalists reported daily about his worsening health. He died on 24 May 1959.

After his death, the media's interest in his story did not wane. Pulitzer Prize-winning journalist Marguerite Higgins wrote a series of articles in the *New York Herald Tribune* based on interviews with people close to Dulles that reported on how he had led his life with bravery, resolve, masculine dignity, and stoicism after learning he had cancer. *Der Spiegel* published portions of the series in an article headlined 'The Man Who Would Not Give Up'.[214] Higgins depicted Dulles as a rational strategist who managed his emotions and pain in his fight against cancer and who struggled to remain lucid and working for as long as possible. Like for Wertenbaker, he wanted to know the 'truth' at all costs in order to remain master of his life and death and be able to make decisions for himself. But according to Higgins, he, in contrast to Wertenbaker, did not reveal his emotions or personal thoughts to anyone, and 'avoided at any time discussing even with his family the fact that he was going to die'.[215] In many respects, this sort of self-control lined up with the image of cancer patients prevalent in films of the era.[216] Following this idealistic depiction of Dulles, media outlets in the early 1960s started reporting more on famous persons' experiences with cancer.[217]

[211] 'Der Tod im Terminkalender', *Der Spiegel* 3 (1960): 48–57, 49.

[212] Barron H. Lerner, 'Politician as Patient: John Foster Dulles Battles Cancer', in *When Illness Goes Public: Celebrity Patients and How We Look at Medicine* (Baltimore: Johns Hopkins University Press, 2009), 81–99.

[213] Alvin Shuster, 'Dulles' Surgery Removed Cancer', *New York Times*, 5 November 1956, 1.

[214] The series was titled *How Secretary Dulles Faced Death* and comprised three articles printed in the *New York Herald Tribune*: Marguerite Higgins, 'How Secretary Dulles Faced Death, Part 1: Battled Disease as Job Intruder', *New York Herald Tribune*, 26 July 1959, A1; 'How Secretary Dulles Faced Death, Part 2: Dulles' Strong Will Helped Battle Disease', *New York Herald Tribune*, 27 July 1959, 7; 'How Secretary Dulles Faced Death, Part 3: Dulles Fought for Comeback' *New York Herald Tribune*, 28 July 1959, A4.

[215] Higgins, 'Dulles' Strong Will'.

[216] Higgins, 'Battled Disease as Job Intruder'.

[217] For instance, Jürgen Thorwald's sixty-eight-part series *Aller Ruhm auf Erden* (*All the Fame on Earth*) in the entertainment paper *Quick* (1959/61).

Literature, too, jumped into the debate on talking about cancer diagnoses. Heinz G. Konsalik's novels about the Second World War had made him one of the most popular authors in West Germany. He also wrote a novel about the fate of cancer patients; first serialized in the *Revue*, it was published as a book in 1961.[218] The plot of *Diagnose Krebs* (*Diagnosis: Cancer*) revolves around Dr Hanser's empathic, passionate search for new, holistic therapies for his terminally ill patients. Konsalik also described the hopes and fears of cancer patients and their loved ones. The protagonist does not withhold diagnoses from any of his cancer patients, because he thinks that knowing the truth will strengthen their will to survive and their resolve to radically change their diet, exercise routines, time management, and disposition.

In a highly emotional scene towards the end of the novel, he reiterates this conviction. Talking to the fiancé of his esteemed assistant Dr Marianne Pechel, he justifies why he told her not only her diagnosis, but the grim prognosis of the metastases on her cerebral membrane.[219] Her fiancé, Dr Wüllner, asks desperately: 'Is it really not possible to operate?' Dr Hansen responds with a lengthy medical explanation that concludes with the exchange:

> 'An operation would no longer help!'—'And... you want to tell Marianne that?'—'Yes.'—'So clearly? So cruelly?'—'It must be, Wüllner.'—'It will just accelerate everything....' Hansen shook his head. 'Perhaps I know Marianne better than you in this respect. She will clench her teeth and fight.'—'Against what?'—'Against hopelessness. Against fear.' He quietly added: 'Much is already won when one can die with composure....'[220]

The doctor was adopting an idea that had been discussed in theological and philosophical debates on hope and hopelessness: the idea that knowledge of one's approaching death could mobilize the will to live and that people could recover hope or even invoke a new type of hope in a situation of seeming hopelessness.

The spread of this idea spurred a number of cancer patients to speak out about their experiences and offer themselves as witnesses of the power of hope. Most of these early autobiographical narratives shared the belief that hope not only helped patients deal with the effects of cancer. They also asserted that without hope, the body would become 'hopeless' and thus that generating 'authentic' hope was integrally necessary for survival. The stories' authors avowed a kind of commitment to both the existential, theological side of hope and the psychosomatic side of hope, describing the decision to recount their experiences as a final act in their

[218] *Revue*, nos. 15 to 34 (1961).
[219] The author uses the term 'Hirnhaut-Melanoblastom', likely meaning meningioma.
[220] Heinz G. Konsalik, *Diagnose Krebs* (Munich: Lichtenberg, 1964), 144–5. The novel had multiple print runs. The 6th and, for a time, last edition was pressed in 1983. The later editions appeared under the title *Die Begnadigung* (*The Pardon*).

fight against cancer. Here, too, the trend originated in the United States and Great Britain, where psychosomatic concepts were embraced much earlier than in West Germany.

Probably the earliest autobiographical narrative of this type was a book published in the United States in 1952 by a woman named Edna Kaehele. Still in her 30s, Kaehele was a single mother of four from Denver who worked as a local reporter but was otherwise unknown to most people. Over a span of one hundred and fifty pages, she narrated how she was diagnosed in July 1946 with such a severe case of cervical cancer that doctors believed she had less than six months to live. The doctor's openness with her prognosis was a purely practical decision, as he wanted to allow her to determine who would take care of her young children after she passed. But despite this shattering diagnosis, she outlived the prognosis by more than twenty-two years.[221]

Her book *Living with Cancer*, published six years after her diagnosis, was a testament to the possibility of continuing to live with an incurable case of cancer. She conceived the book as a manifesto for her certitude that hope and overcoming fear were decisive factors in the fight with cancer.[222] She wrote that her illness confronted her with the bitter realization that everyone around her believed she had no chance of being cured, a problem amplified by her doctor's own doubts that she would ever recover. She pointedly wrote:

> The conscientious doctor makes an examination, performs a biopsy, and gives up before he opens his mouth to further intimidate the cowering wretch on his table. 'Six months', he says, and in six months more or less the obliging patient lies down and dies, never having known that he could do anything else. It is a form of modern-day voodooism, performed by medicine men in sterile white coats fearfully lacking in imagination.... Nobody sends humorous cards to the cancer victim. With cancer, you are already dead; and who toasts a corpse, even though that corpse is unfortunately still housed in a living body?[223]

As she explained in the introduction to her book, this experience motivated her to overcome her reluctance to publicly discuss her diagnosis.[224] She intended the autobiographical text to serve at once as a messenger of hope and as a self-help book for people with cancer who wanted to hear not more expert medical knowledge, but the personal experiences of others.[225] While her style was met

[221] 'Cancer Victim Writes Book "Sealed Orders"', *Sunday Chronicle: North Jersey's Only Weekly Pictorial Magazine* 31, 18 October 1959, 9. Edna Kaehele died in 1969: https://www.findagrave.com/cgi-bin/fg.cgi?page=gr&GRid=99402500.

[222] Edna Kaehele, *Living with Cancer* (London: Victor Gollancz Ltd, 1953), 75–7.

[223] Ibid., 13–14 and 60.

[224] Ibid., 17–18.

[225] And, shortly after the publication of her book, she founded a self-help organization called Cancer Courageous. By 1955, it had branches in twenty states. See Mary Margaret M'Bride, 'They've Survived Death', *Los Angeles Times*, 7 March 1955, B6.

with acclaim in the United States, West Germany was less enthusiastic. The German translation of the book was mostly overlooked by the media. But the publication of the Agnes Karll Verband, an association that promoted the professionalization of nursing, recommended Kaehele's book to all nurses who cared for cancer patients because the author's 'trust that emanates from her affirmation of fate... [will] touch every woman who is struggling to cope with her situation'.[226]

Thus, some readers in the early Federal Republic of Germany were indeed interested in the stories of cancer survivors who sought to offer their own experiences as examples of hope and serve as guides to others on their way to recovery. However, it is unclear why no similar books were written by German cancer patients until the late 1960s. After all, in the United States and Great Britain, Edna Kaehele was by no means the only patient who had made her story public.[227]

Moreover, some American and British cancer survivors founded groups and associations that visited cancer patients at hospitals in order to talk about their discharge from the hospital and assuage their fears about returning to 'normal' life. And many appeared in campaigns to confirm that doctors were not telling fairy tales when they informed their patients they might yet be cured. Associations like Reach to Recovery, founded by breast cancer patient Terese Lasser in 1952/3; the Ostomy Association of Boston, founded in 1952 as a self-help organization for colon cancer patients; and Cancer Anonymous, founded in 1955 by Brian Hession, an Anglican pastor with cancer—all called on doctors to inform patients about their diagnosis, because only then, they asserted, could patients actively engage in their own recovery and chart their own individual path back to everyday life. Just as important in the activists' work was their growing conviction that the chances of curing cancer were becoming more realistic.[228]

After voicing some initial reservations, doctors and, above all, nurses, supported these organizations. The American Cancer Society (ACS) also began thematizing cancer treatments and post-treatment care in its campaigns for the first time. For instance, *After Mastectomy*, a film produced by the ACS in 1958, discussed breast prosthesis, helpful exercises, and the counselling services of Reach to Recovery.[229]

In the 1950s, West German health policy also began addressing rehabilitation in general and post-treatment care for cancer patients in particular. However, cancer awareness films and pamphlets created by the Krebsgesellschaft (German

[226] M. Z., 'Edna Kaehele', *Die Agnes Karll-Schwester* 8, no. 11 (1954): 303.

[227] David Cantor, 'Before Survivorship: The Moment of Recovery in Twentieth-Century American Cancer Campaigns', *Social History of Medicine* 27, no. 3 (2014): 440–65, https://doi.org/10.1093/shm/hkt100.

[228] Maren Klawitter, *The Biopolitics of Breast Cancer: Changing Cultures of Disease and Activism* (Minneapolis: University of Minnesota Press, 2008); Cantor, 'Before Survivorship', 461; Brian Hession, *Determined to Live* (London, 1956).

[229] Cantor, 'Before Survivorship', 451–8.

Cancer Society) and the Gesundheitsmuseum Köln (Cologne Museum of Health) did not discuss them. They continued to give the impression that every cancer patient could simply return to their old lives after operation or radiotherapy. Thus, they effectively remained silent about the side effects of cancer therapies and the possibility of relapse and metastases. The choice not to enlighten people about these issues was informed by the old conviction that it could trigger irrational fear of cancer among the population, who would then ignore early symptoms and, as a consequence, take advantage of early detection measures only after it was already too late. These arguments recycled conceptions of fear from the Weimar era—a sort of 'fear of fear' that also underwent a renaissance in other parts of early West German society.[230] Moreover, the trend is a further indicator of how psychoanalysis and psychosomatics, both of which understood speaking about fears to be palliative, did not have nearly as broad an influence in West Germany as they did in the United States.[231]

In short, cancer patients in West Germany could not count on support from a network of post-treatment care organizations of the type that had been established in the United States and Great Britain. But this in itself does not explain why patients in West Germany only went public with their concerns relatively late. Even when they did begin to do so in the late 1960s, the hesitation to publicly represent oneself as a former cancer patient seems to have remained considerable. Oftentimes, patients were not the ones who took the initiative to speak out. Instead, young doctors or journalists aware of the American and British organizations sought out people open to discussing their experiences in a public forum; some wagered that the stories might be able to give early detection campaigns a more hopeful visage.[232] Still, the first West German cancer patients who did speak or write about their stories often did so under a pseudonym or hid their faces.[233]

Many were flatly shy about speaking about personal matters in public. They also feared that others might avoid them and their families if word got out that they had suffered from cancer. The fear of being excluded on account of having (had) cancer was evidently greater in West Germany than in the United States or Great Britain. The discrepancy may have been an aftereffect of National Socialism, which maligned cancer with antisemitic language as a form of 'degeneration' while

[230] Biess, '"Everybody Has a Chance"'.

[231] Hitzer, 'Oncomotions', 163–9; Hitzer and León-Sanz, 'The Feeling Body and Its Diseases', 89–91.

[232] See Elisabeth Keller's statements in the documentary TV episode 'Ich hatte Krebs' (I Had Cancer) discussed below.

[233] Elisabeth Keller initially published her story under the pseudonym Anni David in the Austrian paper *Neue Illustrierte Wochenschau*, and then with the same pseudonym as a book: Anni David, *Trotz allem—Hoffnung. Tagebuch einer Krebskranken* (Mödling: St. Gabriel-Verlag, 1968). Only for the publication of the book in West Germany a year later did she reveal her real name: Elisabeth Keller, *Ich habe den Krebs überwunden. Aus dem Tagebuch einer Mutter* (Munich: Gilt, 1969). In 'Ich hatte Krebs', as well, two of the interviewed persons concealed their identities.

executing euthanasia programmes rooted in the ideology that the lives of potentially incurable cancer patients were 'not worth living'.

East German media lacked public autobiographical accounts until well into the 1970s. Centred on the individual, their experiences, and their 'bourgeois' self-identity, the genre contradicted the collectivist ideals propagated by the GDR government in the 1950s and 1960s. Perhaps, too, East German health policy-makers were anxious about the critical potential of personal accounts of cancer therapy. Letters to the East German Ministry of Health reveal that patients and their loved ones were uproarious about hospitals' insufficient facilities and the quality of treatment in East German oncology clinics. Indeed, many wanted to undergo treatment outside the GDR.[234] Author Brigitte Reimann, who had breast cancer, wrote in her diary in 1968: 'Day after tomorrow I have to go to the hospital [in Hoyerswerda]—and what a hospital! Ugly, dirty, rundown. I cried just seeing the hallway.' The passage stems from the 1998 edition of her diary. In the edition published in 1983, the passage read differently: 'I was supposed to have an operation tomorrow in Hoy[erswerda], but when I saw the hospital, I broke down completely. I have never before seen such a dirty, gloomy, scruffy hole.'[235]

Aleksander Solzhenitsyn impressively demonstrated how critiques of health-care could be extrapolated into an attack on the communist political system. In his two-volume novel *Cancer Ward*, he rendered in literary form his experiences of cancer treatment at a hospital in Tashkent in the 1950s. The book not only picked apart how the socialist economic system had left the Soviet cancer clinic sorely ill-equipped to provide adequate care. It also detailed the web of lies, complicity, and favouritism at the clinic, which in his eyes defined the Soviet system as a whole. The novel was banned in the Soviet Union and the GDR, but it circulated as samizdat and copies were smuggled into the West.[236]

In contrast, Christa Wolf's novel *The Quest for Christa T.*, whose protagonist suffers from leukaemia, was allowed to be published in the GDR, but only after Wolf made some concessions to the censors.[237] They chastised the novel for not sufficiently criticizing Christa T.'s individualism and withdrawnness, which they suggested might have been accomplished by adding a character who could serve as a 'positive' example.[238] Reviewers and fellow authors could not agree on whether

[234] Letter from Manfred Sch., Klingenthal, Zollstr. 86, to the Ministry of Health, Berlin, 19 November 1959; Letter from the Fritz R., Bremerhaven, Lilienthalstr. 19, 5 July 1964 to the state councillor; Letter from Fritz R. to the Ministry of Health, 31 October 1964: BArch DQ1 2106.

[235] Brigitte Reimann, *Alles schmeckt nach Abschied. Tagebücher 1964–1970*, diary entry from 18 September 1968 (Berlin: Aufbau-Verlag, 1998), 215; Elisabeth Elten-Krause and Walter Lewerenz, eds, *Brigitte Reimann in ihren Tagebüchern und Briefen. Eine Auswahl* (Berlin: Verlag Neues Leben, 1983), 256.

[236] Alexander Solzhenitsyn, *Cancer Ward*, trans. Nicholas Bethell and David Burg (New York: Farrar, Straus and Giroux, 2015).

[237] Sonja E. Klocke, *Inscription and Rebellion: Illness and the Symptomatic Body in East German Literature* (Rochester: Camden House, 2015), 36.

[238] Angela Drescher, ed., Dokumentation zu Christa Wolf 'Nachdenken über Christa T.' (Berlin: Aufbau, 1993), 31–59.

the novel was a subtle critique of the GDR's authoritarian state and East German society. Some interpreted a connection between Christa T.'s sick body and her social discontent. West German literary critic Marcel Reich-Ranicki put this reading bluntly: 'Let's be clear: Christa T. dies of leukaemia, but she is sick with GDR.'[239] This form of social critique was potent because there was no way to gaslight people into believing cancer did not exist in the GDR. As long as people got cancer in East Germany, the government would have a problem with literary or autobiographical depictions of it as a corporeal reaction to the country's oppressive social environment. Thus, it is no wonder that this kind of connection between disease and society was not established again in books published in the GDR. The only exception were representations of disease as a lingering effect of the damage inflicted by fascism, a plotline one censor suggested Christa Wolf pursue for *Christa T.*[240]

State-controlled East German media tended to focus on the opinions of (potential) cancer patients and non-fictional representations of the doctor-patient relationship. Public health officials conducted surveys and selectively published their results in an effort to signal the state's familiarity with the 'man' and 'woman' on the street. For instance, in 1964, journalists of the widely read weekly *Neue Berliner Illustrierte* (NBI) asked East Germans their opinions about a series of matters related to cancer. They then commissioned two oncologists—director of the Charité's oncology clinic Fritz Gietzelt and Robert Rössle Clinic doctor Gustav-Paul Wildner—to comment on them. It seems that the sample was about one hundred people, meaning that it was not a representative, methodologically sound survey. This suggests that the survey served more as a 'hook' than that it offered any real data about the population's opinions.

'If you had cancer, would you want to know it?' was one of the questions. Editors depicted the responses as 'surprising': sixty-four respondents wanted to know, four were uncertain, and thirty-four were decidedly against knowing. But despite the majority clearly electing to know, Professor Gietzelt held on to his view that doctors in the GDR should only communicate cancer diagnoses to patients who refused treatment. For all others, he maintained, doctors should stick to the approach prescribed by medical ethics and medical law: 'The patient must actively participate in their recovery. How can they do that when their optimism is destroyed?'[241] But the NBI journalist responded with some consternation that, if doctors in the GDR generally did not tell their patients their diagnosis and one out of five East Germans got cancer at some point in their lives, then that would mean 20 per cent of the country's population were not correctly informed about the state

[239] Marcel Reich-Ranicki, 'Christa Wolfs unruhige Elegie', *Die Zeit*, 23 May 1969.

[240] Christa Wolf repeatedly thematized the connection between social relations and bodily symptoms in her novels. See Klocke, *Inscription and Rebellion*, 34–71.

[241] Here and the following quotes: Roman Marczikowski, 'Jeder 5. stirbt an Krebs', *Neue Berliner Illustrierte* 35 (1964): 8–13 and 33, 13.

of their health. Gietzelt reassured: 'Trust between doctor and patient must be certain, must be clear. A break in trust making the patient distrustful cannot be allowed.' In plain language, that meant that upholding the 'white lie', as Gietzelt called it, had to be coordinated with everyone involved. Many family members of cancer patients shared this position. For example, in 1968, a machinist from Gera wrote letters to the East German Ministry of Health and Soviet ambassador Peter Abrassimov requesting that his wife be permitted to travel to the Soviet Union for treatment. Although his wife had undergone a mastectomy the previous year and metastases had now appeared, he pleaded at the end of all his letters that responses be sent to his work address; he did not give his home address. He explained that: 'My wife can in no way find out what kind of illness she has.'[242]

Around the same time, two radiologists from Halle inquired into whether the 'white lie' could really succeed in the long term by conducting a survey of doctors, students, and patients. The answer was clear: out of 628 people being treated for cancer in the Halle metropolitan area, two-thirds (412) knew that they were being treated for a malignant tumour. However, a much smaller number (135) had learned of their diagnosis from their doctor. Of the seventeen patients being treated for a benign tumour, twelve believed that they had cancer, which is to say that they had no faith in the soothing, but in their case correct, diagnosis.[243] The authors of the study, Hans-Wolfgang Becker and Hans-Lothar Kölling, drew on these results to criticize their colleagues, 85 per cent of whom declared that they concealed cancer diagnoses from patients when the prognosis was bad.[244] Becker and Kölling judged this reasoning as 'frivolous', because it could 'damage or even undermine the relationship of trust between doctor and patient'.[245]

In the GDR, the practice of rarely telling cancer patients about their diagnosis—and even then only if their chances of recovery were good—seems to have changed little over time. The diaries of Brigitte Reimann again serve as a testament to this. Reimann developed breast cancer in the late 1960s and died in 1973. She feared that she had cancer and a biopsy in the late summer of 1968 confirmed her fears. The doctor at the hospital in Hoyerswerda seems to have told her in straightforward terms that she had cancer and would have to undergo a mastectomy.[246] After the operation at the Robert Rössle Clinic in Berlin, the surgeon ensured her that 'everything was excised' and that she was now healthy.[247] In February 1970, Reimann got an examination after suffering pain in her stomach and back. The doctors told her that she had a tumour in her stomach, 'probably benign', and that

[242] Letter from Comrade Fr. to Comrade Abrassimov, Gera, 22 February 1968, BArch DQ 1/3272, 21–3.

[243] Hans-Wolfgang Becker and Hans-Lothar Kölling, '"Schonendes Betrügen?" Ermittlungen zur Frage der Aufklärung bei Geschwulstleiden', *Nova Acta Leopoldina* 28, no. 168 (1964): 3–18, 12.

[244] Ibid., 9 and 11. [245] Ibid., 17.

[246] Reimann, *Alles schmeckt nach Abschied*, entry from 11 September 1968, 215.

[247] Ibid., entry from 1 or 2 October 1968, 217.

there were no metastases in her spine.[248] They explained the back pain as a slipped disc, and when she was sent back to the Robert Rössle Clinic for radiotherapy, the doctors there stuck to the story.[249] But she had her doubts and wrote in her diary: 'Sometimes I think that in truth I have cancer or a similar abomination, I can guess it from all kinds of suggestions and the "I cannot tell you" and the high R dosage [radiation dose].'[250]

Author Maxie Wander, who was born in Austria and lived in the GDR, had a similar experience when she went to the Charité in the autumn of 1976 to have a lump in her breast examined. The doctor told her that her tumour was concerning and she would have to have an operation, but that this did not mean 'that you have cancer'.[251] After undergoing a mastectomy, Wander asked the doctor about her diagnosis, to which the latter responded: 'It was not cancer, but trouble spots that were very scattered and that tend to reproduce themselves. Radiotherapy must be done out of precaution.' Wander commented in her diary: 'Naturally, she is lying.'[252] The distrust pushed her to open the sealed referral when she needed to have liver problems examined in July 1977. The doctor's letter made clear that she suspected the author had metastases in her liver. Officially, though, Wander was told she had a chronic infection—'allegedly', she wrote with scepticism.[253] However, two months before her death, when she regularly had to undergo chemotherapy, she wrote: 'What confuses me—the certificate of illness I got still has the diagnosis number for cancer....'[254] But the doctors consistently told her that her cancer had been cured. Thus, shortly before her death, she seems to have moved from clear scepticism to uncertainty about the true diagnosis.

Around this time, some East German clinics were shifting their approach to talking about cancer diagnoses. For instance, a year before Maxie Wander's death, radiologist Roland Jacob was promoted to head doctor of the radiotherapy clinic at the hospital in Berlin's Buch section. Jacob decided that doctors should speak to patients before the beginning of their treatment and inform them that they had a 'malignant tumour'.[255] Still, he wanted to avoid the word 'cancer'. He thus recommended that doctors respond to the question of whether it was cancer by asking the patient what they understood cancer to be. The stated purpose was to learn about the fears that patients associated with the word 'cancer'. Afterwards,

[248] Ibid., entry from 17 February 1970 and 18 February 1970, 303–4.

[249] Ibid., entry from 9 April 1970, 310.

[250] Ibid., entry from 9 May 1970, 316–17.

[251] Maxie Wander, entry from 10 September 1976, in *Leben wär' eine prima Alternative. Tagebücher und Briefe*, ed. Fred Wander (Munich: dtv, 1994), 14–15. Maxie Wander's diaries were edited and published in the GDR after her death in 1977 by her husband Fred Wander.

[252] Ibid., entry from 17 September 1976, 25.

[253] Ibid., entry from 26 July 1977, 240–2.

[254] Ibid., letter from 22 September 1977, 270–1.

[255] Roland Jacob, 'Die psychische Führung des Krebspatienten', *Zeitschrift für die gesamte innere Medizin und ihre Grenzgebiete* 33, no. 14 (1978): 455–8, 456.

the doctor was supposed to guide the conversation towards potential treatments in order to bolster the patient's hope.[256]

Jacob justified this reorientation by referencing Becker and Kölling's study, the work of Walter Brednow, the work of Heidelberg-based psychosomatics doctor Richard Siebeck, and the writings of Feifel and Kübler-Ross.[257] He argued that openly discussing the diagnosis with the patient early on would make it easier for them to express their worries, depression, and fears, something that dissembling confidence could not accomplish. Only then, he asserted, could doctors really help dying patients, since in his experience, doctors' willingness to talk was a significant form of support for them.[258] In the previous decades, debates in the GDR on informing cancer patients about their diagnosis had focused on recovery and what was perceived to be the necessity of optimism for facilitating recovery. In contrast, the needs of terminally ill patients were rarely addressed. Jacob's approach explicitly catered to those needs. This placed him among the first generation of doctors and medical ethicists in the GDR who directly grappled with the situation of dying patients and studied how care could be made more humane.[259]

In West Germany, too, the end of the 1970s saw intense engagement with dying and death, discussions that drew on the same American studies quoted by Jacob. However, the West German discourse was, to a large extent, a critique of the modern hospital with its focus on economy and efficiency. At the same time, some people expanded the debate into a broader critique of society.

'The loneliness of the dying' in contemporary times, as sociologist Norbert Elias wrote in 1982, appeared to many not just as an effect of 'the institutionalized routines of hospitals', but also of 'civilization's overgrown taboo on the expression of strong, spontaneous feelings'.[260] This perception fed on arguments formulated during the new social movements of the 1970s, which called for increased social participation and emotional 'warmth', placed primacy on quality of life over the dominant focus on living standards, and questioned the patriarchy. In West Germany, initiatives wanted to change the health system by increasing patients' autonomy and they sharply criticized paternalistic doctors who subordinated patients' subjective sense of their own good to the whirring medical machine. Discontent with hospitals grew out of the perception that the health system was overstrained and in dire need of reform.

Cancer patients' autobiographical accounts of their experiences with the health system took on a more political tone in this context. The first such narratives published in the 1970s were still situated in the discussion on hope and revolved

256 Ibid., 457. 257 See the bibliography: ibid., 458. 258 Ibid., 457–8.

259 Heinz Brandt, Susanne Hahn, and Achim Thom, 'Probleme und Aufgaben der Betreuung Sterbender durch den Hausarzt', in *Grenzsituationen ärztlichen Handelns*, ed. Uwe Körner, Karl Seidel, and Achim Thom (Jena: Fischer Verlag, 1981), 211–32; Kay Blumenthal-Barby, ed., *Betreuung Sterbender. Tendenzen, Fakten, Probleme* (Berlin: Verlag Volk und Gesundheit, 1982).

260 Elias, *The Loneliness of the Dying*, 28.

around illustrating how cancer could be defeated. *Ich habe den Krebs überwunden* (*I Survived Cancer*) was the subtitle of Austrian journalist Elisabeth Keller's *Tagebuch einer Mutter* (*Diary of a Mother*), which was published in 1969 with a preface by Käte Strobel, West Germany's minister of health.[261] An episode of the popular primetime TV show *Gesundheitsmagazin Praxis* (*Health Praxis*) broadcast in April 1970 with the title 'Ich hatte Krebs' (I Had Cancer) ultimately just promoted early detection campaigns. Thus, an offscreen voice towards the end of the film declared:

> People among us. They have defeated cancer and they spoke about it almost as a matter of course in order to spare us outsiders from fear: Early detection is the only promising possibility: for the hope to be able to say after years of uncertainty: I had cancer.[262]

Broken Taboos and Turning Points

Five years later, actress Hildegard Knef wrote with a totally different verve. In 1975, she published a book about her experience with breast cancer, donning it with a title that played on how her doctors had told her about her diagnosis: *Das Urteil* (*The Verdict*).[263] As the media salivated over pre-publication speculation that the book might reveal intimate details, Knef explained in an interview with *Stern* why she decided to write the book:

> I wanted to slaughter a couple of golden calves. First, there's this golden calf, the hospital. I found that it had to be said what kind of hell takes place behind its walls. Why are patients placed under tutelage right at the door, treated like idiots? . . . How the patients are doing doesn't matter. [Interviewer: Which golden calf did you mean again?] The dictatorship of doctors . . . . I think that doctors should regularly consider the extent to which they have succumbed to the standing person's delusions of grandeur. Constantly looking down at people lying down doesn't do them any good . . . . [The media] will accuse me of all sorts of things—that I'm an exhibitionist, a masochist. Why? Because I am attacking a taboo. [Interviewer: Which taboo?] The mystification of cancer. While sex was taboo in my grandmother's time, now dying, death, and cancer are taboo, that is our modern pornography.[264]

261 Keller, *Ich habe den Krebs überwunden*.

262 'Ich hatte Krebs', documentary by Sigrid Schenkenberger, screened on 13 April 1970 as an episode of *Gesundheitsmagazin Praxis*. ZDF-Archiv.

263 Knef, *The Verdict*.

264 Eva Windmöller, '"Ich will mich nicht bedauern". Eva Windmöller interviewt Hildegard Knef', *Der Stern* 19 (1975): 67–72, 67.

This full-frontal attack on modern medicine was not about staking out hope. It was about reclaiming one's subjectivity in the face of the impositions of the 'modern' hospital business. That Knef declared that cancer was a modern taboo is emblematic of a noteworthy shift in what the word taboo meant, because her doctors did not conceal from her the 'verdict', the cancer diagnosis. Instead, according to her account, they told it to her clumsily, hesitatingly, and cloaked in medical jargon, stating: 'It's a carcinoma, about the size of a cherry.'[265] For her, the taboo was the cancer patient themselves, because they were written off as people who merely represented the negation of social expectations of success and ability. As she asserted in the *Stern* interview: 'Whoever is afflicted with it is shut out from our achievement-oriented society, an irritating object that, like with old people, one prefers to sweep away.'[266]

Zurich teacher Fritz Zorn, who, as discussed in Chapter 2, wrote about his experience with cancer in his book *Mars*, posthumously published in 1977, also interpreted his experience in political terms.[267] But his critique targeted 'bourgeois' society and the way it alienated him from his true self and 'real' feelings by teaching him to hide them from others and from himself behind a well-kept façade. He asserted that this degeneration of his authentic self—a concept in vogue at the time—contributed to his cancer. *Mars* became a cult favourite among the alternative scene of the 1980s. It, too, offered a new take on what was taboo, describing 'authentic' emotions as the taboo of a society set on appearances and decorum.

This new thematization of cancer was no longer about dismantling taboos in the doctor-patient relationship. But the politicization of the topic lent greater public resonance to discussions about disclosing and concealing cancer diagnoses. Doctors' approaches to cancer were now grasped as an indicator for how honestly and 'authentically' they treated patients. Did they speak to them as human beings, or just as medical objects? The discussion cast the aporias of silence in ever starker relief, a point well exemplified by a story told by Fritz Meerwein, a trailblazer of Germanophone psycho-oncology. At the beginning of his article 'Bemerkungen zur Arzt-Patientenbeziehung bei Krebskranken' (Remarks on the Doctor-Patient Relationship with Cancer Patients), he narrated:

> A 35-year-old man, father of five children, visited his general practitioner because of upper abdominal pains for the first time when he was 31 years old. A laparotomy occasioned suspicion of a potential pancreas carcinoma. A segmental resection of the tumour was performed; the histology at that time, however, revealed no malignancy.... Four years later and after the birth of his

[265] Knef, *The Verdict*, 5.
[266] Windmöller, '"Ich will mich nicht bedauern"', 69.
[267] Zorn, *Mars*.

> fifth child, the man suffered pain again. A laparotomy reveals a widely metastasized, inoperable pancreas carcinoma.
>
> At the beginning of the clinical presentation, while the patient is not yet present, the lecturer asks the auditorium to feel sympathy with the patient who will now be introduced and to not talk during the discussion. Then the patient was brought into the auditorium where the lecturer briefly presents his anamnesis. He then reassures the man that everything is going to be good again soon and that he wishes him a good recovery. After the patient leaves the auditorium and the lecturer is certain that the door is shut, he explains to his students that the patient's life expectancy is, at the most, six months.
>
> To this, a student wants to know who is responsible for correctly informing the patient about his diagnosis and life expectancy. In his response, the lecturer emphasizes the necessity of putting the patient in an optimistic mood. However, he suggests bringing in the man's wife in order to inform her. He says it is an intrafamilial problem....
>
> Another student knows from his own familial experience that it is enraging for a dying person to learn that he has been lied to by doctors over a long period of time and he tells this to the auditorium. He is interrupted by booing from his fellow students, who are of the conviction that it is not a lie to conceal the truth from a person. They say things have to be differentiated. In a concluding statement, the lecturer underscores the necessity of humaneness when dealing with sick patients.[268]

Whether this scene actually happened or was made up by Meerwein to dramatically illustrate how numerous doctors treated cancer patients is not possible to discern from the article itself. But it is remarkable to what extremes deception was taken in it. Not only did the doctors and nurses know the truth—so did all the students in the lecture hall. They watched from their seats as the patient's cluelessness was presented to them like a stage play and were made privy to his 'death sentence' after his 'exit' from the stage. This theatricality was augmented with boos against the demurring student, like something taken out of a show trial.

Whether fact or fiction, Meerwein and his co-authors certainly selected this scene because it starkly expressed the degrading, condescending nature of deception. This impression is bolstered by the treatment of the student objecting out of personal experience, who is not merely ignored, but aggressively shouted down. But as Meerwein detailed in the run of the article, it suggested that behind the sovereign façade of condescension lurked a fearful defence against the doctor's sense of his own mortality. For Meerwein, this situation represented a

[268] Fritz Meerwein, S. Kauf, and G. Schneider, 'Bemerkungen zur Arzt-Patientenbeziehung bei Krebskranken', *Zeitschrift für Psychosomatische Medizin und Psychoanalyse* 22, no. 3 (1976): 278–300, 278–9.

foundational moment in the split between thinking and feeling, which led the doctor—and people more generally—to 'inauthenticity' in their inner attitude and outward actions.[269] He discarded the dichotomies of inside/outside, feeling/thinking in order to define authenticity as complete concordance with oneself.

Meerwein's analysis was informed by the concept of the authentic self. Other psychotherapists and psychologists as well as activists from the alternative left were formulating this new ideal of a reformed society. They articulated authenticity both as a moral imperative and as a concrete utopia that could be attained by constantly working on oneself.[270] Psychoanalyst Horst-Eberhard Richter, the first professor of psychotherapy and psychosomatic medicine in West Germany, wrote that the inner conflicts of the modern individual were not just a problem for doctors and patients, but represented an illness of all individuals in society.[271] However, seriously ill people were confronted with an existential threat that thrust them out of their everyday lives and routines. While this might have appeared as a burden at first glance, proponents of the universal claim that everyone was in some sense afflicted by inner dividedness thought that it might also offer a chance at renewal. They interpreted the visible illness as a manifest symptom of the more general pathology and thus believed it gave an occasion to 'pose questions about a new meaning of life' or induce the 'rebirth' of a lost 'authentic' life.[272]

But this required the doctor to be 'truthful'. Only then could the patient start working on a 'new beginning'. In contrast to the theological and philosophical discussions of the 1950s and early 1960s, the discourse of renewal and authenticity was not focused on the salubrious effects of (re)vitalizing hope in a situation of hopelessness. Instead, it aimed at overcoming the split between inner life and outer life, between the individual's emotions and her thoughts. The theory rested on the notion that by speaking about repressed emotions, particularly fear, patients would discover in themselves a heretofore unknown power to heal and recover.

This approach was initially spearheaded in West Germany by proponents of person-centred therapy.[273] In 1978, psychologist couple Reinhard and Anne-Marie Tausch began talking about what this kind of therapy might look like on a television show called *Psychotreff* (*Psychology Meeting*); it aired four times a year on the regional public SWR station and was picked up by other regional stations.

[269] Ibid., 288–9.

[270] Sven Reichardt, 'Authentizität als Selbstbeschreibungskategorie im linksalternativen Milieu', in *Die 'andere' Provinz. Kulturelle Auf- und Ausbrüche im Bodenseeraum seit den 1960er Jahren*, ed. Heike Kempe (Konstanz: UVK Verlag), 11–20; Tändler, *Das therapeutische Jahrzehnt.*

[271] Horst-Eberhard Richter, *Die Gruppe. Hoffnung auf einen Weg, sich selbst und andere zu befreien* (Reinbek: Rowohlt Verlag, 1972), 14.

[272] Anne-Marie Tausch, *Gespräche gegen die Angst. Krankheit als ein Weg zum Leben* (Reinbek: Rowohlt Verlag, 1981), 87. On the rhetoric of self-transformation, see Arthur W. Frank, 'The Rhetoric of Self-Change: Illness Experience as Narrative', *Sociological Quarterly* 34 (1993): 41–5.

[273] Tändler, '"Psychoboom"', 82–3.

The show offered viewers the wholly new experience of watching a group therapy session live on TV. They saw how participants spoke about their emotions and psychological pain in order to learn about their 'authentic', healthy self.[274]

While the initial topic were people with mental illness, Anne-Marie Tausch soon shifted her work to cancer patients. She acted as both psychologist and patient, as she was soon diagnosed with cancer herself. In 1981, she published her experiences from both sides in a book titled *Gespräche gegen die Angst* (*Talking against Fear*).[275] Referencing Kübler-Ross, Tausch framed telling cancer patients the truth as an affirmation of a 'philosophy of life' that, to be sure, acknowledged the necessity of survival, but was focused more on the importance of learning how to live 'intensely', 'authentically', and 'self-determined'. This is why her book carried the subtitle *Illness as a Path to Life*.[276] The book meshed well with the works of a number of American psychologists, who also interpreted cancer diagnoses as having the potential to be a 'turning point and new beginning' and offered a guide to 'getting well again' by encouraging cancer patients to get in touch with their own emotions and bodies.[277]

Opinions diverged on what this turning point meant, what it might look like, and which therapies and techniques might best achieve it. But all authors contended that cultivating wholeness was important to piecing together the fragmentation of modern life. Body and mind, thinking and feeling, self and society—they sought to unify these differences with all-encompassing ideas like God, holiness, and the universe. They described becoming whole as an open-ended process: learning to understand one's own emotions and accepting fear were a significant part of it. In the end, they believed this would help people become their own whole, authentic self. Mobilizing inner energies and sowing positive feelings through visualization and conscious emotional 'work' belonged to the standard arsenal of the various streams that flowed into the increasingly popular New Age movement.[278]

Certainly, not all, and not even a majority of cancer patients turned towards New Age philosophy. However, the general notion that being diagnosed with cancer could occasion intense reflection on one's life and emotions struck a chord with many people, as did the concomitant notion that this process of self-evaluation opened the chance to lead a new, more 'authentic' life. Less certain was whether the turning point would necessarily help defeat the illness. But

[274] Thomas von Randow, 'Psychotreff im Fernsehen', *Die Zeit*, 22 September 1978.

[275] Tausch, *Gespräche gegen die Angst*. [276] Ibid., 118, 129, and 177.

[277] O. Carl Simonton, Stephanie Matthews-Simonton, and James Creighton, *Getting Well Again: A Step-by-Step, Self-Help Guide to Overcoming Cancer for Patients and Their Families* (New York: Bantam Books, 1978); Lawrence LeShan, *You Can Fight for Your Life: Emotional Factors in the Treatment of Cancer* (Lanham, MD: Rowman and Littlefield, 1977); and Lawrence LeShan, *Cancer as a Turning Point* (New York: Plume, 1990).

[278] Pascal Eitler, '"Selbstheilung". Zur Somatisierung und Sakralisierung von Selbstverhältnissen im New Age', in Maasen, Elberfeld, Eitler, and Tändler, *Das beratene Selbst*, 161–81.

perhaps that was not the decisive point, even if survival remained of primary importance. At least this was the conclusion reached by American breast cancer patient Treya Wilber in a discussion with her husband Ken, who published the conversation after her death; it was soon translated into German. After Wilber listed everything in her life that might have contributed to her cancer and that she thus wanted to change, both her and her husband arrived at the conviction that there was little evidence that things like expressing heretofore repressed feelings of anger and sadness would really increase her chances of being cured. Wilber experienced precisely this insight as liberating her to act as she saw fit. As her husband told her:

> 'You don't need cancer to tell you what you need to work on. You already know. So let's start. Let's make it a new beginning. I'll help. It'll be fun. Really. Am I getting goofy or what? We could call it Fun with Cancer.' We both started laughing out loud. But that made perfect sense, and I felt a kind of clarity and determination. I wanted—and needed—for this experience to have some meaning and purpose. The only way that could happen with any certainty was for me to act 'as if' it did, to imbue it with meaning through my thoughts and actions.[279]

Seen in this light, concealing a cancer diagnosis from a patient robbed them of the opportunity to reshape their life and come to their 'authentic' self in the time they had left. And it inhibited them from deciding for themselves what kind of treatment they wanted to undergo. This had special weight at a time when many were voicing doubts about conventional medicine and questioning long-standing medical dogmas. Avoiding the despair, hopelessness, and fear that might flow to the surface after learning one had cancer was stripped of its positive connotation. From the perspective of Tausch, Wilber, and others, these emotions were necessary, normal, and capable of being overcome—or at least shouldered—through 'working' on oneself. And, perhaps more importantly, they believed that only by reckoning with and affirming these emotions could the road towards a new beginning be embarked upon.

Talking about Cancer in the Age of Empathy

These new positions altered public perceptions of the debate on concealing or revealing cancer diagnoses to patients. And they impacted medical praxis, too. As an opinion poll conducted by Emnid in 1980 showed, two-thirds of patients in West German clinics were told they had cancer without having to ask. Doctors in

[279] Ken Wilber, *Grace and Grit: Spirituality and Healing in the Life and Death of Treya Killam Wilber* (Boston: Shambhala, 1991), 51.

private practices were more reluctant: they often only informed patients of their diagnosis when explicitly asked.[280] But the trend was clear, as the number of doctors who communicated cancer diagnoses on their own volition consistently rose.[281] There were no comparable surveys in the GDR. However, there is some evidence that a gradual shift occurred in East Germany, too. Beginning in the late 1970s, some prominent doctors voiced public support for telling people their diagnosis and made it policy in the clinics they headed.[282] In West Germany, organizations that stood up for the interests of cancer patients played a significant role in this development. Among them was Deutsche Krebshilfe (German Cancer Aid), which was established in 1974 by Mildred Scheel, wife of then president of Germany Walter Scheel. So too did the self-help groups popping up all over the place. They aimed to remove cancer from the 'taboo zone' and were often supported by doctors in their efforts.[283]

Around the same time period, psycho-oncology gained footing as an independent field of medicine. Beginning in 1978, some initial research on psychosocial care for cancer patients was conducted with funding from the Deutsche Krebshilfe. In 1983, the Deutsche Arbeitsgemeinschaft für Psychoonkologie e. V. (dapo—German Working Group for Psycho-oncology) was founded; in 1988 the Arbeitsgemeinschaft Psychoonkologie (PSO) in der Deutschen Krebsgesellschaft (Working Group Psycho-oncology in the German Cancer Society). Engaged citizens and doctors in the GDR were no strangers to these ideas, a point underscored by Christa Wolf's talk at the 1991 conference of the German Cancer Society. Towards the end of her talk on 'Cancer and Society', she recounted what a friend had told her about their own experience with breast cancer:

> I 'needed' the threat of death in order to risk exposure to situations in which I was fragile, wounded, and vulnerable, and which I would not have allowed otherwise. I was forced to assume total responsibility for the course I took. I discovered in

[280] Folker Kraus-Weysser, 'Nur jeder zweite deutsche Arzt sagt Krebskranken die Wahrheit', *Welt am Sonntag* 28 (1980): 16.

[281] The trend happened in many countries: Jimmie C. Holland, Natalie Geary, Anthony Marchini, and Susan Tross, 'Psychological Issues: An International Survey of Physician Attitudes and Practice in Revealing the Diagnosis of Cancer', *Cancer Investigation* 5, no. 2 (1987): 151–4, https://doi.org/10.3109/07357908709018468.

[282] Jacob, 'Die psychische Führung'; Ernst Günther, 'Das Arztrecht in der DDR und seine Beziehung zur ärztlichen Ethik: Erfahrungen aus dem Umgang mit ärztlichen Fehlleistungen', in *Medizinische Ethik in der DDR. Erfahrungswert oder Altlast?*, ed. Hartmut Bettin and Mariacarla Gadebusch Bondio (Lengerich: Pabst Science Publishers, 2010), 86–93, 89; Susanne Hahn, 'Ethische Fragen und Problemlösungen des Schwesternberufes im DDR-Gesundheitswesen', in Bettin and Gadebusch Bondio, *Medizinische Ethik in der DDR*, 73–85, 78.

[283] See, for instance, the mission of Frauenselbsthilfe nach Krebs e.V. (Women's Self-Help after Cancer). One of the oldest cancer self-help groups in the Federal Republic of Germany, it was founded in Mannheim in 1976: https://www.frauenselbsthilfe.de/verband/wer-wir-sind/geschichte-der-frauenselbsthilfe.html.

myself the belief that it is possible to be deeply close to others only in the face of death.[284]

After 1990, it was consensus in Germany that doctors should tell patients when they were diagnosed with cancer. Multiple official statements declared it to be a right.[285] Since then, the discussion has focused on how best to inform patients that they have cancer. Medical malpractice laws require that doctors educate patients about the risks of various types of treatment and sufficiently document that they have done so. The cases in which a doctor is permitted to consider not informing the patient of their diagnosis are extremely limited.[286]

Moreover, medical schools now train doctors how to sensitively tell patients they have cancer. Two influential models are SPIKES and NURSE.[287] Both strategies promise to help the doctor guide the patient's emotions by breaking the discussion down into individual steps. Medical students and doctors learn them through guidebooks and seminar scripts that lay out how much time should be allotted for the discussion, which type of room should be selected, what hour of the day is best, and which body posture the doctor should assume.[288] Some universities even deploy professional or amateur actors to simulate the strategies and give students the chance to get feedback from fellow students and the actors themselves on how well they perceived, reflected on, and counselled the 'patient's' emotions.[289]

Empathy often figures as the central emotion. By practising empathy, the techniques' inventors advise, doctors will better be able to discern the emotions, thoughts, and inner state of their patients, show understanding, and forge a

[284] Wolf, 'Cancer and Society', 106.

[285] Jörg Gstöttner, *Der Schutz von Patientenrechten durch verfahrensmäßige und institutionelle Vorkehrungen sowie den Erlass einer Charta der Patientenrechte* (Frankfurt am Main: Peter Lang, 2005). The current law is the 'Law on the Improvement of the Rights of Patients', passed on 20 February 2013. See Bundesgesetzblatt Part I, no. 9 (2013), Bonn, 25 March 2013, http://www.bundesaerztekammer.de/fileadmin/user_upload/downloads/Patientenrechtegesetz_BGBl.pdf.

[286] Johannes Lutterbach, Christian Weissenberger, Klaus Hitzer, and Almut Helmes, 'Qui nescit simulare nescit curare—Wer nicht täuschen kann, kann nicht heilen. Anmerkungen zur Aufklärung von Patienten in der (Radio-)Onkologie', *Strahlentherapie und Onkologie* 180, no. 8 (2004): 469–77, 470, https://doi.org/10.1007/s00066-004-1253-y.

[287] SPIKES stands for Setting, Perception, Invitation, Knowledge, Empathy, Strategy, and Summary. NURSE stands for Naming, Understanding, Respecting, Supporting, Exploring. See Robert A. Buckman, 'Breaking Bad News: The S-P-I-K-E-S Strategy', *Community Oncology* 2, no. 2 (2005): 138–42, 139–41. On NURSE, see *Kommunikation im medizinischen Alltag. Ein Leitfaden für die Praxis* (Düsseldorf: Ärztekammer Nordrhein, 2015), 26–7.

[288] Buckman, 'Breaking Bad News', 139–41; *Kommunikation im medizinischen Alltag*, 26–7; Universitätsklinikum Tübingen. Medizinische Klinik, Abteilung Innere Medizin VI, Psychosomatische Medizin und Psychotherapie, *Materialien zum Praktikum Psychosomatische Medizin und Psychotherapie: Leitfaden zur Mitteilung schwerwiegender Diagnosen*, https://docplayer.org/18572092-Materialien-zum-praktikum-psychosomatische-medizin-leitfaden-zur-mitteilung-schwerwiegender-befunde-und-diagnosen-1.html.

[289] W. May, J. H. Park, and J. P. Lee, 'A Ten-Year-Review of the Literature on the Use of Standardized Patients in Teaching and Learning: 1996–2005', *Medical Teacher* 31, no. 6 (2009): 487–92.

human connection. In contrast, they give hope a more ambivalent status. This stems from the recognition of the mistakes doctors can commit when breaking bad news, such as rushing to palliate in order to reduce their own stress or making the prognosis sound better than the diagnosis actually warrants.[290] While hope is oriented towards the future, empathy is generally conceived as an emotion of the present that revolves around the patient's current state of being. Today, empathy features in managers' guides and parenting books. In its popular version, it is often pitched as an important component of successful, 'emotionally intelligent' communication.[291] But in truth, it can be interwoven with a multiplicity of different emotions and interests that might be masked by the rehearsed empathy of a person leading a conversation.[292] Then, the empathy-based discussion strategy can easily slip into becoming a mere emotional *technique*. Some texts on how doctors should communicate with patients explicitly identify this as a danger:

> Techniques alone do not constitute the quality of the conversation; decisive, too, is whether the doctor is experienced by the patient as authentic. Authenticity in the sense of 'coherence' and retaining individuality—even as a professional—results in an essential way from the agreement of content and communication.[293]

But the extent to which straining to be authentic offers a real solution is questionable. After all, can a person not also be 'authentically' emotionless towards a patient? Should the issue not be cultivating an emotional disposition that itself facilitates empathy? Another problem is how to ensure that more than just the technique part of empathetic discussion techniques remain preserved under the economic pressure of everyday clinical practice. The anecdote about the painful experience of Charlotte Link's sister that introduced the chapter is clearly not the end of the long, winding history of speaking and remaining silent, of fear and despair, of hope and empathy.

[290] *Kommunikation im medizinischen Alltag*, 43; Buckman, 'Breaking Bad News', 141.

[291] Goleman, *Emotional Intelligence*.

[292] Rita Gunther McGrath, 'Das Zeitalter der Empathie', *Harvard Business Manager*, 15 September 2014, http://www.harvardbusinessmanager.de/blogs/manager-brauchen-neuen-fuehrungsstil-a-987288.html; Arthur Ciaramicoli, *Der Empathie-Faktor* (Munich: dtv, 2001).

[293] Wolf Langewitz, 'Patientenzentrierte Kommunikation', in *Uexküll. Psychosomatische Medizin. Theoretische Modelle und klinische Praxis*, ed. Rolf H. Adler, Wolfgang Herzog, Peter Joraschky, Karl Köhle, Wolf Langewitz, Wolfgang Söllner, and Wolfgang Wesiack, 7th edn (Munich: Urban & Fischer, 2011), 338–47, 338.

5
Experiencing Cancer

> Considering how common illness is, how tremendous the spiritual change that it brings, how astonishing, when the lights of health go down, the undiscovered countries that are then disclosed, what wastes and deserts of the soul a slight attack of influenza brings to light... when we think of this and infinitely more, as we are so frequently forced to think of it, it becomes strange indeed that illness has not taken its place with love, battle, and jealousy among the prime themes of literature.[1]

> Can't they understand that I'll talk it all to pieces if I have to tell about it. Then it's gone, and when I try to remember what it really was like, I remember only my own story.[2]

Having cancer. Getting cancer. Being sick with cancer. Living with cancer. Dying of cancer. What should I call this chapter? Each expression implies different things, calls up different associations. Each would give the chapter its own tone. Should suffering be its focus, or should distanced, 'objective' perspectives? Can you live a (good) life with cancer? Does the decision between survival and death really determine a person's existence from the diagnosis on? And if so, is it unjustified pessimism or just realism to say that survival comes first, but that death is always the story's endpoint? Couldn't you also say that survival is the end of the story, a ray of hope at the end of the tunnel? But would this then imply that not surviving—dying—is defeat?

There is no satisfactory answer to these questions; no answer that doesn't judge; no answer that is not normative, even though every person confronting cancer should be free to decide what their own priorities are. Thus, I picked 'experiencing cancer'. Doesn't that sound a little banal though? We have lots of experiences, many ordinary, some intense. Some are difficult and leave traces that alter us permanently. For many people, the word 'experience' implies an element of free choice—perhaps a challenge, but at any rate an episode with a clearly defined end that allows us to learn from it and move on. None of this holds for the experience of cancer. Nobody chooses to have this experience, and only very few who go

[1] Virginia Woolf, 'On Being Ill', in *Selected Essays* (Oxford: Oxford University Press, 2008), 101–10.

[2] Tove Jansson, 'The Spring Tune', in *Tales from Moominvalley*, trans. Thomas Warburton (New York: Farrar, Straus and Giroux, 2010), 11.

through it can completely leave it behind and be done with it once and for all. However, the concept of experience also has a broader, more open-ended sense. It encompasses living and dying without prioritizing one over the other or opposing them to one another. It encompasses suffering, pain, and sadness as well as love and the joy of life. And it does so without necessarily prioritizing, valuing, or devaluing one or the other of the range of emotions felt by cancer patients and their loved ones. This is why the chapter is titled 'Experiencing Cancer'.

Still, if I was only interested in emphasizing the open-endedness of experience, I would have stuck to the advice of Snufkin from Tove Jansson's Moomin universe and would have not written the chapter at all. Because every narrative unavoidably organizes and interprets experiences—in short, gives them narrative form—so that the original experience disappears to a certain agree. But narratives are also a way to make the experience one's own, to give it meaning, or to make it more bearable.[3] Narratives involve tone and choices about which events to focus on and which to leave out. They are a way to communicate experiences and make them comprehensible for others and for oneself. Just as stories are shaped by narrative structures and strategies, the experiences that provide their content do not just magically appear. They are conditioned by factors that, to varying degrees, lie outside the control of cancer patients. How cancer was and is experienced is not simply a matter of how the patient chooses to approach it. It is determined by the therapies available at the time, the techniques and practices involved in applying them, the spaces of treatment, and the relations between people and things that, for their part, are shaped by therapeutic 'necessities' and the decisions of policymakers.

This chapter maps out how the spaces that shaped people's experiences of cancer changed over the course of the twentieth century. The analysis of spaces of experience shines light on how the emotions of cancer patients and their loved ones shifted over time, and in turn, on how these emotions mutually determined these broader conditions.[4] So while it does not disclose 'the undiscovered countries' of the experience of cancer, as Virginia Woolf wrote a century ago, it does uncover the structures that formed the basis of subjective inner experience, which, in its individuality, escapes the grasp of historiographical generalization.

The contexts in which cancer was experienced gained definition through the historical rise of the general concept of cancer. Beyond the various types of cancer,

[3] Arthur W. Frank, *At the Will of the Body: Reflections on Illness* (Boston: Houghton Mifflin, 1991); Arthur W. Frank, *The Wounded Storyteller: Body, Illness and Ethics*, 2nd edn (Chicago: University of Chicago Press, 2013); Arthur Kleinman, *The Illness Narratives: Suffering, Healing, and the Human Condition* (New York: Basic Books, 1988).

[4] The concept of 'spaces of experience' (*Erfahrungsraum*) was developed by Reinhart Koselleck. I use it to describe spaces together with the things and practices that constitute them. These complex spaces shaped the experience of patients who were treated inside of them. On Koselleck's concept, see Reinhart Koselleck, '"Erfahrungsraum" und "Erwartungshorizont"', in *Vergangene Zukunft. Zur Semantik geschichtlicher Zeiten* (Frankfurt am Main: Suhrkamp, 1989), 349–73.

the organs affected, the stages of illness, and genetic predispositions, the concept of cancer as such is based on the assumption that cancer is a self-contained, coherent phenomenon. However, it encompasses very different sicknesses: lung cancer and stomach cancer do not just cause distinct symptoms. They cause different types of pain, limit people in different ways, and create different encumbrances in everyday life and social relationships. As a consequence, each type of cancer can evoke different emotional responses. Treating breast cancer with a mastectomy or cervical cancer with radiotherapy are not simply medical decisions. They give rise to therapeutic situations distinct from one another in important ways. Gender differences do not necessarily affect how people experience cancer, but in some contexts, they play a significant role. How advanced a case of cancer is when diagnosed and what the doctor's prognosis is play a part in determining the emotional experience of cancer. Social and economic status can likewise exert a strong influence on how cancer is experienced. And one's geographical location might not only decide over the available treatments, but could also necessitate long trips that might make it impossible to be near family and friends while undergoing therapy.

Many historiographical studies do justice to these differences by telling the story of a specific form of cancer. This follows twentieth-century oncology's categorization of different types of cancer according to the organ affected. But it also lines up with how cancer patients self-identified, which was expressed in the self-help groups that started being organized in the 1950s, first in the United States and then in other Western countries. The wealth of historical studies on breast cancer underscore this point, as women with breast cancer established largescale self-help groups early on, groups that continue to exist today.[5] In recent years, historians have studied other forms of cancer, such as cervical cancer, leukaemia, and lung cancer.[6] Common to all of these studies is their focus on a particular, organ-specific form of cancer and on gender as the primary determinants of how cancer is experienced. As a consequence, they generally relegate other distinctions to secondary status or overlook them altogether. The only two exceptions have been analyses of how age and race have shaped patients' experience of cancer.[7]

This chapter in no way disputes that the location of cancer plays a decisive role in how cancer is experienced; of course, it is enormously important, especially with regard to the history of the body. However, the chapter reconstructs the

[5] See Barbara L. Ley, *From Pink to Green: Disease Prevention and the Environmental Breast Cancer Movement* (New Brunswick: Rutgers University Press, 2009); Klawitter, *The Biopolitics of Breast Cancer*; Lerner, *The Breast Cancer Wars*, 141–95; Ellen Leopold, *Breast Cancer, Women, and Their Doctors in the Twentieth Century* (Boston: Beacon Press, 1999), 153–214 and 223–40.

[6] Carsten Timmermann, *A History of Lung Cancer: The Recalcitrant Disease* (Basingstoke: Palgrave Macmillan, 2014); Löwy, *A Woman's Disease*; Gretchen Krueger, *Hope and Suffering: Children, Cancer, and the Paradox of Experimental Medicine* (Baltimore: Johns Hopkins University Press, 2008).

[7] Krueger, *Hope and Suffering*; Johnstone and Baines, *The Changing Faces of Childhood Cancer*; Keith Wailoo, *How Cancer Crossed the Color Line* (New York: Oxford University Press, 2011).

broader contexts that shaped the experience of cancer beyond specific organs, all while underscoring differences that often ran counter to or alongside what was often seen as the 'natural' categorization of cancers according to body part. Thus, the chapter's goal is to map the shifting historical contexts that to a large degree determined how cancer *as such* was experienced in the twentieth century, even if each different localization was not experienced in the exact same way. Examining the common features of how cancer has been historically experienced opens room for studying a range of other, non-organic factors that defined the experience of cancer, such as socioeconomic status and doctors' judgements about whether a case was curable or not.

Suppressed Fear, Hidden Disgust

Around 1880, when a person with a tumour went to the doctor, the doctor's diagnosis basically had two steps: is it cancer? If yes, can it be operated on? Whether a tumour was considered operable likewise depended on two factors. First, was it even possible to operate in the area where the tumour was located? Second, was the tumour small enough and isolated enough to be totally excised such that no cancerous cells would remain and the patient could still survive the surgery? If surgery was possible, then there was a chance the cancer could be cured.

The practice meant that doctors made an existential judgement very early in the patient's case. A cherry-sized breast tumour? Operable, so potentially curable. A lung tumour? Inoperable, since lung surgery was still in its fledgling years. Patients had to continue breathing on their own during the operation, and the lung could easily collapse the minute the ribcage was opened.[8] Thus, incurable.

This dichotomy of possible cure or inevitable death became slightly less drastic in the early twentieth century. The discovery of radiotherapy fostered new hopes for curing 'inoperable' cases. Radium and x-rays reshaped the conditions of experiencing cancer. Inoperable no longer necessarily meant incurable. The pain, disfigurement, and risk associated with surgery might no longer be the price of a chance at recovery. Could radiotherapy make tumours operable by shrinking them down? Could the chances of a cure be increased by a combination of 'rays and steel'? But there were economic, technological, and medical limits to radiotherapy. Thus, at first, radiotherapy opened a marginal third option between operation and incurability, which left open the big question: what to do with incurable cases?

[8] Timmermann, *A History of Lung Cancer*, 36–49.

Excised: Does Radical Removal Equal Cured?

Most people who suspected they might have cancer went to a general practitioner; women with female-specific symptoms went to a gynaecologist. The doctors listened to their descriptions, manually and aurally examined the affected areas, inspected excretions, or looked into the body's openings with the instruments available at the time. The speculum and, after 1925, the colposcope, enabled doctors to see the cervix. In the nineteenth century, the invention of the endoscope made it possible for doctors to visually examine the outside of the pharynx, stomach, and intestines.

Early detection campaigns at the beginning of the twentieth century repeatedly remonstrated that many patients came to the clinic after it was already too late—whether out of procrastination or because their doctor had hesitated too long to employ diagnostic instruments clearly disliked by patients. Statistics from some clinics evidence that this was not just a scare tactic. They reveal that cancers of the internal organs were often classified as inoperable at the very first diagnostic appointment. In 1903, for instance, a comparison of various clinics in the German Empire found that, in the best-case scenario, only half of all women who entered surgical or gynaecological clinics with cancers of the internal reproductive organs could be operated on.[9] The other half could not, either because the tumour was too large and had already spread into the abdomen, or because their general state of health was too poor to risk an operation. Over the next few decades, these numbers changed little.[10] For patients who entered the clinic with stomach cancer, the outlook was even grimmer. Between 1914 and 1930, 410 patients at the University of Berlin's surgical clinic—one of the most renowned in the German Empire—had been considered operable after undergoing endoscopic and x-ray examination. The published data does not betray how many patients were sent home as inoperable. All 410 patients were brought into the operating theatre, but only about a third of them actually underwent surgery on their tumours. After a look into the abdomen of the other roughly 260 patients, doctors classified them as inoperable. Surgeons saw more possibilities for operating on breast tumours. In the early 1930s, about 90 per cent of women with breast cancer who had come to the large oncological clinics were operated on. This number of 'operable cases' was markedly higher than was true even of patients with skin cancer, which can often be diagnosed by the naked eye.

While early detection campaigns never tired of insisting that the 'procrastination' and 'indolence' of patients and general practitioners were the reason why

[9] Gustav Klein, 'Die operative Behandlung des Gebärmutterkrebses', *Münchener Medizinische Wochenschrift* 50, no. 11 (1903): 472–4, 474.

[10] E. Philipp and P. Gornick, 'Die Behandlung des Gebärmutter- und Scheidenkrebses an der Universitäts-Frauenklinik Berlin (Geh.-Rat Bumm †)', *Münchener Medizinische Wochenschrift* 73, no. 7 (1926): 272–5, 272.

only about 50 per cent of cases of other types of cancer could be operated on, it was unclear if this was true. A study conducted in 1922 asked patients and doctors when they had first noted their symptoms and how much time had elapsed between their first doctor's visit and their referral to the cancer clinic. It showed that about half of all cancer patients entered the clinic no more than six months after they had first registered their symptoms, and some significantly earlier.[11] By any measure, this timespan did not seem extraordinarily long.

So, did patients only notice symptoms once they had become severe?[12] Statistics suggest another, more unsettling explanation. The tumours of those who quickly went to the doctor after noticing their symptoms were in no way always the smallest. As early as 1906, Ismar Boas, a gastroenterologist, shared some dumbfounding findings. Of the 116 cancer patients who had come to him no more than six months after their first symptoms appeared, he could only completely excise about 2 per cent of the tumours. In contrast, of the 127 cancer patients who had delayed their first doctor's visit more than six months after first suffering symptoms, he was able to successfully operate on 6 per cent. Boas might have been particularly struck by this discrepancy because of his specialization, which was uncommon at the time. His observations led him to the conclusion that early diagnosis did not necessarily imply positive prognosis; rather, he wrote that the specific malignity of the tumour was the essential prognostic factor. Hardly any renowned surgeons of the time were convinced. Instead, they surmised that the patients had probably forgotten when their first symptoms appeared or that the anamnesis had not been carefully conducted.[13]

Twenty years later, however, Boas's views began to be vindicated. Contributing to this was accurate follow-up documentation about how long patients remained healthy after their operation. This facilitated better assessments about the effectiveness and safety of different surgical methods and allowed clinicians to compare surgery and radiotherapy. One finding stuck out in particular: among those who came to the doctor within three months of their first symptoms were many patients with inoperable tumours.[14]

Even more confounding was the insight that among those patients with tumours seen as operable, the ones who survived the longest were those who only went to the doctor after they had symptoms for a considerable period of time.

[11] Arthur Hintze, 'Wider den Pessimismus in der Krebsbehandlung', *Münchener Medizinische Wochenschrift* 82, no. 6 (1935): 210–13, 211; Wilhelm Anschütz, 'Diagnose und Prognose bei der chirurgischen Behandlung des Magenkarzinoms', *Münchener Medizinische Wochenschrift* 72, no. 1 (1925): 1–4, 2; Theodor Köhler, 'Beitrag zur Operation des Mastdarmkrebses', *Münchener Medizinische Wochenschrift* 69, no. 20 (1922): 738–9.

[12] Hintze, 'Wider den Pessimismus', 211.

[13] Ismar Boas, 'Welche Aussichten bestehen für eine Frühdiagnose der Intestinalcarcinome', *Mitteilungen aus den Grenzgebieten der Medizin und Chirurgie* 15 (1906): 73–88; Anschütz, 'Diagnose und Prognose', 2.

[14] Anschütz, 'Diagnose und Prognose', 2.

Most surgeons believed this only allowed a single conclusion, one that Boas had anticipated in 1906: there were tumours that grew exceptionally fast, while others spread much slower. Doctors treating skin cancer had already realized this, distinguishing between slow-growing, late metastasizing basal-cell carcinomas and rapidly metastasizing squamous cell carcinomas. Surgeon Karl Friedrich Steinthal's classification, widely used after 1905, also differentiated between slow- and fast-growing breast tumours; however, he understood them as successive stages of one and the same type of cancer.[15]

Thus, when patients sought out the clinic at an early stage, it was often because their tumour grew rapidly and therefore caused graver pain. Surgeon Wilhelm Anschütz lamented that with some cases of cancer, doctors 'probably always come too late'.[16] The lay public did not hear much about these debates, which cast serious doubts on the early detection campaigns' supposedly indisputable message. Laypeople thus continued to be burdened with the belief that anyone whose tumour could not be operated on at the beginning of their illness were themselves responsible for being 'too late'.

Some types of cancer were in and of themselves more or less inoperable, because the affected organ was either too important, could not be bypassed through procedures like an intestinal stoma, or because the risk of surgery was so great that doctors were only willing to take it in exceptional cases.[17] Thus, well into the 1930s, surgeons remained powerless when they uncovered tumours of the oesophagus, bronchia, lungs, or bladder. In such cases, the only possibilities were to remove the tumour endoscopically through electrocoagulation—i.e., by destroying it with electricity—or to send the patient to the radiologist. Small brain tumours were indeed operated on, but patients or their loved ones often refused the procedure because of its known risk of complications and high mortality rate.[18]

All other types of cancer were considered theoretically operable. Because cancer was defined as an illness that began in individual cancer cells and only later spread out into the blood and lymph streams, doctors deemed it prudent to excise not only the visible tumour, but also some tissue surrounding it. This practice was intended to ensure that no isolated cancer cells invisible to the naked eye were left behind. Moreover, lymph nodes in the proximity of the tumour were also viewed as vulnerable. Clinicians debated whether they should always be removed or only

[15] Karl Steinthal, 'Zur Dauerheilung des Brustkrebses', *Bruns' Beiträge zur klinischen Chirurgie* 47 (1905): 226–39, 233–4.

[16] Anschütz, 'Diagnose und Prognose', 2.

[17] Arthur Hintze, 'Welche Faktoren bestimmen die Prognose des Karzinoms?', *Münchener Medizinische Wochenschrift* 82, no. 8 (1935): 283–6, 284.

[18] This is evidenced by a survey of patients' files from the neurology clinic of the University of Heidelberg's hospital between 1920 and 1939, UAH, preliminary signature: Acc. 30/01, new: L-V (Neuro).

when they were swollen. Some believed that nearby muscle, tendons, and fatty tissue should also be extirpated.

Described as 'radical' at the time, these techniques had been developed in the late nineteenth century. Among them was the so-called Wertheim operation. Named after Austrian gynaecologist Ernst Wertheim, it involved cutting open a female cancer patient's abdomen in order to be able to see her insides and, if necessary, to remove the connective and fatty tissue around the uterus as well as the lymph channels and nodes. In 1897, Zurich surgeon Carl Schlatter conducted the first gastrectomy, in which a man's cancer-ridden stomach was entirely removed and the oesophagus connected to the small intestine. The resulting ersatz stomach made it possible for the man to consume food.[19] In 1882, American doctor William Stewart Halsted invented a method of operating on breast cancer that entailed not only amputating the breast, but also the large breast muscle that extends to the upper arm; he later expanded the technique by removing the small breast muscle and the lymph nodes below the armpit.

In Germany, though, the 'radical' methods did not gain the kind of widespread application that they did in the United States. One reason was the establishment of radiotherapy in the German Empire—and in Europe as a whole—as a serious alternative to surgery.[20] Radiotherapy had two apparent advantages over surgery, and particularly its more invasive forms. It was, at least in the short-term, much less dangerous, as nobody died immediately after radiation treatment. In comparison, up into the 1940s, between 10 and 50 per cent of patients who underwent the more radical forms of surgery died either during or in the days after the operation. Second, radiation initially left few visible traces. Some tumours on the skin's surface even healed without scarring, while radical operations permanently marked the patient's body.

Against this background, surgeons had to prove that surgery would offer significantly better chances of survival over the long term, and they had to carefully assess which risks and potential disabilities caused by the operation were acceptable. Thus, early on, surgeons began gathering statistics on how long patients lived after a given type of surgery. They generally defined a patient to be 'cured' if they lived five years after the operation, because they had observed that after this period, only few people developed relapses at the site of the surgery or metastases in other parts of their body.

The notion that German surgeons' more conservative approach stemmed from them placing more value on the female breast seems doubtful, especially since mastectomies were usually part of even the milder surgical methods. Indeed, there is evidence that for German doctors, the potential increase of a patient's survival

[19] Carl Schlatter, 'Über Ernährung und Verdauung nach vollständiger Entfernung des Magens beim Menschen', *Bruns' Beiträge zur Klinischen Chirurgie* 19 (1897): 757–76.

[20] Lerner, *The Breast Cancer Wars*, 35.

chances outweighed any concerns about the loss of the breast. One example is a statement made by Arthur Hintze, director of the X-Ray and Radium Institute of the Surgical University Clinic of Berlin and, after 1935, deputy director of the Allgemeines Institut gegen die Geschwulstkrankheiten (General Institute against Tumorous Diseases). In a list of organs he considered operable because they could be dispensed with, Hintze wrote that there were some organs 'the loss of which brings not inconsiderable negative physical or psychological consequences (sex organs, rectum); with others, the loss really only has negative cosmetic consequences, such as the female breast'.[21] Hintze did not believe that living through a mastectomy could be difficult, because the scar could be covered over, whereas incontinence, impotence, or the inability to bear children could, he thought, lead to social exclusion or stigmatization.

But the publications of early detection campaigns almost never discussed operations' effects and potential complications. Similarly, they did not inform people about the choice between different types of surgery and radiotherapy—not to speak of saying anything about their chances of success, something that doctors themselves disagreed about. Rather, the images they used showed empty operating rooms; the controversial 1930 film *Krebs* was the first to depict a patient being operated on (Fig. 17). Pictures of cancer patients cured by surgery were lacking entirely, while before-and-after photos of skin cancer patients healed by radiotherapy were regularly printed (Fig. 18).

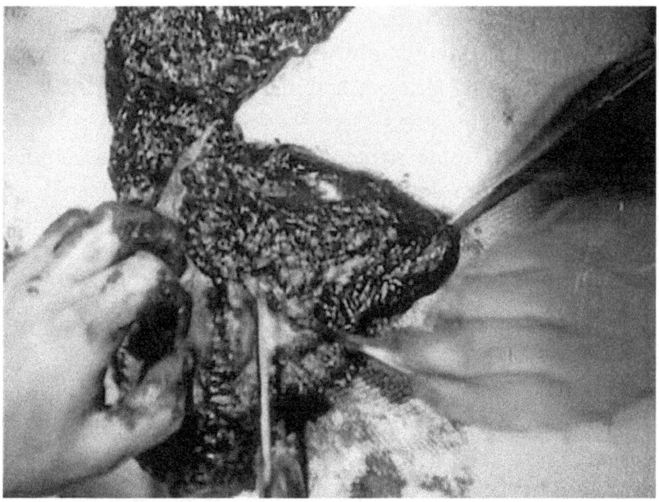

Fig. 17 Image of operation. Still from the film *Krebs* (*Cancer*, 1930).

[21] Hintze, 'Welche Faktoren', 284.

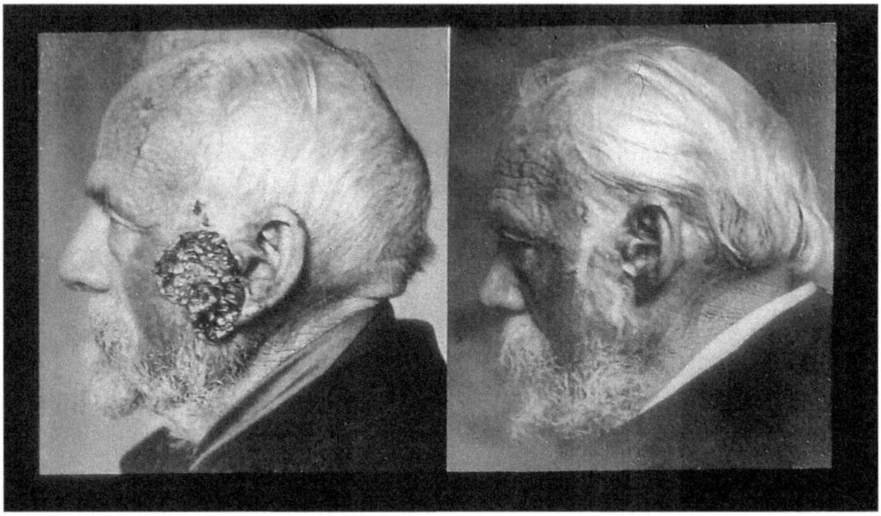

Fig. 18 Skin cancer patient before and after radiotherapy: Lichtbildreihe DHMD (1929).

However, there are indices that patients knew more than campaigns wanted to tell them. For instance, in 1922, Otto von Franqué, a gynaecologist and the president of the University of Bonn, told his colleagues:

> For the mental life and the feeling of health of some patients, it is indeed better when they have the certainty that the sick organ has been entirely removed: despite the statistics that show that radiotherapy alone has a similar or even higher cure rate, the remaining uterus will negatively affect the mental equilibrium of some patients more seriously and their fear of relapse will be greater.[22]

The passage implies that some patients knew that relapses could occur after treatment, even though this knowledge was not communicated by the early detection campaigns. The fact that many cancer patients chose to have their uterus removed instead of undergoing radiotherapy—which, at least on the surface, seemed less dangerous—suggests that they knew that the mortality rate of this type of surgery had sunk dramatically since the beginning of the 1920s. Nevertheless, such operations were anything but routine procedures at the time.

There are few first-hand accounts from the first half of the twentieth century that detail patients' thoughts and feelings upon entering the surgery department. However, it is possible to reconstruct the paths they travelled and the spaces, procedures, and therapeutic instruments that they encountered. For most

[22] Otto von Franqué, 'Wie soll man den Uteruskrebs behandeln?', *Münchener Medizinische Wochenschrift* 70, no. 21 (1923): 676–87, 677.

oncological operations, patients had to report to the clinic a few days beforehand. In line with their position in the field of medicine itself, the surgery clinics were often at the centre of hospital campuses. They were almost always multi-story buildings. In 1927, Munich-based surgeon Albert Krecke tried to put himself in his patients' shoes, writing:

> The long, often 100-meter or longer bare corridors evoke an oppressive feeling of barrenness. Upon entry, the visitor is received by the singular hospital air, which is a strange mixture of Lysol, iodoform, steam, and worse. Across from the entrance, large and small signs inform one that this is the way to the operating theatre. If even one patient is being carried in or out on a stretcher, then the new arrival is thoroughly filled with feelings of aversion.[23]

In this account, the surgical clinics' 'barracks-like' size and architecture were enough to intimidate. Everything that hinted at the coming operation amplified feelings of fear and anxiety: the smell of disinfectants, the signs, and the sight of patients prepped for operation or unconscious patients being carried out of the surgical theatre. Krecke wanted to counter this by keeping out of sight anything that might remind patients of the surgery they were about to undergo. He believed the lack of premonition would ensure they entered the surgical theatre in a calm state. One of his recommendations was not to place cancer patients together in the same room, and in particular not new patients with those who had already been operated on, because, he claimed, the latter would find 'satisfaction in representing to the new patient the discomforts and pains of operation in the worst possible light'.[24] The strategy would not have been difficult to carry out, since cancer patients were a small minority in surgical clinics, the majority being comprised of patients there for broken bones and other injuries, hernia, appendicitis, amputations, and benevolent tumours.

In Krecke's ideal clinic, neither doctors nor nurses were supposed to tell cancer patients what they were about to go through. Thus, like many of his colleagues, Krecke only informed his patients which organ was going to be operated on—not, however, how the operation would proceed and what kind of damage it might leave behind. Moreover, diagnostic instruments of the time did not always allow surgeons to know in advance exactly how extensive the planned operation would end up being. For instance, if the clinician suspected a woman had breast cancer, the surgeon would generally excise a tissue sample from the suspicious lump during the operation and have it analysed by a pathologist while the patient was still anesthetized. If the pathologist returned and said it was cancer, the surgeon

[23] Albert Krecke, 'Über die seelische Schädigung des chirurgischen Kranken', *Münchener Medizinische Wochenschrift* 74, no. 5 (1927): 197–201, 198–9.
[24] Ibid., 199.

immediately amputated the breast.[25] At smaller clinics that lacked the facilities for rapid histopathological analysis, doctors treating a potential breast cancer patient judged by sight during the operation whether they thought the tumour was malignant. For most cases of stomach, colon, cervical, and uterine cancer, too, x-rays often did not reveal enough to determine how and if the tumour should be operated on. Thus, not a small number of these operations began with a so-called test laparotomy, in which the abdomen was opened so that the doctors could take a diagnostic look at the state and size of the tumour. Only then did they decide how the operation should proceed. Even though surgeons often did not know exactly what the operation would involve before they started, the complications that it would have for the patient were, for the most part, predictable. But in order not to frighten patients, most doctors remained silent about them. Krecke wrote succinctly on this point:

> If it is foreseeable that an artificial rectum will have to be implanted after an operation on the rectum, one should not terrify the patient with this knowledge. The patient always imagines the situation to be much more terrible than it actually is; afterwards, everybody comes to terms with the fact.[26]

Krecke conveniently ignored that patients had little choice but to 'come to terms' after the fact, because in his medical doctor's mind, there was no alternative to a radical rectal operation if it promised even the slightest hope of recovery. This minimal chance of curing the patient and prolonging their life seemed to him categorically more desirable than life with a tumour and intact rectum, which would ultimately lead to a painful death.

But suppressing information about the potential side effects of an operation served not only to soothe patients' fears so that they would consent to surgery. It was also supposed to help them calmly shoulder the preparations for the operation.[27] Patients usually began staying at the clinic one or two days before surgery. If they were going in for a stomach or colon operation, bowel preps intended to empty out the digestive tract as much as possible were necessary. Before oral surgery, the teeth were thoroughly cleaned and teeth with cavities removed. On the day before the operation, patients only received liquid nourishment, had a thorough bath, and were shaven around the body part to be operated on.

An hour or two before the operation, patients were brought into the surgical theatre's waiting room, which was separated by gender in order not to encroach upon the dictates of decency. Immediate preparations for the operation were performed in a special space. The primary purpose was to allow the operating

[25] Heinrich Braun, 'Allgemeine Operationslehre', in *Chirurgische Operationslehre*, ed. August Bier, Heinrich Braun, and Hermann Kümmell, vol. 1 (Leipzig: Johann Ambrosius Barth, 1914), 1–150, 27.
[26] Krecke, 'Über die seelische Schädigung', 198.
[27] Braun, 'Allgemeine Operationslehre'.

room itself to be equipped with only the necessary instruments, thus limiting potential sources of contamination and making it easier to maintain aseptic standards. But it had the secondary purpose of keeping the patient from seeing little or nothing of the surgical theatre.[28] Some clinics dressed the patient with a special operating outfit that kept them warm while leaving open the site to be operated on.

The body part was disinfected with substances like soap spirit, iodobenzene, alcohol, or iodine tincture. Then doctors began general anaesthesia. If the patient was very nervous in the preparation space, then they would have been injected with a dose of morphine about an hour before the surgery began and thus would have been half asleep when they were rolled into the operating room.[29] But for small or weakened patients, this was rarely an option, since the morphine could lower their blood pressure and body temperature and thus make it difficult to control the anaesthesia. Excited persons could only be put to sleep with larger-than-normal quantities of aether or chloroform, which could lead to complications in the run of the operation. For these reasons, too, clinics did their utmost to calm patients' nerves before the operation.

The advent of asepsis (germ-free space) made it necessary to convert many operating theatres in the early twentieth century. While at the end of the nineteenth century, operations often still took place in amphitheatre-like spaces in front of students, after 1900, operations were almost always performed in separate operating rooms. Special, often smaller rooms were designed for the treatment of patients with inflammations or infections on the body part to be operated on in order to prevent new infections from endangering the success of the aseptic operation. The trend saw large operating rooms being reserved exclusively for aseptic operations, such as at the surgical clinic in the Moabit section of Berlin (Fig. 19).

Anaesthesia, in either liquid or gaseous form, was often administered through a mask that was placed over the patient's nose and mouth. The mask made most patients feel like they were suffocating; doctors generally tried to distract them from this discomfort by slowly counting.[30] Thus, while many patients were already unconscious before being brought into the operating room, some were still awake as they were placed on the operating table and strapped down before the anaesthesiologist began their work. These patients saw the operating room, which, after the turn of the century, was usually entirely tiled and had large windows and an overhead lamp to provide adequate lighting.[31]

If the patient was still awake, they saw the surgeon dressed in a cap, surgical mask, gown, and perhaps expensive, reusable rubber gloves, the wearing of which

[28] Krecke, 'Über die seelische Schädigung', 200.
[29] Braun, 'Allgemeine Operationslehre', 45.
[30] Krecke, 'Über die seelische Schädigung', 200; Braun, 'Allgemeine Operationslehre', 47.
[31] Braun, 'Allgemeine Operationslehre', 2–3.

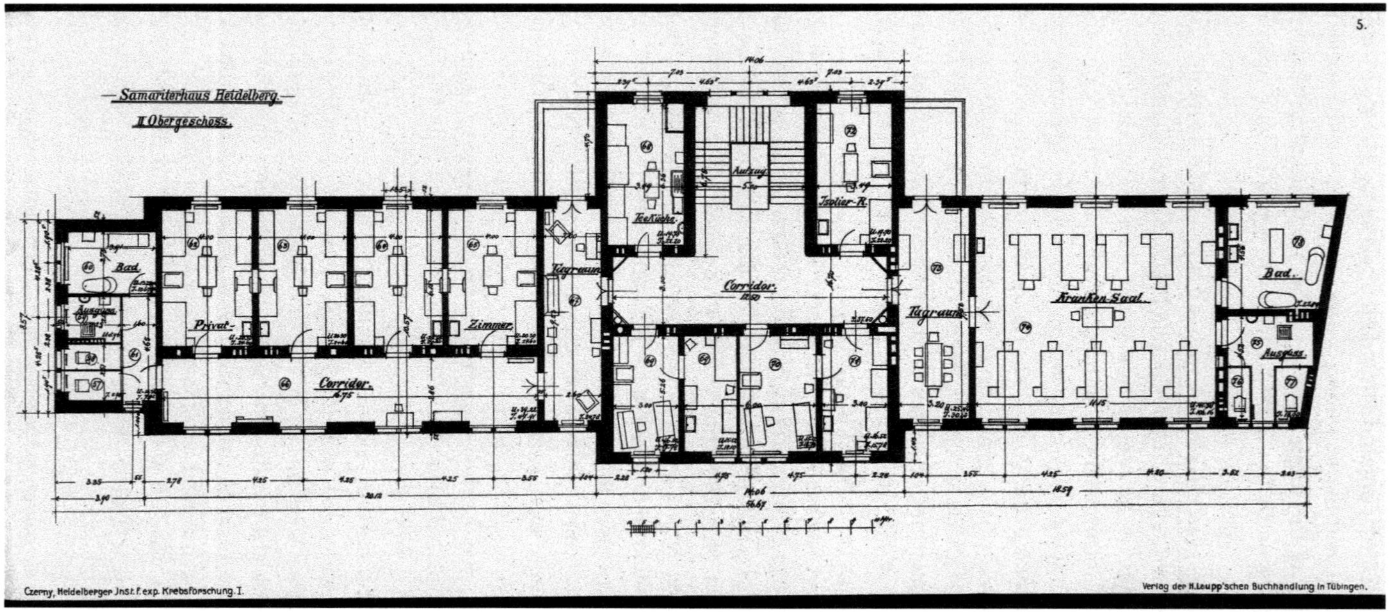

Fig. 19 Floor plan of a typical hospital ward at the Moabit Hospital (1896).

was still a matter of debate among doctors even after 1900.[32] At the latest, this was when general anaesthesia began. Surgery textbooks advised that the flow of anaesthesia be kept as low and steady as possible in order to avoid complications like respiratory issues, cardiac arrest, and vomiting—and to minimize the risk that the patient would begin to move around or come close to waking up.[33]

Once the operation was concluded, patients who were still asleep were brought back into the ward, as special rooms for waking up had not yet been implemented. If patients could not afford a first-class room for themselves, they awoke in a long, high-ceilinged ward with twenty or more beds. Most patients had to lie in bed for the first day after the operation and could not receive visitors. But after the second day, many could move some or even stand up. This represented a shift away from nineteenth-century best practices. By the beginning of the twentieth century, surgeons realized that leaving the sickbed early could facilitate recovery and reduce the risk of lung infections, ileus, and persistent vomiting.

Sepsis was another serious danger. In the nineteenth century, doctors immediately changed out the patient's bandages after the surgery and then regularly swapped them thereafter in order to identify infections before they could get out of hand. But with the advent of antisepsis, surgeons discovered that replacing wound dressing could itself be a source of infections; accordingly, they waited a while after surgery before changing the bandages and then did so less frequently. Surgical incisions on the belly or breast often had to be hooked up to a drain in order to push out discharge. Sometimes, particularly after extensive operations on breast cancer, the surgical wound was so large that it had to be patched up with a piece of skin taken from the thigh or buttocks. This procedure could not always be performed during the first operation and thus made a second one necessary. Patients often only discovered the extent of the 'damage' caused by the operation when their bandages were changed for the first time. While bandages were being changed, patients' beds were commonly blocked off from others' view with screens.[34]

When the patients saw their wounds, it was often the first time they realized what they had lost, because, as discussed above, they were usually told little about the operation and its risks before undergoing it. This was particularly an issue after operations on breast tumours, since the actual diagnosis of cancer was made during the operation itself. After the operation, the wound was covered with a thick layer of bandages, so that only during the first change of bandages did patients grasp that their breast had been amputated. A handful of women sued

[32] Thomas Schlich, 'Negotiating Technologies in Surgery: The Controversy about Surgical Gloves in the 1890s', *Bulletin of the History of Medicine* 87, no. 2 (2013): 170–97.

[33] Braun, 'Allgemeine Operationslehre', 48–9.

[34] Krecke, 'Über die seelische Schädigung', 201.

their doctors in the 1920s and 1930s because they refused to 'come to terms' with the shock of having had a mastectomy without their consent.[35]

Other patients only understood the operation's effects after they were released from the hospital. For instance, some who had a colorectal tumour removed had to live with an intestinal stoma. Depending on exactly where their tumour was and thus the section of colon or rectum removed, they might not be able to control bowel movements and flatulence. Incontinence could be somewhat managed by adhering to a strict diet and flushing with an enema once a day. In many surgeons' estimation, most patients were 'wholly satisfied' with this state of things, noting: 'Uncomfortable for them is just their inability to hold back flatulence, which has made socializing impossible for them.'[36] Doctors regretted such social exclusion, but viewed it as acceptable in the face of a lack of alternatives.

Gynaecologists reacted similarly to women who complained about the restriction or loss of their sex lives after their uterus was removed. Walter Stoeckel, a gynaecologist based in Berlin, wrote to his colleagues:

> The vulva has been reconstructed completely back to normal, but the vagina is without exception seriously shortened, so that cohabitation can no longer be carried out in a satisfying fashion. One tends to place little weight on this detriment in light of the usually advanced age of the patient and in consideration of the serious ailment to be combatted. But in practice, things are entirely different. First, many women are not yet old, but are between 30 and 40 years old, and are thus sexually active and often also have high standards. Thus, as laypersons, they are not attuned to the fact that their health was and is in such danger that no price is too high to retain it and no abstinence too great; eventually, marital life ends with brutality and inconsiderateness from the husband, who seeks sexual pleasure elsewhere. Whence it comes that women who have undergone radical operations—whom the surgeon must wish well and from whom he expects gratefulness—are terribly unhappy, curse the day of the operation, and live with thoughts of suicide.[37]

Two different lines of reasoning are discernible in Stoeckel's argument. On the one hand, there was the perspective of the doctor, which deemed any price worth paying to save the patient from certain death from cancer. Dying from cervical cancer could be especially painful and, because of the foul-smelling excretions that

[35] See, for example, 3rd Civil Law Panel, Decision from 1 March 1912, III. 231/11, 1.

[36] Köhler, 'Beitrag zur Operation des Mastdarmkrebses', 739.

[37] Walter Stoeckel, 'Die vaginale Radikaloperation des Collumkarzinoms', *Zentralblatt für Gynäkologie* 1 (1928): 39–63, 57.

could appear in later stages, especially awful.[38] On the other hand, there was the perspective of the patient, which Stoeckel seemed to view with confoundment. The patient might have had no notion of what dying from cervical cancer looked like, was not involved in deciding which surgical method would be used, was usually not informed about its potential consequences, and only 'discovered' these consequences after the operation.

For a doctor to assume or even acknowledge the patient's grief would have required them to relativize the assumptions of their profession and grapple with what the patient's 'quality of life' might be after surgery. At the time, few surgeons were concerned with such questions. Their confidence had been boosted by the medical advances of the nineteenth century and, in particular, the considerable expansion of surgical methods. They viewed themselves as medical experts and wanted to make full use of their knowledge and techniques. Meanwhile, non-surgical methods of treating the pain and other issues caused by cancer remained limited. In cases where a cure seemed out of reach, many doctors thought there was little they could do. But they were forced to address the question when a patient experienced relapse or metastases in the weeks, months, or years after undergoing surgery.

Surgeons knew from their meticulously gathered statistics that the majority of cancer patients would have relapses or metastases at some point after their operations. And they also knew that even these statistics painted an all too optimistic image of the chances of full recovery, because they themselves had removed from their datasets patients whose whereabouts were unknown, even though they assumed that most such patients had passed away.

In order to identify relapses and metastases early on, patients were scheduled for regular post-operation check-ups. They were told that new, initially benign tumours could develop in the area of their body that had been operated on. Opinions diverged on how often such check-ups should take place and when recovery should be considered definitive, thus making further check-ups superfluous. Some doctors had their patients come in once every four months during the first year after surgery, others once every two months over a period of two years. Most ended the exams at the latest after five years, which statistics suggested was a milestone representing full recovery. Only a few thought exams twice a year were necessary after that.[39]

[38] Richard Kurt Kepp, 'Die Behandlung unerträglicher, durch Genitalcarcinome hervorgerufener Schmerzen mit paravertebralen und präsacralen Alcoholinjektionen', *Archiv für Gynäkologie* 174, no. 3 (1942): 620–66, https://doi.org/10.1007/BF01961038.

[39] Transcription of a conversation between the general secretary of the Reichsauschuss Felix Grüneisen, Prof. Dr Schroeder, Kiel, ministerial director Dr Dammann, and ministerial advisor Dr Taute, Berlin, 12 May 1930, BArch R 1501/126321, 122–3; Arthur Hintze, 'Röntgen-Radium-Institut Berlin', in *Unsere Erfahrungen in der Krebsbekämpfung und unsere Erfolge in der Krebsbehandlung in 20-jähriger Tätigkeit*, 4. BArch R 1501/126319, 228.

Thus, long after it was completed, the operation continued to be an everyday part of patients' lives. The visible, tangible scars and disabilities were one part of this, while post-operation check-ups regularly confronted patients with the question as to whether and to what extent they would ever recover.

When relapses or metastases were found, the patient crossed an invisible barrier. They went from being a person whom the doctor hoped could be cured of cancer, to being an incurable patient whose treatment the doctor believed only served to prolong life and ameliorate pain and symptoms. Relapses and metastases were seldom operated on because medical knowledge of the time observed that new relapses usually appeared shortly after operating on one, sometimes even before the surgical incision had healed.

In a few cases, though, surgeons did operate on them. Sometimes, they just did it as one final attempt to restore 'the cruelly destroyed hope' of the patient who believed they had been cured by the first operation. For their part, surgeons had a tough time admitting that their patient no longer had a chance.[40] In general, though, treatment after the discovery of relapses was geared towards keeping symptoms in check. One occasion when a second operation was more common was when tumours blocked the stomach or intestines and thus complicated digestion or defecation; the section of stomach or intestine was then either removed or bypassed. Sometimes tumours caused pain because they put pressure on the surrounding tissue, and in these cases, too, surgeons sought to help by removing parts of the tumour. There was a third, yet less common case when doctors reached for the scalpel after operating on a cancer patient: when every attempt at pain management failed, they placed the patient under local anaesthesia and performed a cordotomy, which involved cutting through spinal nerves to reduce or even stop pain.[41] In 1912, neurologist Otfried Forster conducted the first cordotomy in Germany. But the procedure was risky. More than 10 per cent of patients died a few days afterwards, and the nerves responsible for movement were often severed, thus temporarily or permanently paralyzing the patient's legs.[42] For these reasons, cordotomies were only an option for bedridden cancer patients who were considered incurable.

But surgeons viewed their true mission as curing patients. Moreover, after the advent of various disinfection techniques, instruments, and substances, their expenses had ballooned, placing them under economic distress. Thus, most surgeons refused long-term treatment of relapsed cancer patients.[43]

[40] Walter Stoeckel, *Lehrbuch der Gynäkologie*, 2nd edn (Leipzig: Hirzel, 1928), 421.

[41] Wilfried Witte, 'Schmerz in Deutschland. Die Geschichte der Schmerztherapie in Deutschland im 20. Jahrhundert unter besonderer Berücksichtigung der Zeit von 1945 bis 1990' (habilitation diss., Charité Berlin, 2014), 71–3.

[42] Demetrius Philippides, 'Über die Chordotomie bei Karzinomkranken', *Monatsschrift für Krebsbekämpfung* 12 (1944): 66–70, 69; Otfried Foerster, *Der Schmerz und seine operative Bekämpfung* (Halle: Buchdruckerei des Waisenhauses, 1935).

[43] Vinzenz Czerny, 'Aus meinem Leben, herausgegeben und mit Anmerkungen versehen von Wilfried Willer', *Ruperto Carola* 11, no. 14 (1967): 3–25, 21.

Radiotherapy, though, seemed to offer a small chance of recovery for patients with relapses and was at least able to temporarily stop the tumour's growth. This alternative form of treatment made it easier for surgeons to turn patients away, because it signalled to both patient and doctor that there was still hope.[44]

Radiotherapy: Hope for Inoperable Patients

Maintaining hope was of great importance for doctors, a point evidenced by the 1913 annual conference of the Deutsche Gesellschaft für Gynäkologie (German Gynaecological Association) in Halle. The year's main topic was the influence of heart and kidney conditions on pregnancy, birth, and the postnatal period.[45] Unexpectedly, however, a completely different topic captured everybody's attention: research on radiotherapy for cervical and uterine cancer, which was presented by Alfred Döderlein, director of the University of Munich's women's clinic, and Bernhard Krönig and Carl Joseph Gauß, both from Freiburg's women's clinic. Years later, professor of gynaecology Walter Stoeckel described the scene:

> Still today, I can remember the excitement in the room as the representatives of Freiburg's women's clinic concluded their presentation after reporting on initial successes. Everyone discussed wildly. A very well-known surgeon jumped up, red in the face, and shouted with pathos: 'Yesterday was the last day I pick up a knife! Never again will I take it in my hands!' Dignified men embraced. A lecturer who sat behind me declared in celebration: 'The danger of cancer is banished, humanity can breathe!' Never before, it seemed, had a method been available that had such a strong capacity to destroy cancerous cells.[46]

The doctors' delirium over radiotherapy only makes sense in historical context.[47] Cervical cancer was one of the most common forms of cancer at the time. It afflicted many young women and mothers, and it often led to a particularly painful death. Hysterectomies, which were extremely risky, were the only known treatment for it. But now, it seemed as if it could be cured without danger. Even more, the 'death sentence' of being inoperable was put out of force, as Döderlein's assistant Ernst von Seuffert wrote in 1914.[48]

[44] Arthur Hintze, 'Die Prognose des Karzinoms nach den Erfahrungen der Bierschen Klinik', *Münchener Medizinische Wochenschrift* 82, no. 5 (1935): 163–6, 166.

[45] L. Fraenkel, 'Zum Hauptthema des XV. Kongresses der Deutschen Gesellschaft für Gynäkologie', *Monatsschrift für Geburtshülfe und Gynäkologie* 37, no. 5 (1913): 663–7, https://doi.org/10.1159/000290821.

[46] Walter Stoeckel, *Erinnerungen eines Frauenarztes*, 2nd edn (Leipzig: Hirzel, 1980), 86.

[47] Ibid., 114.

[48] Ernst von Seuffert, 'Heutiger Stand, Probleme und Grenzen der Strahlenbehandlung des Krebses', *Strahlentherapie* 4 (1914): 740–84, 741.

Fascination with new therapeutic technologies reached a new level, because before this event, doctors had almost only had success irradiating surface tumours. In contrast, deeper tumours could not be irradiated without causing severe burns, because the radiation came from the outside and thus had to penetrate the skin and healthy tissue, which harmed them while at the same time diminishing the radiation's strength before it reached the tumour inside the body. That this was potentially fatal was evidenced by isolated experiments on irradiating uterine, stomach, and colorectal cancer conducted in Germany, France, Great Britain, Sweden, and the United States.[49]

The primary difficulty was to determine a dosage of radiation that would both eliminate the tumour while causing minimal damage to healthy tissue. But knowledge about the relation between radiation intensity and its biological effects was murky, thus making it difficult to precisely measure the necessary dose. Technology to set how much radiation hit the tumour had also not yet been developed. In the era before dosimeters, doctors simply irradiated until they could see the desired effect or until the skin reddened, which meant that the patient had already suffered burns. Though in some cases the burns quickly healed, in others, they had potentially fatal long-term effects. Additionally, the first x-ray machines were not able to continuously produce radiation of consistent quality and quantity, so that the radiation intensity regularly fluctuated during sessions.[50]

During the first decade of the twentieth century, medical doctors, physicists, and electrical engineers throughout Western Europe and North America worked on a solution to this issue. Their labour resulted in the invention of various types of dosimeters, new units of measurement for dosages, and different models for gas-free x-ray tubes, which would make it possible to better control the radiation.[51] Despite this progress, the question of how to irradiate tumours deep inside the body with adequate intensity but without damaging the skin remained a problem. Krönig and Gauß seemed to have solved it. And it was this proposed solution that they presented to the gynaecologists from the German Empire, Austria, Great Britain, and Sweden at the conference in Halle in 1913.

First, they developed an aluminium filter that concentrated the rays while at the same time protecting nearby skin from errant radiation. Second, they created a novel system of irradiation that protected the skin by targeting multiple overlapping fields

[49] Cantor, 'Cancer', 553.

[50] Wolfgang Frobenius, '"Gestern habe ich zum letzten Mal ein Messer angefasst!" Die Strahlentherapie auf den BGGF-Tagungen von 1912 bis 1939', in *Herausforderungen. 100 Jahre Bayerische Gesellschaft für Geburtshilfe und Frauenheilkunde*, ed. Christoph Anthuber, Matthias W. Beckmann, Johannes Dietl, Fritz Dross, and Wolfgang Frobenius (Stuttgart: Thieme, 2012), 60–86, 63–5; Caroline Claire Scanlan Murphy, 'A History of Radiotherapy to 1950: Cancer and Radiotherapy in Britain 1850–1950' (PhD diss., University of Manchester, 1986), chs 4.4–4.5.

[51] Simone Gleßmer-Junike, 'X-Strahlen, Radiometer und Hauteinheitsdosis. Die Entwicklung der Messverfahren und Maßeinheiten für Röntgenstrahlung in der medizinischen Physik von den Anfängen bis zur internationalen Standardisierung' (PhD diss., Universität Hamburg, 2015).

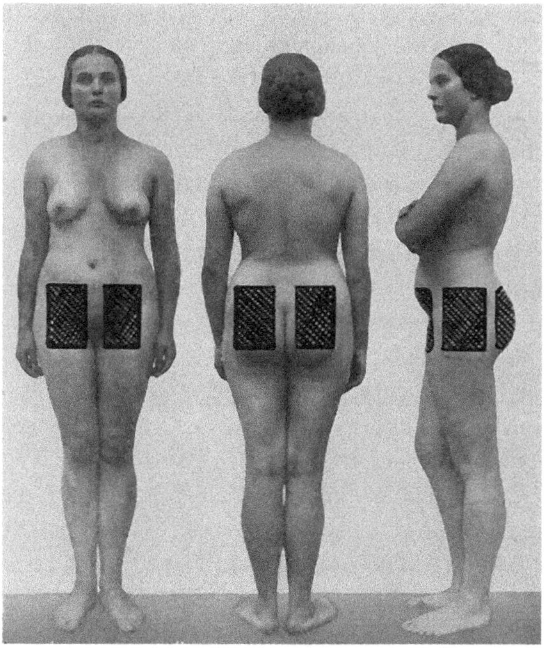

Fig. 20 Technique of overlapping irradiation, University of Berlin women's clinic (1928).

on the body so that the overlapping points received more radiation than the surrounding skin. This technique was improved after the First World War by sending the radiation from various positions, as the illustration of the method used at the University of Berlin's women's clinic in Figure 20 shows.[52]

Radiologists also invented a technique for irradiating tumours in the abdominal area at close range, either by placing the radioactive substance into capsules and implanting the capsules into the area near the tumour or by running radioactive gases or salts through needle-like catheters. Small lead plates fixed with a resinous compound were used to protect healthy tissue. These new technologies and improved machines made radiotherapy—with x-rays, radium, or mesothorium—into a standard component of cancer treatment in the 1920s and thereafter.

However, many surgeons stopped greeting radiotherapy with the same enthusiasm they had shown in 1913. Radiology began establishing itself as its own field of medicine, which raised the question: would surgeons, gynaecologists, and other specialists continue to be the standard bearers of cancer treatment, or would radiologists, with their expert knowledge and expensive equipment, assume the lead role and bring all aspects of treatment together at centralized institutes? This

[52] C. J. Gauß, ed., *Lehrbuch der Strahlentherapie*, vol. 4, parts 1 and 2: *Die Strahlentherapie in der Gynäkologie* (Berlin: Urban & Schwarzenberg, 1929), 261–70.

competition between disciplines, which was just as much about power and influence as it was about the benefits of each form of treatment, played out in many European countries and in the United States. It reappeared in Germany regularly all the way into the 1950s, because the established medical disciplines and their respective trade groups, which were dominated by surgeons, hindered efforts at widescale centralization of the type that had succeeded, for instance, in Sweden with the founding of the Stockholm Radiumhemmet.[53]

But the radiology departments established in Germany in the 1920s and 1930s were separated from their respective hospital's surgery department, both spatially and, to a certain extent, organizationally. For instance, the surgical clinic at the University of Berlin had already set up its own X-Ray and Radium Institute in 1910, which gained more independence in the Weimar Republic. While officially headed by August Bier, the director of the surgical clinic, its everyday affairs were for all practical purposes run by Arthur Hintze after 1927. In 1926, Hans Holfelder took the reins at a radiology institute that belonged to the University of Frankfurt's surgical clinic.[54] Thus, there were, if informally, some efforts at centralization, because only the radiotherapy departments at large clinics possessed the powerful machinery and adequate quantities of radium and mesothorium necessary to be able to effectively irradiate carcinomas and sarcomas.[55]

The main reason for this were the enormously high prices of radioactive substances. Radium is extracted from uranium ore. At the time of its discovery, it was a rare element. The only known source of radium before 1900 was in the Bohemian town of Jáchymov, then a part of Austria-Hungary. After scientists realized that it could be used in radiotherapy, the price on the world market increased exponentially.[56] In 1911, another source was discovered in Colorado, bringing the price down a bit. More enduring downward pressure on the price occurred in 1922 after abundant sources of uranium were found in what was then the Belgian colony of Congo.[57] But Germany had no radium stores in its own territory, forcing its clinics to purchase the element on the international market. For this reason, German radiologists often employed mesothorium, a less stable radioactive substance discovered by

[53] Ton van Helvoort, 'Scalpel or Rays? Radiotherapy and the Struggle for the Cancer Patient in Pre-Second World War Germany', *Medical History* 45, no. 1 (2001): 33–60.

[54] On Holfelder's work during the Nazi period, see Katja Weiske, 'Hans Holfelder—Radiologe in Frankfurt, Nationalsozialist, Gründer des SS-Röntgensturmbanns', in *Mengele, Hirt, Holfelder, Berner, von Verschuer, Kranz: Frankfurter Universitätsmediziner der NS-Zeit*, ed. Udo Benzenhöfer (Münster: Klemm & Oelschläger, 2010), 43–60.

[55] Letter from Dr Frik of the X-Ray Institute to the Board of the Moabit Hospital, Berlin, 17 August 1928, LAB A Rep. 003-04-03, no. 143, 63–9.

[56] Helvoort, 'Scalpel or Rays?', 40; A. Döderlein, 'Röntgenstrahlen und Mesothorium in der gynäkologischen Therapie, insbesondere auch bei Uteruskarzinom', *Monatsschrift für Geburtshülfe und Gynäkologie* 37, no. 5 (1913): 553–93, 579, https://doi.org/10.1159/000290814.

[57] Rainer Kalsch and Zbynek Zeman, *Urangeheimnisse. Das Erzgebirge im Brennpunkt der Weltpolitik 1933–1960* (Berlin: Ch. Links, 2013), 51–69; Rudolf Th. von Jaschke, 'Allgemeine gynäkologische Therapie', in Rudolf Th. von Jaschke and Otto Pankow, *Lehrbuch der Gynäkologie*, 5th edn (Berlin: Springer, 1933), 171–237, 230.

Otto Hahn in 1907. Mesothorium was a by-product of incandescent gas mantle production and was obtained from Brazilian monazite sands. In contrast to radium, mesothorium's short half-life meant its therapeutic efficacy diminished after about two years, necessitating that it be regularly replaced.[58] And the production of mesothorium was by no means cheap, either. In 1913, one milligram of mesothorium cost between 160 and 200 marks.[59]

On the one hand a matter of economics and on the other a matter of occupational politics, this complex situation had two immediate consequences for patients. First, in order to receive effective radiotherapy, patients had to go to a large clinic. For many, this required long-distance travel and a lengthy stay in an unfamiliar city if they received outpatient treatment. Moreover, they had to find a way to pay for the expensive treatment.

Ferdinand Blumenthal, director of the Institute for Cancer Research at Berlin's Charité hospital, calculated the average costs for radiotherapy in 1921/2 in a report to the hospital's leadership:

> Consider that a sick person who visits the cancer institute and who generally can only do so with an accompanying healthy person needs about 60 marks each way for travel expenses. This makes it difficult for patients of lesser means who do not have statutory health insurance to be treated here. Let us assume that they need to undergo six sessions of radiotherapy. The travel costs alone would then be 480 marks. At the rate paid by health insurance, the six sessions would cost about 2,000 marks.[60]

Blumenthal was drawing attention to the fact that radiotherapy was inaccessible for many. This healthcare gap became larger after the end of the First World War, as incomes in Germany sank, inflation took hold, and many people suffered from asset loss in the wake of the war. Statutory health insurance only covered the costs of medical consultation and hospital treatment.[61] As a rule, they did not pay for travel and accommodation for outpatient treatment, which represented an insurmountable financial barrier for many, especially because the sick pay distributed by the insurers only amounted to half of the recipient's normal income.[62]

[58] Jaschke, 'Allgemeine gynäkologische Therapie', 230.

[59] Helvoort, 'Scalpel or Rays?', 41.

[60] It is unclear whether Blumenthal falsely calculated ($6 \times 60 = 360$) or if he actually meant eight sessions or eighty marks for the one-way trip. See Ferdinand Blumenthal, Report on the Institute for Cancer Research, Berlin, 27 October 1922, 129, HU Archiv Charité-Direktion, 951, 124 and 126–30.

[61] Wolfgang J. Mommsen, 'Sozialpolitik im Deutschen Reich', in *Geschichte der Gesundheitspolitik in Deutschland*, ed. Wolfgang Woelk and Jörg Vögele (Berlin: Duncker & Humblot, 2002), 51–66; Franz Knieps and Hartmut Reiners, *Gesundheitsreformen in Deutschland. Geschichte—Intentionen—Kontroversen* (Bern: Huber, 2015), 51–70.

[62] In 1925, workers' average actual wages were eighty-one marks per week. In Berlin in 1924, office workers earned on average between 161 and 301 marks per week depending on their industry. See Dietmar Petzina, Werner Abelshauser, and Anselm Faust, *Sozialgeschichtliches Arbeitsbuch*, Vol. 3: *Materialien zur Statistik des Deutschen Reiches 1914–1945* (Munich: Beck, 1978), 98 and 100.

Moreover, only 30 per cent of the population were members of the statutory insurers at the time, which meant that many received neither coverage for healthcare nor sick pay.[63] Only in 1930 did legislators make membership for an insured person's family members a standard service of statutory health insurance.[64]

And not all workers and employees were eligible for statutory insurance. Thus, they either had to pay for everything out of pocket or had to purchase private insurance.[65] Not covered by statutory insurance were the self-employed, lawyers, architects, doctors, businesspeople, and civil servants. Before the First World War, people in these groups were often able to pay the costs of hospital treatment themselves and thus did not purchase private health insurance. After 1918, many businesspeople could still afford radiotherapy by themselves, but this did not hold for the majority of the self-employed and civil servants. Thus, after 1923, many entered into private insurance plans, but not all could afford the premiums. Moreover, some private insurers required co-pays, which often made radiotherapy a serious financial burden for middle-class patients. Blumenthal observed that in such cases, many patients' families opted against radiotherapy 'if we cannot promise [them] with great probability to cure the patient or significantly improve their health'.[66]

But those with statutory insurance could incur financial difficulties, too, because the insurer could refuse to pay for parts of treatment or cancel their coverage. Beginning in 1903, the public health insurance corporations had been required to pay for twenty-six weeks of treatment along with sick pay. But radiotherapy, which usually necessitated multiple sessions, could last longer than that. Additionally, it was common for workers with cancer to take sick leave for a year. Many had a hard time finding new employment afterwards, especially since their ability to work was not seldom limited as a consequence of treatment. These patients were 'pushed out' of the health insurance system just like those who doctors predicted from the very beginning would no longer be able to work. For all of these people, even the 'secondary costs' of radiotherapy were unaffordable, not to speak of the treatment itself, because people who would not be able to return to work were no longer covered by statutory insurance. Only one path to accessing radiotherapy remained open for such patients: if they were lucky, they could be placed in one of the limited number of cost-free beds. But

[63] Petzina, Abelshauser, and Faust, *Sozialgeschichtliches Arbeitsbuch*, 28 and 156.

[64] Claus Wendt, *Krankenversicherung oder Gesundheitsversorgung? Gesundheitssysteme im Vergleich*, 3rd edn (Wiesbaden: Springer VS, 2013), 92.

[65] Petra Baier, *Der Basistarif der privaten Krankenversicherung* (Karlsruhe: Verlag Versicherungswirtschaft, 2012), 42–9; Margarete Wagner-Braun, *Zur Bedeutung berufsständischer Krankenkassen innerhalb der privaten Krankenversicherung in Deutschland bis zum Zweiten Weltkrieg* (Stuttgart: Franz Steiner Verlag, 2002), 151–93.

[66] Ferdinand Blumenthal, Report on the Institute for Cancer Research, Berlin, 27 October 1922, 129, HU Archiv Charité-Direktion, 951, 124 + 126–30.

conditions applied there, too, because clinics preferred to give them to patients whose cases were of interest for their research.[67]

When the first radiotherapy departments were established in the early twentieth century, it was impossible to foresee how rapidly technology would develop. Thus, they were often more or less provisionally 'annexed' to hospitals. But the space afforded them soon proved too small. In the 1920s and 1930s, new radiotherapy institutes were constructed—or at least planned, since actual construction plummeted during the Second World War—to do justice to the increased application and importance of radiotherapy for cancer treatment.

A paradigmatic example of the new radiology departments was the Werner-Siemens-Institut für Röntgenforschung am Krankenhaus Moabit/Berlin (Werner Siemens Institute for Radiological Research at the Moabit Hospital, Berlin). It was set up in 1924 through a contract between the city of Berlin and Siemens & Halske, an electrical engineering firm that was part of the Siemens industrial conglomerate. This made its technological infrastructure superior to many of its peers: the contract stipulated that Siemens & Halske would supply all equipment free of charge in exchange for access to data about the clinical use of their products there.[68]

The Werner Siemens Institute was housed in wards 17, 18, and 19 at the Moabit Hospital. The three buildings were connected by passages that enabled doctors and nurses to walk from the diagnostics section to the treatment section to the administrative section without ever having to go outside.[69] The institute did not have a main entrance for patients. Outpatients entered through the door of the diagnostics building, situated at the north of the complex, and waited in a small room together with patients who had been sent there for x-ray exams. The waiting room had a single window and wooden benches lining two sides. Because of the limited space, there was no separate waiting room for bedridden patients. They were brought to the treatment building either from the radiology department's own wards or from other parts of the hospital; they entered through doors in the passages between the three buildings. There was no real separation between

[67] Letter of the administrative director of the Charité to the Reichsminister of Science, Education, and National Culture, Berlin, 11 January 1939, BArch R 4901/1341, 1.

[68] Similar collaborations had happened between the women's clinics of the university hospitals in Munich and Freiburg and the company Reiniger, Gebbert & Schall, which later merged with Siemens to form Siemens-Reiniger. See Wolfgang Frobenius, *Röntgenstrahlen statt Skalpell* (Erlangen: Universitätsbund Erlangen-Nürnberg, 2003), 103–4; Carl Stein, 'Das Werner-Siemens-Institut für Röntgenforschung', *Polytechnisches Journal* 339 (1924): 243–5; Thomas Meier and Volker Taenzer, 'Das Werner-Siemens-Institut für Röntgenforschung im Krankenhaus in Moabit', in *125 Jahre Krankenhaus Moabit 1872–1997*, ed. Städtisches Krankenhaus Moabit (Berlin: Weidler, 1997), 119–22.

[69] Stein, 'Das Werner-Siemens-Institut für Röntgenforschung'; Letter from Dr Karl Frik to the board of the Moabit Hospital, Berlin, 27 March 1934, LAB A Rep. 003-04-03, no. 158, 1; Letter from Dr Frik to the Tiergarten district administration, Berlin, 25 January 1936, LAB A Rep. 003-04-03, no. 159, 29–31.

patients undergoing diagnosis and those undergoing treatment. The stretchers carrying patients there for an exam were placed in the hallway of the diagnostics building, while those of the patients there for treatment were placed in the somewhat wider, draughty, unheated connecting passage. One half of this connecting passage was reserved for men, the other for women, with each half providing easier access to the respective bathroom. This situation was not uncommon at the time, but in 1935/6, it sufficiently irked the institute's director, Karl Frik, that he sent a complaint to the Tiergarten district administration stating that these conditions for 'the sick ... can no longer be tolerated'. His note that many foreign researchers who visited the institute also found it reprehensible assisted in the complaint's success. Blueprints for a new building were drawn up, which was supposed to be completed in time for the scheduled (but ultimately never convened because of the war) 1940 International Radiology Conference in Berlin.[70]

But the institute's halls and small waiting room were a sad place in another respect. Patients with operable tumours who came for radiotherapy before or after their surgery saw here, perhaps for the first time, patients who were suffering from relapses and metastases despite having already undergone operations, and patients whose cancer was so advanced that radiotherapy was merely palliative. These patients were weak, pale, and suffering severe pain. Some had visible tumours. Some had ulcerating cancer wounds that emitted a penetrating, noxious smell. Thus, people who had just been diagnosed with cancer saw in these hallways and waiting rooms the most damning manifestation of the loss of hope for a cure. And even though not all patients at the radiology clinic had cancer, there were more cancer patients gathered in this relatively small space than at any other hospital station. This experience likely shook the healthier patients' willingness to buy into the (self)-deceptive narrative of hope.

Radiotherapy treatment took place in the middle building, the hallway of which did not contain any stretchers. Probably the first thing that struck patients entering the building was the singular odour. The most common technique for producing radioactive beams—including that used by one of the three x-ray machines at the Moabit clinic—emitted ozone and nitrous oxide. Alongside their unpleasant smell, exposure to these gases over a longer period could irritate the nose and throat and cause other respiratory problems.[71] The rooms themselves were austerely furnished. In the middle of the room were the patient's cots; above them hung the x-ray machines, which drew power from a high-voltage transformer in the basement. One of the radiotherapy rooms contained a moveable tube that allowed radiation to be directly aimed at a specific body part

[70] Statement on the Reduced Need for Space in the Proposed New Building of the X-Ray Institute (appended to the application from 25 January 1936), composed by Frik, LAB A Rep. 003-04-03, no. 158.

[71] F. Dessauer and M. Brenzinger, 'Röntgenapparate und Röntgenröhren', in *Die wissenschaftlichen Grundlagen der Strahlentherapie*, ed. Hans Meyer (Berlin: Urban & Schwarzenberg, 1925), 361–434.

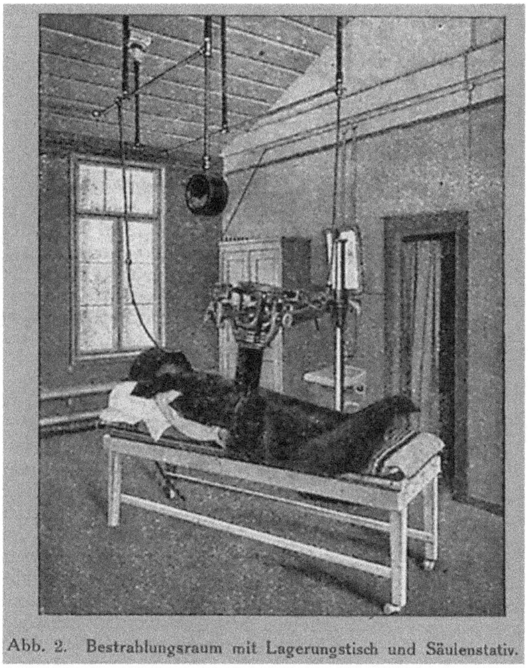

Fig. 21 Treatment room of the Werner Siemens Institute for Radiological Research (Berlin), 1924.

(Fig. 21). Because the tube emitted errant radiation, patients wore lead coverings for the entirety of the radiotherapy session that only left the target open. To protect patients' heads, some clinics used a lead helmet with a 'window made of lead glass; because anxious patients become much calmer when they can see the tube during the procedure'.[72] The radiological assistants who operated the machines either stood behind a sort of screen or worked in a separate control room with a window, enabling them to intervene if the patient moved during the treatment, which could last between thirty to sixty minutes.[73]

A second treatment room contained an immobile x-ray machine enclosed in sheet lead. It only emitted beams through an aperture. This allowed the radiology assistant to stand next to the patient, who did not need to be covered with a lead vest and could thus breathe and see better (Fig. 22). This more modern machine likely reduced 'the mysterious impression of a darkroom' and was therefore less likely to make the patient feel 'uncanny', as Heinrich Cramer wrote in 1935 about

[72] Alexander Lorey, 'Der Röntgenstrahlenschutz', in Meyer *Die wissenschaftlichen Grundlagen der Strahlentherapie*, 1101–22, 1103–4.

[73] 'Die Eröffnung des Werner-Siemens-Instituts für Röntgenforschung im Städtischen Krankenhaus Moabit, Berlin', *Klinische Wochenschrift* 3, no. 19 (1924): 863.

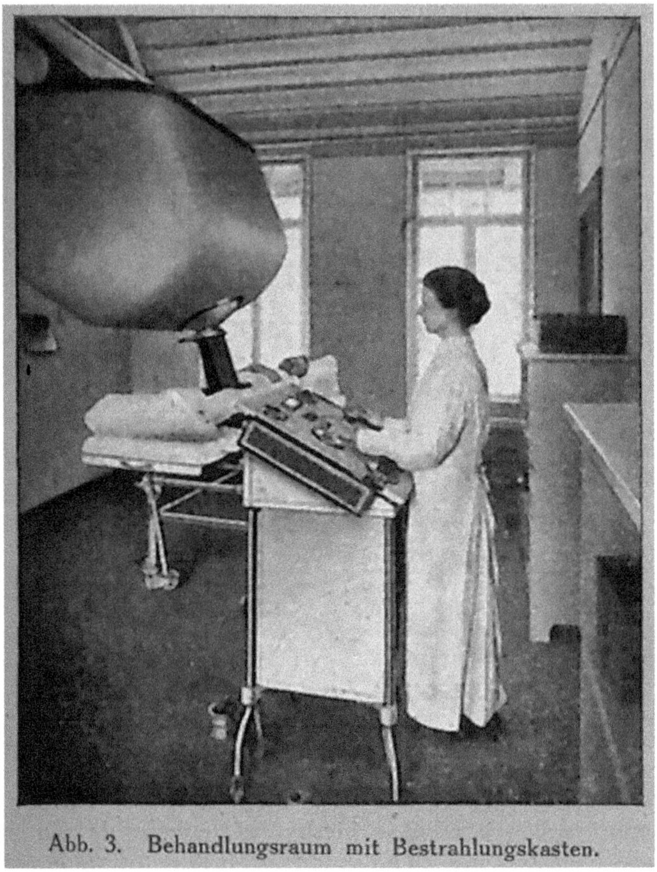

Fig. 22 Treatment room of the Werner Siemens Institute for Radiological Research (Berlin), 1924.

the radiotherapy institutes of the past in order to underscore the advantages of the new radiotherapy clinic that he was planning.[74]

After undergoing radiation therapy, outpatients had to remain at the clinic for a few hours and were then allowed to go home. Bedridden patients were carried into the gender-separated wards of the Werner Siemens Institute, which each contained nineteen beds. A total of fifteen beds were reserved for cancer patients.[75] The procedure was repeated for a few successive days until the (first) series of radiotherapy treatments was concluded.[76] The institute's lack of space forced its

[74] Heinrich Cramer, 'Das neue Röntgeninstitut im Rudolf-Virchow-Krankenhaus, Berlin', *Zeitschrift für das gesamte Krankenhauswesen* 31, no. 10 (1935): 221–6, 221.

[75] Bruno Harms, 'Sechzig Jahre Krankenhaus Moabit: Entwicklungsgeschichte des ersten Berliner städtischen Krankenhauses', *Zeitschrift für das gesamte Krankenhauswesen* 28 (1932): 197–201, 199.

[76] Stoeckel, *Lehrbuch der Gynäkologie*, 2nd edn, 458.

directors to make the abnormal decision to conduct mesothorium and radium treatment in the wards, too.[77] But this ultimately conflicted with rules on the use of radium that were issued by Berlin's municipal authorities in the mid-1930s.[78]

A prime example of how the other most prominent form of radiotherapy—brachytherapy, or the insertion of radium capsules at the site of the carcinoma—was practiced in interwar Germany could be found at the Rudolf Virchow Hospital in northern Berlin.[79] As discussed above, because of the high price of radium and mesothorium, hospital administrations were greatly concerned that their stores might be lost or stolen. Moreover, radiologists knew that exposure to radioactivity was a health hazard. Thus, hospitals prescribed in detail the conditions under which radium and mesothorium capsules could be implanted.

Like at many other radiotherapy clinics in Germany, the Rudolf Virchow Hospital had a special 'radiation room' where radium was both stored and inserted in capsules into patients' bodies.[80] When patients entered the space, they were often in a medically induced twilight state, because the insertion of radium was painful and sometimes the surface of the tumour had to be removed through electrocoagulation or with a sharp surgical instrument before radium capsules could be inserted.[81] Then the doctor placed radium tubes or needles as close to the tumour as possible and fixed them to the body with gauze and pins. To protect healthy tissue, they fastened small lead plates with a resinous compound to surrounding body parts.

When inserting radium capsules and setting the protective lead plates, doctors had to be careful not to damage tissue, because this could lead to infections and high fevers. The most common complications of radium therapy, they could be fatal and thus often necessitated that the treatment be ended prematurely. For this reason, nurses had to check patients' temperature regularly, because if peritonitis developed, the patient's fate was, as one gynaecologist wrote in 1933, 'usually one that is hopeless and ends with death'.[82]

After the radium capsule was set, the patient had to remain as still as possible for the duration of the treatment. This ensured that the capsule did not become displaced, which could reduce its therapeutic effectiveness or damage healthy tissue. The demand posed a considerable challenge for patients, because a single session could last two or three days, during which they could not leave the room or

[77] Letter from Dr Frik to the Tiergarten District Administration, Berlin, 25 January 1936, 5. LAB A Rep. 003-04-03, no. 159, 29–31.

[78] Letter from Dr Frik to the Hospital Board, 5 December 1935, LAB A Rep. 003-04-03, no. 143, 36.

[79] Hans Meyer, ed., *Lehrbuch der Strahlentherapie*, 5 vols (Berlin: Urban & Schwarzenberg, 1925–9).

[80] Letter from the Berlin Magistrate to the Board of the Moabit Hospital, Berlin, 7 July 1923, A Rep. 003-04-03, no. 143, 43; Draft of Rules for the Storage and Treatment of Radioactive Substances at the Moabit Hospital, composed by Dr Frik, Berlin, 14 October 1931, LAB A Rep. 003-04-03, no. 143, 116–18; Stoeckel, *Lehrbuch der Gynäkologie*, 2nd edn, 461–3.

[81] F. G. Dietel, 'Die Strahlenbehandlung der Uteruskarzinome an der Universitäts-Frauenklinik Heidelberg (mit einer Statistik der Jahre 1913–1924)', *Strahlentherapie* 46 (1933): 201–72, 217.

[82] Ibid., 250.

receive guests.[83] They were cared for by a specially trained nurse who was personally responsible for watching over the radium or mesothorium to ensure it did not get lost or stolen. Thus, the nurse had to lock the door when she left the room. If the patient had to go to the bathroom, they had to use a bedpan or chamber pot in the nurse's presence. If the patient was receiving treatment in their rectum, vagina, or urethra, the nurse was obligated to check if the radium capsule was still in the right place before she emptied out the waste. If the patient wanted to write a letter, the nurse had to first let the head nurse inspect it to ensure that the expensive radium was not being smuggled out.

Post-treatment, patients had to stay at the hospital for a few days, because most had fevers and doctors had to guard against peritonitis, regardless of whether the patient was bedridden or not.[84] Like patients who had undergone x-ray treatment, they suffered from a 'hangover' with nausea and vomiting. Many felt dizzy and weak, had a lack of appetite, and could not sleep.[85] Moreover, almost all radiotherapy patients had diarrhoea and a constant need to go to the toilet. While the 'hangover' generally subsided quickly after treatment with radium capsules, the aftereffects of x-ray therapy could linger for weeks in some cases. One of the causes was the ozone and nitrous oxide exhausted by the machines. This problem was more or less resolved by the use of stable tubes with protective lead coverings, which many clinics, including the Werner Siemens Institute, implemented. Thus, in the run of the 1930s, the intensity and duration of 'x-ray hangovers' subsided.[86]

Days after treatment, many patients' skin reddened, swelled up, got infected, and itched; they suffered stabbing pain and hair loss. A month or more was often needed for these problems to recede, leaving behind a darkened spot on the skin that faded with time. Only a few patients escaped these side effects, which depended on the radiation dosage as well as individual factors that doctors were not always able to explain.[87]

Some patients treated with x-rays had markedly more severe skin damage, even when they followed the doctor's advice by applying Vaseline or a special lotion and avoiding potentially irritating clothing like corsets or suspenders. Some patients formed fluid-filled blisters that burst after two or three months, causing extreme pain and leaving behind scars. But the scarred skin remained dry, brittle, and sensitive, because the sweat and sebaceous glands were permanently destroyed; often, the tissue contracted. During the early days of radiotherapy, some of

[83] W. Rieder, 'Vermeidung der Allgemeinerscheinungen nach Röntgentiefenbestrahlung (Röntgenkater)', *Strahlentherapie* 12 (1921): 573–84, 574; Dietel, 'Die Strahlenbehandlung', 250.

[84] Stoeckel, *Lehrbuch der Gynäkologie*, 2nd edn, 464; O. Strauß, 'Schädigungen durch Röntgen- und Radiumstrahlen', in Meyer, *Die wissenschaftlichen Grundlagen der Strahlentherapie*, 979–1060.

[85] Otto Pankow, 'Strahlentherapie', in Jaschke and Pankow, *Lehrbuch der Gynäkologie*, 5th edn, 196–237.

[86] Pankow, 'Strahlentherapie', 210–18 and 234–5; Stoeckel, *Lehrbuch der Gynäkologie*, 2nd edn, 464–6.

[87] Walter Stoeckel, *Lehrbuch der Gynäkologie*, 11th edn (Leipzig: Hirzel, 1947), 519–20.

these skin lesions did not heal at all. The tissue ultimately necrotized, leaving skin transplants as the only option. However, such serious aftereffects became less common in the run of the 1920s, because improved technology, including filters, dosimeters, and better irradiation methods, generally were able to prevent third-degree burns.

Brachytherapy patients, in contrast, did not suffer from skin lesions, but they did have to endure very painful bloody diarrhoea that lasted for days. In a few cases, pain caused by infections or ulcers in the intestines, bladder, or vagina appeared months after treatment. Potentially fatal intestinal obstruction was another possible side effect.

The development of fistula between the colon and vagina or bladder and vagina was even more feared and was not directly correlated with the radiation dosage. It could lead to incontinence, inflammation of nearby skin, a high risk of infection, and serious pain. Surgery was often of no use, and the same held for standard methods of pain management; poor hygienic conditions in many patients' homes made the odour given off by the fistula difficult to control.[88]

Still, a large number of women and men 'only' experienced less severe after-effects, like the aforementioned 'hangover', radiation dermatitis, or a painful urge to defecate or urinate. But these issues, too, were felt by many to be serious burdens, so that they 'only begrudgingly and dejectedly' submitted themselves to a second round of radiotherapy when their doctor thought it necessary.[89] The majority of women who underwent radiotherapy for cervical cancer refused to attend both post-treatment exams and further radiotherapy sessions. One explanation favoured by some doctors was that the women's symptoms, such as post-irradiation bleeding, had stopped, and that they thus believed they were healed and did not want to pay for transportation to the clinic.[90]

At home, irradiated patients as well as those who had surgery could expect little post-treatment help. Some received financial assistance from their insurer or charity organizations to help pay for the special diet prescribed by their doctors or for help around the house, and a few were sent to take the waters. But whether a patient got such assistance often depended on the doctor's assessment of the likelihood that they would be able to return to work.[91]

Considering the many sanatoriums for tuberculosis patients that existed at the time, it seems at first glance somewhat surprising that there was such a dearth of

[88] Pankow, 'Strahlentherapie', 234–5.

[89] Hans Müller, 'Zur Allgemeinbehandlung röntgen- und radiumbestrahlter Patienten', *Strahlentherapie* 69, no. 1 (1941): 175–8, 175.

[90] Stoeckel, 'Die vaginale Radikaloperation', 57.

[91] Rules for the Provision of Assistance to Cancer Patients für die Gewährung von Beihilfen Krebskranker (established by the Brandenburgische Bezirksarbeitsgemeinschaft für Krebsbekämpfung), Berlin, 9 October 1937, BArch R 36/1391; Transcription of a conversation between the general secretary of the Reichsauschuss Felix Grüneisen, Prof. Dr Schroeder, Kiel, ministerial director Dr Dammann, and ministerial advisor Dr Taute, Berlin, 12 May 1930, BArch R 1501/126321, 122–3.

post-treatment care for cancer patients. Tuberculosis patients not only enjoyed more support from the state; many private initiatives, too, spearheaded fundraisers for their welfare. These initiatives had usually been started in the late nineteenth century and thus might have been more firmly established in the philanthropic economy, while similar initiatives for cancer patients lacked such solid roots. However, many doctors surmised that two other factors were responsible for the comparatively punier willingness to help cancer patients. First, most people believed cancer was incurable, while tuberculosis had shed this reputation, even though many were still dying from it. Thus, doctors conjectured that people's reasoning might have been something along the lines of: in a time of financial insecurity, why support expensive treatment for people who are consigned to die anyways and who will thus no longer contribute to the economy?[92]

Second, many people erroneously believed that most cancer patients were either old or poor. In this prejudice, too, the patient's 'economic value' played a defining role.[93] There was some evidence for both suspicions. Statistically speaking, more seniors did indeed get cancer, and there was at least one visible form of cancer that afflicted the rural population much more frequently than the middle class: skin cancer. But, as discussed in Chapter 3, early detection campaigns criticized both of these popular fallacies.

Alongside these reasons, there was likely a third that was not openly discussed because it implicated the attitude of medical professionals: Cancer patients were often not gladly seen in clinics and at home. Many people believed that cancer was contagious and thus were afraid of having contact with cancer patients. Similarly, many people, including family members, felt disgust towards cancer patients. For instance, in 1909, a man wrote to the Königlich-Preußische Institut für Infektionskrankheiten (Royal Prussian Institute for Infectious Diseases) to ask if there was any way they could help his 55-year-old mother, who had late-stage uterine cancer. After receiving a negative reply, he wrote again with an undertone of despair:

> Furthermore, I would be very grateful if you could also tell me if there are any disinfectants that can eliminate the vexing odour that constantly surrounds my sick mother and that truly poisons the air in the room; some doctors who I have asked for advice on this point were not able to give me a disinfectant.[94]

Not every tumour exuded odour, and those that did were often at an advanced stage. Moreover, beginning in the 1920s, brachytherapy could, at least

[92] Stoeckel, 'Die vaginale Radikaloperation'.

[93] Dr Klose, head of the Kiel municipal health department, 'Bekämpfung der bösartigen Geschwülste. Carcinom und Fürsorge', *Deutsche Zeitschrift für öffentliche Gesundheitspflege* 5–12, special edition (1929): 229–37, 230–1, BArch R 86/2584.

[94] Letter from Otto J. to the Royal Prussian Institute for Infectious Diseases, Dresden, 27 August 1909, BArch R 86/2763.

temporarily, lessen it in many cases. But the smell seemingly triggered an almost irrepressible disgust in many people that exceeded that evoked by the 'disfigurations' caused by cancer. Accordingly, doctors reported that some relatives did not welcome family members returning home from the clinic with advanced cancer. Indeed, many doctors expressed sympathy with this act of rejection.[95]

Because doctors and nurses also disliked having cancer patients in their wards. This did not just derive from the relatively new definition of hospitals as sites of curing, a point underscored by an article published in 1941 in the journal *Strahlentherapie* (*Radiotherapy*) by the head doctor of Tübingen's gynaecology clinic, August Mayer:

> But isolation is necessary, because the awful stench emanating from the decomposing tumour and the great unrest of terminally ill patients bother other patients and interrupt their sleep. Providing sufficient care at home almost always encounters the most serious difficulties.[96]

This position cannot be explained entirely by the crisis situation caused by the war, as similar statements can be found as early as 1933.[97] Even patients complained in letters about the smell.[98] In 1936, Karl Frik, leader of the Werner Siemens Institute for Radiological Research, applied for funding for small sickrooms, reasoning: 'Additionally, housing cancer patients in wards causes all kinds of difficulties that I do not want to describe in detail.'[99] What he meant is made clear by a statement that was composed by surgeons and internists at the Moabit Hospital two years earlier:

> Because of their serious disfigurations, awful smells, [and] numerous deaths, cancer patients [are] such a distressing encumbrance for other patients who come to the clinic that total spatial separation must be demanded, even of the entrances to the department, even if all are housed in the same central building.[100]

A complaint written in 1935 by the husband of a woman with cancer demonstrates that cancer patients could not always count on understanding from nurses, either:

[95] Design of a Care Centre for Cancer Patients by Ernst von Leyden, submitted on 15 July 1904 to the Royal Charité board, HU Archiv Charité-Direktion, 955, 3.

[96] Mayer, 'Die Entwicklung unserer Therapie beim Uterus-Kollumkarzinom', 25–6.

[97] Blumenthal, 'Die Organisation der Krebsbekämpfung', 810 and 820; 'Organisation der Krebsfürsorge. Bericht über die Sitzung eines zusammengesetzten Ausschusses des Landesgesundheitsrates am 31. Mai 1930', *Veröffentlichungen aus dem Gebiete der Medizinalverwaltung* 32, no. 6 (1930): 635–94.

[98] 'The Current Embarrassments at Station 18 of the Moabit Hospital', sent to the board of the Moabit Hospital, care of Dr Praeprer, by former patient Franz Sch., Berlin-Borsigwalde, 25 October 1927, LAB A Rep. 003-04-03, no. 114, 14–15.

[99] Letter from Dr Frik to the Tiergarten District Administration.

[100] Memorandum for the Establishment of a Central Radiology Institute at the Moabit Hospital, Berlin, 2 May 1934, Board of the Moabit Hospital, LAB A Rep. 003-04-03, no. 158, 4–8.

> She [the letter's author's wife] complained constantly about the most awful pains in her breast and external pains in the breast-belly-back, could not ingest any food, and constantly vomited green bile. Twenty days passed without any measures being undertaken against this state of health—neither from the doctor nor the head nurse! The moaning and sighing of my wife were called by the head nurse those of 'a weak person'—indeed, every sigh of the seriously ill woman was called weak—and as something unbefitting of a hospital.[101]

But where were cancer patients supposed to go when they were seen as incurable, when they were perceived as nuisances and burdens in the large wards, when hospital administrations pressed to free up beds intended for curable patients?

Spaces of Hope, Spaces of Dying

Caring for cancer patients posed a significant challenge for family and loved ones. If the tumour was open, it had to be regularly cleaned and bandaged.[102] Advice literature recommended burning the bandages after changing them out, because adequate disinfection was impossible at home. Internal tumours often secreted pus and discharge. They often bled, and if the bleeding was not stopped quickly, the patient could bleed to death, meaning that a patient prone to bleeding could not be left alone at all. Because of the danger of infection, the literature advised that cancer patients should always have their own bed. But the cramped living conditions of many working-class families made fulfilling this dictate impossible, so that family members had to share a bed with their sick relative despite the unsettling smell. Author Hans Frick, who was born to a working single mother and grew up in poverty, recounted such an experience years after the fact. During the Second World War, his grandmother fell ill with cancer and died. He wrote:

> My grandmother's state of health worsened noticeably. Her last bit of energy was exclusively used in resisting me when I tried to make her get up when the [bomb] alarms went off.... I was constantly subjected to my grandmother's wish to die. I started to get revenge against her by often *forgetting* to give her food.... In the last years of the war, my mother allowed me to sleep on a mattress in the kitchen. She had grasped that she could no longer expect me to lie between her and her cancer-sick, stinking mother.[103]

[101] Complaint from Eugen K. to the Hospital Director Dr Burghardt, Neukölln, 1 July 1935, LAB A Rep. 003-04-03, no. 114.

[102] Gertrud Dewitz, 'Krankenpflegerin in Potsdam, Zur Pflege Krebskranker', *Deutsche Krankenpflege-Zeitung* 6, no. 16 (1903): 243–5; 'Für die Beratung und Pflege Krebskranker', *Zeitschrift für das Krankenpflege-, Bade- und Massagewesen* 2, no. 5 (1934): 63.

[103] Hans Frick, *Die blaue Stunde* (Berlin: Aufbau, 1978), 44–5 (emphasis in original).

The passage indicates that someone had to prepare food for cancer patients when they were no longer capable of doing so themselves. Moreover, people with cancer that affected their digestive system, mouth, or oesophagus could only eat food in pureed or liquid form. Adults in working families could not perform these tasks, because they generally could not miss work. Serious disabilities and conditions, like an ileostomy or intestinal stoma, gastric feeding tube, fistula, or grave pain, could all overtax family members' abilities to care for the patient, especially if they were poor. Assistance from a nurse or house doctor did not necessarily relieve this issue.[104] In principle, caring for a cancer patient at home was only possible if the family had sufficient money to give the person their own room and pay for a caretaker. Working-class families usually did not have the means, nor did those from the petit bourgeoisie.

Thus, many families could not or did not want to let relatives with cancer stay with them if their doctors did not think they had a chance at being cured. In principle, hospitals should have received incurably ill cancer patients. In early modern times, hospitals gave shelter to various groups, including impoverished seniors, houseless families, chronically ill persons, and seriously and terminally ill people who could not be cared for at home.[105] In the run of the nineteenth century, the broadly oriented institution turned into a medical establishment dedicated to treating acutely sick people. Terminally and chronically ill persons were no longer served. Some modern hospitals did care for terminally ill patients, often as a reaction to public pressure campaigns. But hospital administrations were generally against it.[106] At the same time, some municipal governments, religious congregations, and private philanthropists built care centres for terminally ill people, such as the Incurabelnhaus in Augsburg (1718), the Unheilbarenhaus in Bamberg (1806), and the Armen Kranken Versorgungshaus of Bamberg's Catholic hospital (1821).[107]

In most cities, however, the 'old' asylums remained the only places where terminally ill cancer patients could go for care. In the 1920s, the municipal administrations that ran their cities' hospitals made it policy to send 'patients who cannot be released to home care' to asylums after the briefest hospital stay possible.[108] Transferring terminally ill patients to asylums as early as possible also allowed doctors to keep the fatality numbers in their sections or hospitals low, as

[104] Hermann Weber, 'Behandlung inoperabler bösartiger Geschwülste durch den Hausarzt', *Zeitschrift für ärztliche Fortbildung* 36, no. 10 (1939): 289–94, 291–2.

[105] Artur Dirmeier, *Organisierte Barmherzigkeit. Armenpflege und Hospitalwesen in Mittelalter und Früher Neuzeit* (Regensburg: Pustet, 2010); Hans-Peter Rhomberg, *Das Hospital. Heil- und Pflegestätten im Wandel der Zeit* (Lindenberg: Kunstverlag Fink, 2015).

[106] Michael Stolberg, *Die Geschichte der Palliativmedizin. Medizinische Sterbebegleitung von 1500 bis heute*, 2nd edn (Frankfurt am Main: Mabuse, 2013), 197–202.

[107] Stolberg, *Die Geschichte der Palliativmedizin*, 206–7.

[108] Letter from the Mayor of Berlin to the City's Centrally Administered Hospitals and Clinics, Berlin, 11 November 1931, LAB A Rep. 003-04-03, no. 60, 169–70.

these numbers were more and more read as indicators of the quality of medical care provided by an institution.[109]

Patients and their families often vigorously resisted plans to send them to an asylum. Just the mention of the name 'Siechenhaus' (infirmary, asylum) was for most people equivalent with being dispatched to die.[110] Because municipalities often centrally organized the transfer of patients to asylums, patients could end up far away from their home in other parts of the city or on the city's outskirts.[111] But doctors, too, criticized the practice, because asylums and alms-houses did not have the facilities to adequately care for cancer patients.[112]

Berlin's standard procedure for transferring patients to asylums was representative of practices throughout Germany. In the 1920s, the city's health administration directed all hospitals to send all terminally ill patients who could not be cared for at home to the city's Hufeland Asylum, which had a special annex for incurable patients.[113] Constructed between 1886 and 1889 as the Friedrich Wilhelm Asylum, the building complex was originally considered a 'model institution' for caring for and housing poor people and seniors. Because it was almost always at capacity, a new building was added in 1897.[114] Consisting of two hospital buildings, two infirmaries, an administration building, multiple buildings for cooking, laundry, and the like, and a morgue with a small chapel, the complex was located on a large piece of property between Prenzlauer Allee, Fröbelstrasse, Diesterwegstrasse, and Stargarderstrasse in the Prenzlauer Berg district. The asylum initially had beds for 1,246 people; by the early 1920s, it had expanded to over 1,400.[115] Most rooms contained four beds, while the infirmary rooms generally had six beds. There were also a few two-bed rooms, and each building had two large wards for ten or eleven beds, multiple bathrooms, and a recreation

[109] Stolberg, *Die Geschichte der Palliativmedizin*, 198.

[110] Transcription of Circular Part VII/1934, 34, no. 69, 6 February 1934: 'Weiterverweisung siecher Hilfsbedürftiger an die Hospitäler zur Vermeidung der Aufnahme in die Krankenhäuser' (Referring infirm needy persons to the asylums to avoid their intake in hospitals), LAB A Rep. 003-04-03, no. 115, 122.

[111] Klose, 'Bekämpfung der bösartigen Geschwülste', 237.

[112] [Ferdinand] Blumenthal, 'Gründung und Aufgaben der Krebs-Institute', *Sonderdruck. Archiv für Soziale Hygiene und Demographie* 3, no. 3 (1928), BArch R 1501/126318, 48–9.

[113] Georg Wolff and Alfred Jahn, 'Die Sterblichkeit an Tuberkulose und an Krebs in Beziehung zur sozialen Struktur der Berliner Bevölkerung', *Archiv für soziale Hygiene und Demographie* 7, no. 6 (1932): 461–77; *Pamphlet for Intake and Station Doctors*, 1930, LAB A Rep. 003-04-03, no. 33, 19–28; Georg Wolff, 'Das Verhalten der Krebssterblichkeit in Berlin', *Deutsche Medizinische Wochenschrift* 58, no. 30 (1932): 1173–5, 1175.

[114] Architekten-Verein zu Berlin und Vereinigung Berliner Architekten, ed., *Berlin und seine Bauten*, vol. 2 (Berlin: Ernst Verlag, 1896), 471; Barbara Jakoby, 'Das Hospital und Siechenheim Fröbelstraße (1889–1934)', in *Prenzlauer, Ecke Fröbelstraße. Hospital der Reichshauptstadt, Haftort der Geheimdienste, Bezirksamt Prenzlauer Berg 1889–1989*, ed. Berlin-Brandenburgische Geschichtswerkstatt (Berlin: Lukas Verlag, 2006), 25–49.

[115] Architekten-Verein, *Berlin und seine Bauten*, 471–4; Zentrale für private Fürsorge, ed., *Die Wohlfahrtseinrichtungen von Groß-Berlin nebst einem Wegweiser für die praktische Ausübung der Armenpflege in Berlin. Ein Auskunfts- und Handbuch*, 4th edn (Berlin: Springer, 1910). On the bed numbers around 1920, see Jakoby, 'Das Hospital und Siechenheim Fröbelstraße', 41.

room on each floor for non-bedridden patients. Thus, the spaces were in no way worse than what many residents—or at least those who came from working-class families—were accustomed to at home. However, the mere fact that the asylum was located across the street from a shelter for houseless persons that was designed by the same architect with a similar external appearance ensured that the social status of its residents was seen as being not much higher than that of the unhoused.

Residents received—free of charge—food, clothing, medicine, and medical treatment from doctors employed by the hospital, but in exchange they only retained a small amount of whatever pension money they might have been entitled to.[116] In other respects, too, they had to accept considerable limitations on their personal freedom and property rights. They were not permitted to bring their own furniture, pillows, or blankets; incoming and outgoing packages were searched by the hospital administration; sleeping hours for the non-bedridden patients were set. If they wanted to leave the campus, they had to ask for permission in writing. Bedridden cancer patients were probably hurt by the short visiting hours more than anything else. While visitors were initially welcome every day between two and four o'clock in the afternoon, the hours were gradually curtailed in the run of the 1920s. By May 1934, they had been cut to Wednesdays and Saturdays from two to four o'clock.[117]

Berlin's central health department also thought the restrictions went too far, because they gave the 'character of the asylums as public institutions' a bad reputation.[118] The asylum's administration justified the rules by pointing to the overloaded Hufeland Asylum, where there was not enough personnel to care for the many 'most seriously ill patients' and where every visiting day, they alleged, caused 'disturbances' and 'disorder', thus creating another burden for the already overburdened nurses and doctors.[119] Under these conditions, empathetic, attentive care was impossible, which is underscored by the fact that mobile patients had to help bathe and feed their gravely ill roommates.[120] The situation was disappointing for new arrivals, because hospital staff had given many of them 'grand promises' that were supposed to help them overcome their 'aversion towards treatment at the asylum'. They were told not only about 'trained care personnel' and 'special facilities' for the care of cancer patients, but also about the very comfortable furnishings: 'cushy chairs, your own headphones, much better care,

[116] Zentrale für private Fürsorge, *Die Wohlfahrtseinrichtungen von Groß*-Berlin, 62; Jakoby, 'Das Hospital und Siechenheim Fröbelstraße', 37–8.

[117] House Rules for the Patients at the Hufeland Asylum, dated 31 May 1934, LAB A Rep. 003-04-13, no. 35, 75–81.

[118] Letter from Berlin's Central Health Department to the Hufeland Asylum, Berlin, 21 September 1934, LAB A Rep. 003-04-13, no. 35, 90.

[119] Statement of the Asylum Leadership, dated 2 November 1934, LAB A Rep. 003-04-13, no. 35, 91–2.

[120] Jakoby, 'Das Hospital und Siechenheim Fröbelstraße', 37.

and much more' were, it was said, standard at the Hufeland Asylum.[121] Although some of the deceived patients fell into a rage, they could alter their situation little, because hospitals refused to take back cancer patients from the asylums.

This did not change when the Hufeland Asylum moved its 707 bedridden and 621 mobile patients in March 1934 to the former Genesungsheim Buch (Buch Recovery Home), which was part of a hospital complex that had been built in an outlying district of Berlin in the late nineteenth century.[122] From then on, terminally ill cancer patients from all of Berlin's hospitals were sent to Buch and thus away from the city, where they were housed together with tuberculosis patients and mentally ill persons. Alongside the Hufeland Asylum, male cancer patients could be sent to the Asylum Buch West (Dr Heim Asylum), women to the Ludwig Hoffmann Asylum in the same district. When the Second World War began, asylum care suffered further setbacks, because inner-city hospitals were handed over to the Wehrmacht and the patients housed at them were also sent to the Buch asylums.[123] In March 1941, the Hufeland Asylum moved to a different building at the Buch complex, which had been vacated after the psychiatry patients living there were sent to be murdered at other medical centres as part of the Aktion T4 euthanasia programme.[124] At the new location, the number of nurses consistently dwindled. The situation worsened further after the building had to be repurposed as a bomb shelter once the Allies started air raids on Berlin in 1943, forcing the asylum to move again to yet another site in the faraway Buch district. The number of deaths at the asylum rose continuously during the war, from 362 (1938) to 722 (1940) and, finally, 2,705 (1942). Whether a kind of 'silent' euthanasia through starvation was responsible for this increase, as was true of some other asylums, is impossible to tell from the preserved records.[125] Beginning in 1943, numerous patients were moved to places that could not provide adequate care. As one female patient wrote in a complaint, an 'appalling number of women were thrown in a pile' there and had to figure out how to survive on their own.[126]

Outside of asylums, there were few institutions in Germany in the first half of the twentieth century where terminally ill cancer patients could receive medical care. For the majority of dying cancer patients, these places were out of reach and thus played no concrete role in their personal experience of the illness. However, they were known not only among researchers. Many considered these institutions to be places of hope as well as of despair and abysmal suffering: hope for breakthrough discoveries in cancer research, hope for first-class medical treatment, and hope just because

[121] Transcription of a Letter from the Board of the Hufeland Asylum to the Berlin Central Health Department, Berlin, 24 September 1934, LAB A Rep. 003-04-03, no. 114; Transcription of Circular Part VII/1934, 34, no. 69, 6 February 1934.

[122] Horst-Peter Wolff and Arno Kalinich, *Zur Geschichte der Krankenhausstadt Berlin-Buch*, 2nd edn (Frankfurt: Mabuse, 2006), 111–18; Jakoby, 'Das Hospital und Siechenheim Fröbelstraße', 33.

[123] Wolff and Kalinich, *Zur Geschichte der Krankenhausstadt Berlin-Buch*, 118.

[124] Ibid., 128–33. [125] Ibid., 136. [126] Ibid., 137.

they accepted terminally ill cancer patients—which is also why they were seen as sites of profound despair, because in hardly another place did so many terminally ill cancer patients lie side by side in such large numbers.

These places were Heidelberg's Samariterhaus (Samaritan House), which was opened in 1906 as part of the town's Institut für experimentelle Krebsforschung (Institute for Experimental Cancer Research), and the clinical station of the Berlin Charité Hospital's Institut für Krebsforschung an der I. Medizinischen Klinik zu Berlin, which opened in 1903 and was also known as the Krebsbaracke, or cancer pavilions, because of its architecture. Both establishments grew out of renewed public interest in cancer, which mixed concerns about increasing rates of cancer with hope for the development of more effective treatments. In contrast to many of the long-existing English and French cancer hospitals, Heidelberg's Samaritan House and Berlin's cancer pavilions were explicitly conceived of as clinical divisions of research institutions.[127] This had two consequences. First, both were constructed on the edges of the respective city's university hospital campus. Second, both had laboratories where scientists experimented not only with chemicals and human tissue, but also on animals. Thus, in Heidelberg, a number of stalls were set up in the old cigar factory behind the clinic, while stalls were built behind the Berlin clinic later on.

The institutes' connection to the university hospitals determined not only their geographic location, but also, to a certain extent, their organizational position. The professors of the established clinics exerted themselves to ensure that the new cancer institutes did not take any patients that they could have treated themselves. Thus, in their first years, both institutes were not allowed to receive patients directly, but only when they were transferred to them from other clinics.[128] It is unsurprising that they were mostly sent patients considered to be incurable.[129]

Vinzenz Czerny, the first head of the Samaritan House, and Ernst von Leyden, the first director of the institute in Berlin, had both founded their clinics with the aim of giving incurably ill patients a place to receive medical care while at the same time teaching young doctors the 'difficult art' of treating them.[130] However, neither institute was supposed to be wholly reserved for terminally ill patients,

[127] Voswinckel, *Erinnerungsort Krebsbaracke*; Ulrike Scheybal, 'Krebsforschung in der Zeit des Nationalsozialismus unter besonderer Berücksichtigung des Allgemeinen Instituts gegen die Geschwulstkrankheiten' (PhD diss., Leipzig University, 2000), 9–10 and 12–28; Hellmann-Mersch, *Institutionen zur Krebsforschung und Krebsbekämpfung in Deutschland*, 115–50; Rahel Neubert, 'Das Institut für experimentelle Krebsforschung', in *Die Universität Heidelberg im Nationalsozialismus*, ed. Wolfgang U. Eckart, Volker Sellin, and Eike Wolgast (Heidelberg: Springer, 2006), 959–74; Cornelia Lindner, 'Vinzenz Czerny (1842–1916). Leben und Wirken des Heidelberger Chirurgen und Krebsforschers im zeitgeschichtlichen Kontext' (PhD diss., Heidelberg University, 2007), ch. 4.

[128] Czerny, *Das Heidelberger Institut für experimentelle Krebsforschung*, 10.

[129] Ibid., 11; Copy of a Letter from Blumenthal to the Board of the Charité, dated 15 March 1928, HU Archiv, Charité-Direktion, 951, 237.

[130] Vinzenz Czerny, 'Über die Pflege unheilbarer Krebskranker', *Die Krankenpflege* 1 (1901/2): 289–304, 296.

because if they were, Czerny forewarned, the hope of both patients and medical personnel would be endangered. As he wrote in 1912:

> I believe that one should not exclusively take incurable carcinomas and sarcomas in a cancer institute . . . , so that the establishment does not become defined with the character of an asylum and so that the cured cases will help sustain the courage and hope of the patients and the care personnel's eagerness to work. Because it should not be forgotten how depressing and debilitating a ward full of dying people can be for doctors and nurses. Doctors and nurses must themselves have hope in order to be able to remain optimists and sustain hope even for the despairing patients.[131]

Thus, alongside palliative radiotherapy and experiments with various medicines, the Samaritan House had its own surgery room so that operable patients could also be treated at the clinic. Moreover, the institute had a comfortable atmosphere that unmistakably distinguished it from an asylum.

The 900,000 marks that Czerny had raised to establish the clinic made this all possible. Donations came from 163 people, including members of the Rothschild and Krupp families, Czerny's colleagues, and a few 'small donors'.[132] The Grand Ducal Government of Baden donated a piece of property worth almost 290,000 marks where a three-story building with two wings was built. The building was customized to the cancer institute's needs and its furnishings went 'somewhat beyond the standard of other local clinics'.[133]

The interior design was intentionally open and inviting. All rooms and hallways were designed in various colours by Karl Eyth, a professor of applied arts in Karlsruhe; the colours of the walls and linoleum flooring were harmonious, and many rooms had decorative tiling. Even the three large third-class wards with their outsize windows had an uncustomarily high-quality design and only had nine beds (Fig. 23), making them small in comparison with similar wards in other hospitals. Near the three wards was a spacious recreation room where non-bedridden patients could congregate and even play the piano.

The first and second floors of the east wing each had four two-bed rooms for wealthier self-paying patients or those with private insurance, and each floor had its own recreation room. Thus, the Samaritan House had a total of sixteen beds for private patients, twenty-seven beds for patients with statutory health insurance, and two beds in isolated rooms for the most seriously ill or dying patients.

[131] Czerny, *Das Heidelberger Institut für experimentelle Krebsforschung*, 12.

[132] Ibid., 11 along with the list of donors on pages 55–7.

[133] On the cancer institute's financial situation see ibid., 47–54 (quote on page 50), and Robert Koch, 'Die Ätiologie der Tuberkulose', in *Die Ätiologie und die Bekämpfung der Tuberkulose* (Leipzig: Thieme, 1912), 10–38, 15.

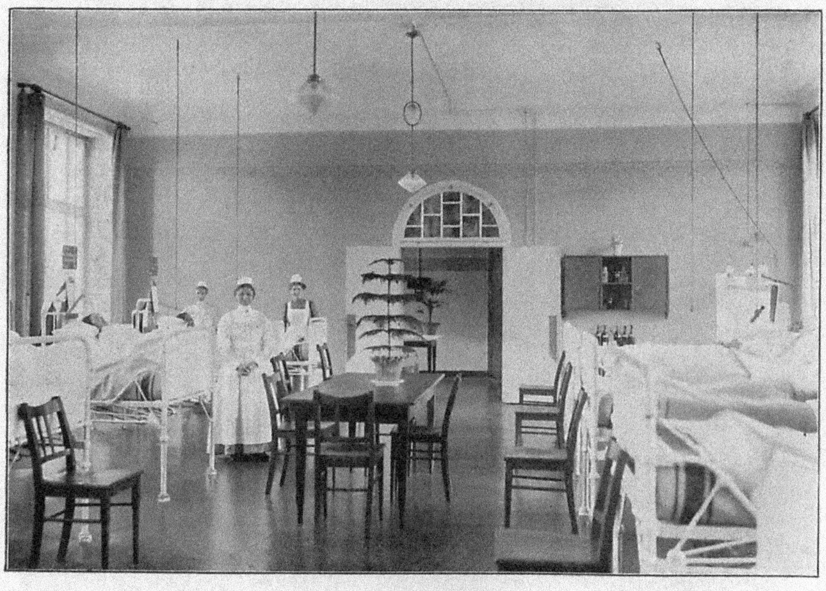

Abbildung 11.

Fig. 23 Third-class ward at the Samaritan House in Heidelberg (1912).

The Samaritan House's comparatively large number of private patients increased revenues and made possible its relatively high standard of care. At the same time, the layout was specially designed to fit Czerny's wishes for the clinic. He did not want it to be an asylum for indigent patients but wanted to offer incurable patients from the upper classes a place to live and die with cancer, a place where the hope for a cure and competent care would be fostered (Fig. 24).

Things were completely different at the Institute for Cancer Research in Berlin. Like its counterpart in Heidelberg, it was founded on the initiative of a renowned doctor, internist Ernst von Leyden, and a high-ranking government official, Friedrich Althoff. But it was financed entirely by the Prussian Ministry of Culture.[134] And because doctors at the city's flagship hospital, the Charité, were sceptical about the need for a special oncology institute, it was considerably more modest than the Heidelberg clinic.[135] The ministry was only willing to dole out 65,220 marks for the construction of the building, the interior design, equipment,

[134] Atzl and Helms, *Die Geschichte der Deutschen Krebsgesellschaft.*

[135] Voswinckel, *50 Jahre Deutsche Gesellschaft für Hämatologie und Onkologie* (Würzburg: Murken-Altrogge, 1987), 55–7.

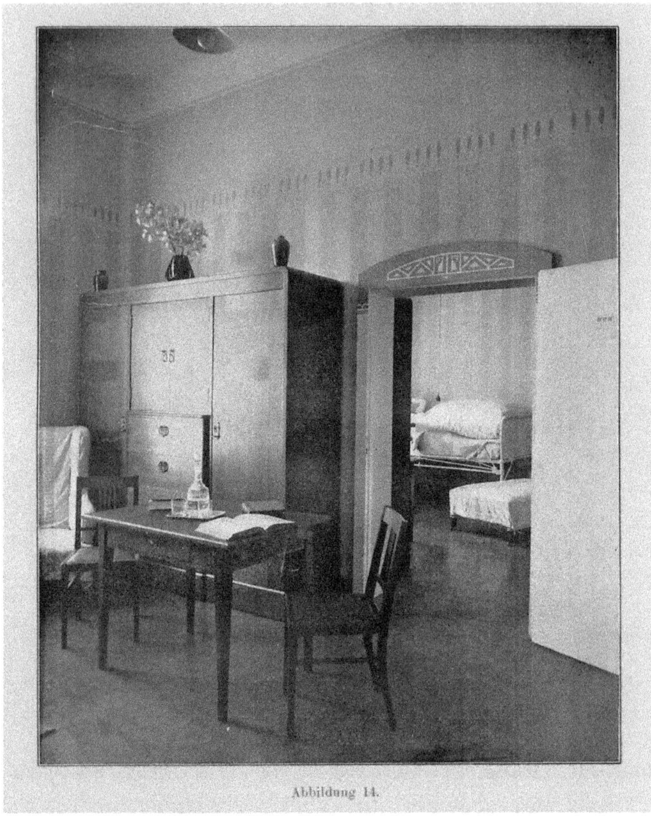

Fig. 24 A room for self-paying and privately insured patients at the Samaritan House in Heidelberg (1912).

and the yard.[136] The money was enough for two roughly 158-square-metre buildings for patients as well as a small laboratory building.[137]

The pavilion-style architecture of the 'cancer pavilions' did not yet evoke the kind of negative connotations it would acquire over the next one hundred years in Germany. In the last third of the nineteenth century, this type of building was viewed as an alternative to the poorly ventilated, poorly lit wards of old. Nevertheless, pavilions were generally constructed for two reasons: as military hospitals that could be quickly and cheaply built and then easily disassembled later, and as hospital divisions for infectious diseases, because the pavilion form made it easy to separate infected patients from one another and to air out the

[136] Ibid., 18.

[137] The size was calculated on the basis of the blueprints: Ernst von Leyden and Ferdinand Blumenthal, 'Die Abteilung für Krebsforschung an der I. Med. Universitätsklinik', *Charité-Annalen* 28 (1904): 36–44, 37.

rooms.[138] Thus, people living around 1900 probably associated the pavilion-style architecture with temporariness and separation. Indeed, at the Berlin cancer clinic, the cancer patients' proximity to the clinic for tuberculars on the one side and the quarantine pavilion on the other certainly bolstered this impression.

The facilities and design of the bare buildings aligned with medical and hygienic standards of the time, but 'avoided all superfluous luxury', as Ernst von Leyden defensively wrote in 1904 in the *Charité-Annalen* (Fig. 25).[139] Keeping the number of beds in the 71-square-metre wards of both the male and female pavilions relatively low was, in his eyes, not a superfluous luxury. Each could hold eight patients, while both buildings had two so-called isolation rooms for seriously ill patients. It was better staffed than many other sections of the hospital, but considering the intensive care that it was tasked with providing, this also did not seem like a luxury to Leyden. Each building employed an overnight nurse for its total of ten patients. The simple furnishings were tailored to the practical needs of medical care and little more.[140]

For well-off self-paying or privately insured patients, the cancer pavilions were thus only a last resort when no other form of care was possible. In 1915, though, the cancer research institute opened a well-equipped radiotherapy section with the help of donations, leading doctors to send patients who were seen as still having a chance at being cured. Because there was no space to expand the cancer pavilions or build an annex, the clinic's then acting director Ferdinand Blumenthal decided to have an outpatient radiology clinic constructed at a different property far away.[141] In contradistinction to the layout of the Heidelberg clinic, this decision drew a more or less clear line between curable and incurable cancer patients.

Thus, the cancer pavilions remained the place where terminally ill and dying cancer patients were treated and cared for (Fig. 26). Alongside palliative radiotherapy, they received medication to manage pain and anxiety and help them sleep; their wounds were cleaned and dressed; and tumorous lesions were flushed out with zinc chloride solution in order to prevent and combat infections. Many nurses found caring for patients at the cancer pavilions almost unbearable and few worked there by choice. In order to fill the positions, nurses from other sections of the Charité hospital were forced to take shifts there as a punitive measure—a situation that certainly did not promote devoted, attentive care.[142]

Many patients, and particularly those emaciated and weakened by lengthy radiotherapy, were given arsenic solutions that had long been in use to strengthen

[138] Voswinckel, *50 Jahre Deutsche Gesellschaft für Hämatologie und Onkologie*, 3–10.

[139] Leyden and Blumenthal, 'Die Abteilung', 37.

[140] Ibid., 37 and 39–40.

[141] Evelyn Hoeppner-Salazar, 'Krebsforschung und Krebsbekämpfung in Berlin bis zum Jahre 1945' (PhD diss., Freie Universität Berlin), 56–8; Memorandum on the Research Activities of the University Institute for Cancer Research at the Charité between 1917–20, HU Archiv, Charité-Direktion, 951, 56–67.

[142] Prof. Auler's Response to Martha H.'s Complaint in a Letter to the Administrative Director of the Charité, Berlin, 30 October 1942, HU Archiv Charité-Direktion, no. 2724, 183.

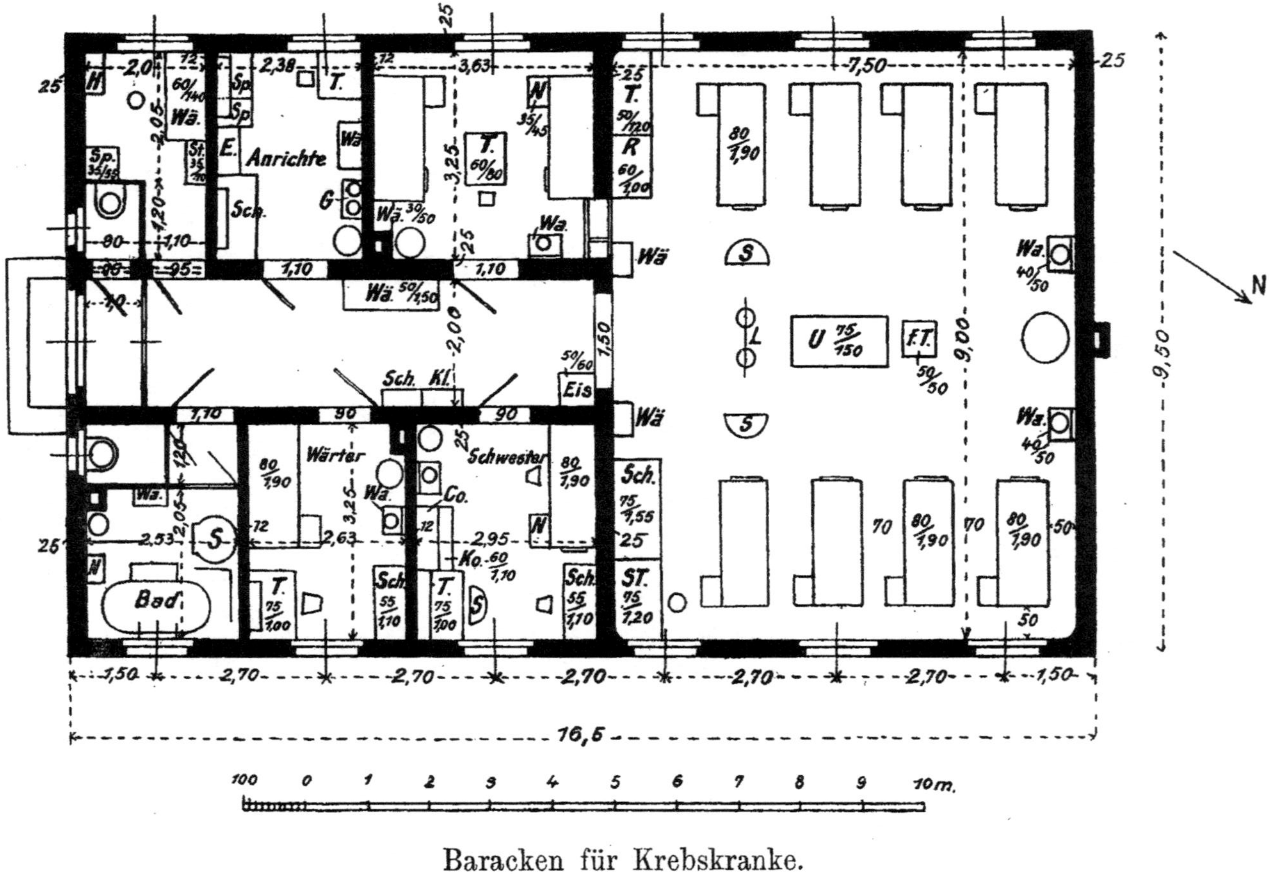

Fig. 25 Floorplan of the ward of one of the cancer pavilions (1910).

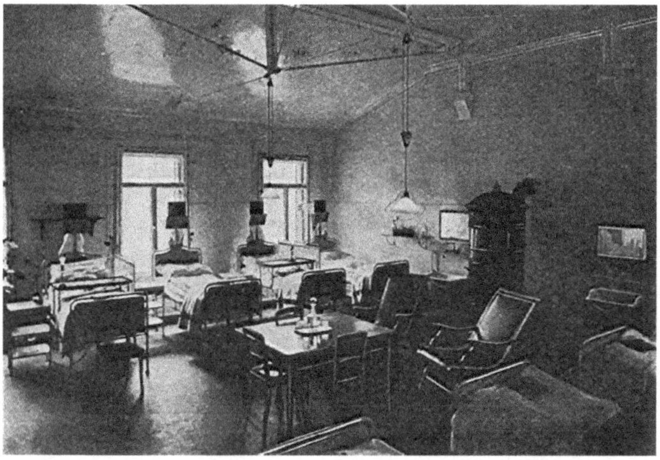

Fig. 26 View of the ward of one of the cancer pavilions (1910).

the body. They also received new, as yet untested substances like metallic salts and selenium compounds that had been shown to diminish tumours in animals. The clinic also experimented on its patients with so-called serum or vaccine therapy, in which they were injected with extracts of their own or another person's tumour or infectious discharge in the hope that this would jumpstart the immune system or 'immunize' the body against the development of relapses and metastases.[143]

Experimenting with new treatments on 'hopeless' patients was widespread practice at research-focused clinics.[144] It was legal so long as doctors believed that the treatment would increase the patient's chances of improving. And without a doubt, many doctors at the institute for cancer research had humanitarian motives. However, 'moribund' cancer patients were welcomed in the cancer pavilions precisely because they were, as Blumenthal put it in a 1928 letter to the Charité hospital's directors, 'valuable for our research'.[145] It is difficult to determine how seriously doctors and scientists took the dictate to apply a new therapy only when it had a somewhat realistic chance of helping the patient. The difficulty is not just a matter of historical research, as the doctors themselves likely found it hard to definitively distinguish between 'attempt at treatment' and 'human experiment'. Doctor and patient could both perceive an almost futile attempt at treatment as a sign of hope that, as Czerny wrote, 'if one method fails, a

[143] Memorandum on the Research Activities of the University Institute for Cancer Research at the Charité between 1917–1920; Hans Auler, 'Über die Wartung und Behandlung Krebskranker', *Monatsschrift für Krebsbekämpfung* 3 (1933): 101–5.

[144] Hellmann-Mersch, *Institutionen zur Krebsforschung und Krebsbekämpfung in Deutschland*, 145.

[145] Copy of a Letter from Blumenthal to the Board of the Charité, 15 March 1928, HU Archiv, Charité-Direktion, no. 951, 237.

new one is still at hand that bolsters their [the patients'] courage and makes the harrowing suffering more bearable'.[146]

But patients faced the danger that the experiment would have the opposite effect of that intended, hurting them instead of helping them. For this precise reason, Robert Dax, head doctor at the hospital in Munich's Schwabing district, was interrogated by the Bavarian Ministry of the Interior in 1933. He admitted to having injected preagonal patients with a serum that caused 'turbulent reactions' and ultimately led to their deaths—a procedure that Dax promised to refrain from in the future.[147] This experiment on dying patients clearly transgressed the boundaries of what could reasonably be called an attempt at treatment. The guidelines adopted in Prussia in 1931 were unmistakable on this point: 'Experiments on dying patients are not compatible with the principles of medical ethics and are therefore not permitted.'[148]

There is considerable evidence that patients were aware of such experiments and feared becoming objects of them themselves at Berlin's Institute for Cancer Research. In 1912, Czerny reported that publicly insured patients whose doctors wanted to transfer them to the Samaritan House protested because they 'believed they would have to serve as objects of experiment'.[149] By 1935, the Nazis' racist policies had led to the dismissal of almost all doctors at Berlin's cancer pavilions. With them went the institute, which was to be replaced by a new Allgemeines Institut gegen die Geschwulstkrankheiten (General Institute against Tumorous Diseases). The Nazi paper the *Völkische Beobachter* justified the plan to the public by thumping on these fears:

> At the new institute, 300 beds are available to sick persons, who will receive adequate treatment and need not have any fear that they might be objects of experiment here; because in National-Socialist Germany there is no such thing anymore.[150]

Whether the *Völkische Beobachter* journalist was expressing his own rejection of human experiments here in the year 1935 is hard to say. Certain is that the argument was driven by the cynical antisemitic attempt to defame the Institute for Cancer Research. The quote also implies that such fears existed in society. These fears were not entirely unfounded, since the institute did test new forms of treatment on human subjects. However, preserved documentation makes it

[146] Czerny, *Das Heidelberger Institut für experimentelle Krebsforschung*, 11.

[147] Prof. Dr R. Dax, head doctor of the surgery department of the Schwabing hospital, to Dr Viernstein of the Bavarian Interior Ministry in Munich, dated 11 August 1933, BArch R 86/4136.

[148] Guidelines for New Treatments and for Scientific Experiments on Humans, decreed by the Prussian Minister of Welfare Hirtsiefer, 11 June 1931, LAB A Rep. 003-04-03, no. 137, 147–8.

[149] Czerny, *Das Heidelberger Institut für experimentelle Krebsforschung*, 10.

[150] 'Das neue Berliner Zentral-Krebsinstitut', BArch R 86/2764.

difficult to discern whether they clearly overstepped the bounds of medical ethics, like the case in Munich, or whether they were always conducted with the patient's consent and a genuine belief that they might have a salubrious effect.[151]

Patients' experiences were not just shaped by fears about what might happen to them at the clinic, though. They were also formed by the everyday reality of the clinic that played out before their eyes. In 1912, poet and doctor Gottfried Benn described what he saw when he first entered the cancer ward as a young doctor in the then controversial poem 'Man and Woman Walk through the Cancer Ward':

> The man:
> This row here is made up of collapsed wombs.
> And this row is made up of collapsed breasts.
> Bed stinks by bed. The nurses change each hour.
>
> Come, you may safely draw back this cover.
> Observe, this knob of fat and fetid pus,
> that was once large to some man or other
> and signified passion and athomeness.
>
> Come and observe this scar upon the breast.
> Do you feel the rosary of softened knots?
> Yes, touch it. The flesh is soft and feels no pain.
>
> Here, this one bleeds as from thirty bodies.
> No man on earth has so much blood.
> This one here first had
> a child cut out of the cancered womb.
>
> They are left to sleep. Day and night—New ones
> are told: here one sleeps one's way to health—for
> Sunday visits they're made a little brighter.
>
> Only a little nourishment is taken.
> The backs are sored. You see the flies. Sometimes
> the nurse washes them. As one washes benches.
>
> Here the land is swirling up around each bed.
> Flesh subsides to soil. Red heat dies off.
> Sap starts to trickle. The earth is calling.[152]

[151] There is evidence that Berlin's university oncology clinic conducted experiments on terminally ill cancer patients. See BStU, MfS-HA IX/11, RHE 25/87, vol. 2, 180–1, and Alexander von Schwerin, 'Prekäre Stoffe. Radiumökonomie, Risikoepisteme und die Etablierung der Radioindikatortechnik in der Zeit des Nationalsozialismus', *NTM: Zeitschrift für Geschichte der Wissenschaften, Technik und Medizin* 17, no. 1 (2009): 5–33, 23, https://doi.org/10.1007/s00048-008-0324-z.

[152] Gottfried Benn, 'Man and Woman Walk through the Cancer Ward', in J. M. Ritchie, *Gottfried Benn: The Unreconstructed Expressionist* (London: Oswald Wolff, 1972), 107. Ritchie translates

Benn detailed the impressions of a male doctor whose gaze reduces the women in the ward to their cancer-ridden body parts as he describes these impressions to the woman mentioned in the title, who remains silent throughout the poem. Visual and olfactory traces of decay are so dominant that the personhood and subjectivity of the living women disappear behind them. It is hard to interpret whether Benn was giving artistic expression to his own perspective or trying to illustrate that of what he saw as a typical male doctor. This difficulty is compounded by the personal context in which he wrote the poem: At the time, his mother, with whom he was very close, was dying of breast cancer at home under extreme pain because her husband, Benn's father, would not allow her to take morphine.[153]

In contrast to Benn's narrative, though, doctors at Berlin's cancer pavilions did indeed wonder about how patients processed the atmosphere of decay surrounding them, an atmosphere that also occupied considerable space in doctors' accounts from the clinic's early years.[154] Ferdinand Blumenthal, who did his utmost to provide patients with a comfortable space, perceived with particular insight how much the situation in the pavilions burdened patients.[155] In a letter he wrote to the Charité's administration in 1928, he complained:

> The severity of the individual cases has the consequence that in the wards, deaths occur more often than at a clinic that also treats people with more hopeful illnesses. We have no spaces to isolate the dying patients in time. This makes it difficult to prevent patients from sometimes having the feeling that they will soon die. As this is in reality true for many cases, it represents an inhumane hardness to embitter the rest of the lives of these poor, hopeless patients with this knowledge. Additionally, the disease often necessitates large bandages, and because there are no separate bandaging rooms in the wards, each patient has to be bandaged in the presence of the others. This seriously depresses a few very sick patients, because the similarity of the illness allows them to draw direct conclusions about how their illness will turn out.[156]

In order to provide terminally ill and dying patients space for themselves, Blumenthal requested that a new pavilion be built with space for ten beds each for women and men, with the difference that it only contain one- or two-bed

'Krebsbaracke' as 'cancer ward'. It is not clear whether Benn ever visited Berlin's 'Krebsbaracke', translated in this book as 'cancer pavilions' because of their pavilion-style architecture and layout. On the issue of whether Benn visited the clinic, see Voswinckel, *Erinnerungsort Krebsbaracke*, 146–7.

153 Yahya Elsaghe, *Krankheit und Matriarchat. Thomas Manns Betrogene im Kontext* (Berlin: de Gruyter, 2010), 107.

154 Hans Hirschfeld, 'Euguform, ein neues Desodorans', *Berliner Klinische Wochenschrift* 56 (1919): 1189.

155 Letter from Blumenthal to the Prussian Minister for Science, Art, and Cultural Education, Berlin, 19 September 1925, HU Archiv, Charité-Direktion, 951, 224.

156 Copy of a Letter from Blumenthal to the Board of the Charité, 15 March 1928, HU Archiv, Charité-Direktion, no. 951, 237.

rooms. Blumenthal's demand fit with contemporaneous standards. For instance, when plans were being drawn up for a new radiological institute in Berlin's Moabit section, the lead radiologist, Karl Frik, also called for a separate room to be built for dying patients.[157] Like Blumenthal, Frik's primary motivator seems to have been consideration of the patients who were not (yet) dying; he was less concerned with the wishes of dying patients themselves. At other clinics during this period, dying patients were 'hidden' by placing screens around their beds and removing their bodies under a sheet as soon as they passed away.[158]

Blumenthal's request thus appeared justified, but the hospital administration rejected it in order to avoid further fragmenting the institute, which was already scattered among multiple buildings. The administrators were concerned that they would lose control over the now internationally renowned institute, which had a tumultuous financial history. Since 1915, it had only received inadequate funding from the state. Blumenthal filled the gap with donations, which were enough to expand the institute. By the 1920s, the clinic was, in a sense, a private institution. This was reversed when the government took it over in 1929, which fuelled hopes that its architecture and layout would be improved.[159]

But when the Nazis seized power, the situation at Berlin's cancer clinic rapidly declined. The antisemitic Law for the Restoration of the Professional Civil Service caused twelve of the thirteen doctors at the institute, including its director Ferdinand Blumenthal, to be fired or forced to resign.[160] The only remaining doctor, Hans Auler, was promoted to acting director of an institute that now really only existed on paper. This presented an 'opportunity' to reorganize cancer research and treatment in Berlin, which various groups immediately leapt upon. Ideas included retaining and expanding the institute at the Charité, making it into a subdivision of the surgery department under the leadership of Ferdinand Sauerbruch, and moving it to one of the other radiology centres in Berlin at either the Moabit Hospital, the Rudolf Virchow Hospital, or the Cecilienhaus women's clinic, which specialized in the treatment of women with breast cancer, cervical cancer, and uterine cancer.[161]

After lengthy negotiations, Berlin's health administration decided in late June 1935 to open a new Allgemeines Institut gegen die Geschwulstkrankheiten (General Institute against Tumorous Diseases) at the Rudolf Virchow Hospital,

[157] Statement on the Reduced Need for Space in the Proposed New Building of the X-Ray Institute.

[158] Instructions for the Care Staff at the Municipal Health Facilities, Berlin, 14 October 1911; Deputation for the Municipal Health Facilities and Public Healthcare, Selberg; Guideline for the Care Staff in the Municipal Health Facilities [Special Reproduction from the Circular Part VII, no. 171, dated 21 June 1930], LAB A Rep. 003-04-03, no. 114, 4–8 and 40–2.

[159] Voswinckel, *50 Jahre Deutsche Gesellschaft für Hämatologie und Onkologie*, 61–2 and 75–81; Hoeppner-Salazar, 'Krebsforschung', 56–60.

[160] Voswinckel, *50 Jahre Deutsche Gesellschaft für Hämatologie und Onkologie*, 82–95 and 134–5.

[161] Scheybal (2000), 16–25.

which would hold one hundred beds in two radiotherapy departments.[162] It was endowed by Adolf Hitler with a 'Führer donation' of 50,000, and later 100,000 Reichsmarks. The original Institute for Cancer Research did not become a part of this new institute, nor was it disbanded. Instead, it was, as Ferdinand Sauerbruch had desired, brought under the wings of his surgery clinic at the Charité.[163] These decisions had far-reaching consequences for the terminally ill and dying patients at the cancer pavilions. Racist, antisemitic pseudoscience and territorial struggles between surgeons and radiologists were two serious problems. They were exacerbated by the decision to take the institute in a new direction. Arthur Hintze, one of the newly appointed directors, wrote:[164]

> The idea of an institute for cancer treatment is not new, but the spirit with which I want to fill this institute is: orienting the compass towards the curing of the sick.... The institute will be a research establishment; it should not be a centralized receptacle for all kinds of cancer patients that other hospitals want to get rid of.[165]

But if the 'compass' was supposed to be directed towards curing patients, what happened to incurable patients for whom the new General Institute against Tumorous Diseases did not want to become a 'receptacle'? The cancer pavilions at the Charité remained responsible for these patients, while at the same time having diminished resources to care for them. As early as November 1934, Dr Adam, who had become the ward's lead doctor, complained:

> The situation at the Ca-pavilion, station 3, is such that it does not seem fitting to continue to use it to house patients. Irrespective of the fact that it is unbearable for the medical sensibility to place seriously ill patients in such wholly inadequate surroundings, the technical difficulties of caring for patients are such that regular business is only possible with serious effort and then only in mediocre fashion. Adequate heating for the coming winter will be very difficult in the sick wards. It is already such that the rooms are either too cold or too warm.[166]

But although the influential surgeon Ferdinand Sauerbruch formally led the institute and supported Adam's suggestions for improvement, conditions for the terminally ill cancer patients were in no way bettered over the following years.

[162] Letter from the Berlin Police Chief (composed by Scholtz) to the Mayor of the Imperial Capital City Berlin, Main Health Department, Berlin, 20 December 1938, LAB A Rep. 003-03, no. 161, 17 front and reverse.

[163] Scheybal, 'Krebsforschung in der Zeit des Nationalsozialismus', 26.

[164] Ibid., 46–7.

[165] Quoted in ibid., 89.

[166] Letter from Dr Adam, Radiology Department of the University Institute for Tumorous Diseases at the Charité to the Board of the Charité, Berlin, 20 November 1934, HU Archiv Charité-Direktion, no. 2724, 28–9.

Instead, the institute began an odyssey through various new spaces, forced to move multiple times because the buildings it was using were needed for purposes seen as more urgent. First, it moved from the cancer pavilions into the third floor of a Charité building located at Robert-Koch-Platz 3. But in 1936, it had to move to the second floor because the space on the third was needed as nurses' quarters. In August of the same year, it had to move again to an empty building on the Charité campus. In late 1939 or early 1940, that building was slated for demolition, and so the division for seriously ill patients moved back to Robert-Koch-Platz, now to the first floor. But again, it had to leave and arrived at Luisenstrasse 2, probably in early 1942.[167]

Thus, while much money was spent on the new cancer treatment centre at the Rudolf Virchow Hospital in order to produce research and improve care for cancer patients seen as curable, the responsible authorities were unwilling to grant sufficient space and funding to the clinic for incurable and dying cancer patients. This had been true well before the war. For the period during the war, two complaints preserved in the archives reveal what this situation might have meant for patients. In June 1940, a civil servant named Dr Josef M. from southern Berlin described in a long letter to Bernhard Rust, Reichsminister of Science, Education, and National Culture, how his wife had experienced her cancer treatment during the twenty days she spent at the clinic at Robert-Koch-Platz:

> Even entering the place must appal the patient, it is a real dungeon they're being brought into here.... There is no elevator, just a small spiral staircase that the patients either have to drag themselves up with difficulty or must be carried up with great care.... The toilet in the men's section can only be reached by passing through the common bathroom for all genders. In front of this bathroom is the only space where the people who have fallen victim to their illness can be kept until somebody comes and picks them up.... The switchboard does not have labels so that the nurses might see who called. The effect of this is that the nurses must unnecessarily go from room to room and thus unnecessarily disturb the patients. How often it occurred that my wife, after just having fallen asleep, was awoken by a nurse asking her if she had just rang.... There is not even the barest recreation room for patients who are not bedridden, and there is absolutely no

[167] The available archival sources make it difficult to reconstruct the relocations and their destinations precisely. In her dissertation, Scheybal writes that the section had already moved in 1933 to a ward at the skin clinic on the second floor of the building at Robert-Koch-Platz 3. In 1937, she writes, it moved, together with the radiology department, into the building of the Strassmann Clinic at Schumannstrasse 18. See Scheybal, 'Krebsforschung in der Zeit des Nationalsozialismus', 26. Voswinckel, *50 Jahre Deutsche Gesellschaft für Hämatologie und Onkologie*, 90 also references the move to the Strassmann Clinic, which had recently been expropriated from its owners. However, this contradicts the content of Hans Auler's writing from 16 July 1940, the patients' complaints quoted here, and the response to them from the doctor of the city's health department from 3 October 1942. Auler's text informs the account of the relocations given here. According to him, only the radiology department moved to Schumannstrasse 18, not the section for severely ill patients.

> attempt in these spaces to offer the patients and their caretakers even a bit of comfort and accommodation.[168]

In a statement to the Charité's board of directors, Hans Auler noted that many patients had filed similar complaints and he confirmed that all of Dr M.'s criticisms were true.[169] But his proposals on how to improve the situation were ignored. In July 1942, Martha H. from Kleinmachnow, a small town outside of Berlin, wrote to Reich Health Leader Leonardo Conti in order to report on the 'very ugly conditions' at the clinic at Luisenstrasse 2, where she had spent eight weeks as a patient:

> The very deficient rooms—it is an old building with a heating oven—let in little light and air. The women's rooms have direct access to those of the men. The tobacco smoke of the men penetrates the fairly large cracks in the doors, which is almost unbearable for me, especially at night when some men smoke when they cannot sleep. It is also unbearable that less sick patients have to lie in the same rooms as seriously ill and dying patients. The pestilent smell of the final stage of this serious illness does not facilitate health. I have only been able to sleep somewhat with a moist handkerchief over my face. A patient with a stomach illness next to me often vomited because of the disgust caused by the bad odour. Ventilation is made very difficult because of the heavy blinds.[170]

A medical inspector from Berlin's health department wrote a report on 3 October 1942 in which he corroborated the complaints and called the 'treatment division of the institute, as it is now, a cultural disgrace'. But the police correspondent, a high government official and medical officer named Dr Franz Redeker, dismissed the whole thing as a conspiracy set up by Hans Auler. He told Reich Minister of the Interior Wilhelm Frick: 'Naturally, such unproductive statements only hinder the war effort.'[171] And so, things remained miserable and 'ugly' at the Station G IV until it was evacuated—probably together with the surgical clinic—to Berlin's Buch section to escape Allied bomb raids.

This marked the end of the history of Berlin's Institute for Cancer Research. Established in 1903 with great hopes and exceptional engagement, the institute

[168] Copy of a Letter from Ministerial Offical Dr Josef M., Bismarckstr. 19, Berlin-Lichterfelde, June 1940, to the Minister of Culture, HU Archiv, Charité-Direktion, no. 2724, 100–1.

[169] Letter from Hans Auler to the Board of the Charité, 16 July 1940, HU Archiv, Charité- Direktion, no. 2724, 103–4.

[170] Letter from Former Patient of the Charité Tumour Clinic Martha H. to Reich Health Leader Dr Conti, Kleinmachnow, 22 July 1942, BArch R 4901/1341, 41–2.

[171] Copy of a Letter from the Medical Officer and Head of the Health Department to the Mitte Health Department and the Police Chief of Berlin, 3 October 1942; Copy of a Letter from the High Government Official and Medical Officer Dr Franz Redeker of the Berlin Police Headquarters, Division V, to the Reich Minister of the Interior, 12 January 1943, BArch R 4901/1341, 43–4.

was one of the first that explicitly aimed to care for cancer patients who were seen as incurable. But the end of its story was not entirely unique. A look at the Samaritan House in Heidelberg elucidates that what happened in Berlin was part of a nationwide policy to 'Aryanize' cancer research and treatment, which excluded terminally ill and dying cancer patients. In Heidelberg, too, the director of the Institute for Experimental Cancer Research and the head of the Samaritan House, Richard Werner, was forced into retirement in 1934 by the Nazis' anti-semitic legislation.[172] Former lead doctor Otto Ewald became acting director, but he could not stop the institute from being incorporated into Heidelberg's surgery clinic, just as Berlin's institute was merged with the Charité's surgery clinic. As part of the annexation, the radiotherapy division had to pay the surgery clinic sixty Reichsmarks for every patient who came in for treatment, causing the Samaritan House to lose considerable revenue. Ewald tried to fill the gap by selling some of its radium. Even after the fees were abolished in 1939, though, the Heidelberg institute had to grapple with a series of restrictions and was constantly under-staffed. Though its name was changed to the Czerny Hospital in 1942, it could no longer function as its namesake had envisioned. Like in Berlin, providing adequate care and treatment for terminally ill and dying cancer patients became increasingly difficult.[173] Germany's two clinics dedicated to treating incurable cancer patients offered them the hope that they could spend their final days enjoying good medical care. They had always had to make do with less than desirable financial conditions. But year by year, National-Socialist policies undermined even this barebones economic foundation.

The New Paradigm of Rehabilitation

By the end of the Second World War, hospitals and asylums in Germany were in a desolate state. Many hospitals were partially or completely destroyed, sickbeds were moved to schools, hygienic conditions were catastrophic. Thus, in the first years after the war, authorities prioritized the reconstruction of hospitals at their former locations and treatment for people suffering from a lack of food and diseases like typhus.[174] Medical care for cancer patients was relegated to secondary status, and the lack of adequate facilities for them was hardly discussed by health officials.[175] Thus, it took until the 1950s before cancer treatment started to improve in both East and West Germany.

[172] Neubert, 'Das Institut für experimentelle Krebsforschung', 967. [173] Ibid., 967–9.

[174] Jürgen Wasem, Gerhard Igl, Aurelio Vincenti, Angelika Behringer, Udo Schagen, and Sabine Schleiermacher, 'Gesundheitswesen und Sicherung bei Krankheit und im Pflegefall', in *1945–1949. Die Zeit der Besatzungszonen. Sozialpolitik zwischen Kriegsende und der Gründung zweier deutscher Staaten*, ed. Udo Wengst (Baden-Baden: Nomos, 2001), 464–528, 498.

[175] Wasem et al., 'Gesundheitswesen und Sicherung', 506–7.

However, in the mid-1950s, a topic arrived in health policy discourse in both Germanys that would lastingly change cancer patients' experiences with the healthcare system: rehabilitation and aftercare. Though both states had different reasons and developed different programmes, medical discourse in East and West Germany quickly grasped the process of convalescent patients' recovery after treatment as a problem in its own right. The German discussions were part of a broader international 'moment of recovery', as David Cantor described the two decades between the end of the 1940s and beginning of the 1970s, which also encompassed other European countries and the United States.[176]

Rehabilitation and Silence towards Cancer Patients

In early September 1945, 35-year-old mother of six Elisa R. went to the University of Heidelberg's hospital complaining of pains in her left breast. A few months earlier, right after the end of the war, a small lump had been removed from it and, a month after that, a relapse was excised. The doctors found a relapse again. On 19 September 1945, surgeons removed a 'compact, cherry-sized lump'. A histological analysis identified it as cancer. The doctors thus recommended a mastectomy, which they scheduled for 22 September. Of the operation, Elisa R.'s patient file states:

> Oval cut around the mamma. Dissection of it from the breast wall along with the pectoralis maj. after separating it at the connection with the upper arm. The pectoralis min. is also for the most part removed. The remarkably strong bleeding is stopped. Thorough draining of axillary glands, whereby no enlarged glands are visible. On the lateral thorax surface, the fat tissue is removed as much as possible, because some lumps were found here. Despite strong tension, the skin can be closed over the wound.[177]

In short, the operation was 'radical'. The surgeons amputated Elisa R.'s breast and both breast muscles (*pectoralis major* and *minor*) and removed the axillary glands and the fatty tissue on the side of the chest. The healing process went well, enabling doctors to remove the surgical drain three days later and allow the patient to stand. On 1 October, the doctors took out stitches and irradiated the operated area for the first time. On 11 October, less than three weeks after the operation, the mother of six was 'released home in good shape with smoothly healed wound'. Eight weeks later, she had to come in for a second series of radiation treatment. The files, like many others from the period, contain no

[176] Cantor, *Cancer in the Twentieth Century*.

[177] Patient File Elisa R, UAH, preliminary signature: Acc. 11/02 (Surgery Clinic), 1945, no. 3054.

mention of post-treatment care. In all likelihood, Elisa R. was sent home without further ado after the second round of radiotherapy, where she, perhaps with the support of family and friends, looked after her six children and her household. As a housewife and mother, she was not eligible for a stay at a health resort. But working men and women did not necessarily qualify for post-treatment options, either, because the public insurers did not cover it and there were not enough recovery resorts and aftercare centres.

In the 1950s, doctors and health policymakers in both Germanys began recognizing that the immediate return to 'normal' life after an extended period at the hospital was not just a burden for the patient, but could also compromise the success of the expensive cancer treatment.[178]

And they drew on very similar arguments. First and foremost was the insight that local cancer treatment had to be rounded out with holistic care aimed at bolstering physical and mental defences. This realization was the product of a clutch of observations and discursive shifts. One was the sobering truth that cure rates had not improved much at all since the 1920s, despite all of the therapeutic innovations of the intervening years. Surgery in particular seemed to have reached its limits, as the 'radical' methods could not be taken any further. Things were different for radiotherapy, as megavoltage x-rays had only recently been invented.

However, many oncologists were convinced that the key to long-term recovery was holistic treatment. This perspective harmonized with research on vitamins and hormones that had been conducted since the 1930s in Nazi Germany, the Soviet Union, the United States, and multiple European countries. Meanwhile, research on stress provided verifiable evidence that mental health could influence physical health and the immune system. And statistics gathered by some regional cancer societies established a correlation between the social status of women with cancer and their chances of being cured. This seemed to suggest that quality nourishment, low levels of physical and mental stress, access to paid assistance, and a lack of worries about one's finances and the future of one's family played a significant role in convalescence.[179]

Society's new interest in aftercare for cancer patients was more comprehensive than it might seem at first glance. Efforts to provide aftercare had long been limited to local initiatives. The primary hindrance to broader, more organized actions was many doctors' and health policymakers' belief that cancer patients would not be able to return to work permanently, and thus that it was not 'worth

[178] Copy of a Statement on Rehabilitation for Women with Cancer, signed Hanke, undated [1957], BArch DQ1 6120; German Central Committee for Fighting Cancer and Cancer Research (President Prof. Dr Heinrich Martius, MD), Memorandum on the Care and Economic Security of Cancer Patients, Göttingen, July 1958, 3–4, BArch B 142/410, 412–18.

[179] Johannes Kretz, 'Die gegenwärtigen Aufgaben der Krebsbekämpfung', *Der Krebsarzt* 10, no. 1 (1955): 209–17, 216–17; Heinz Kirchhoff, 'Der Einfluß sozialer Faktoren auf Ablauf und Heilung des Genital-Karzinoms der Frau', *Deutsche Medizinische Wochenschrift* 79, nos. 31/2 (1954): 1153–5, https://doi.org/10.1055/s-0028%961119330.

it' to expend resources trying to reintegrate them into working life. After 1945, doctors did not necessarily become more optimistic, but they generally thought it less acceptable to exclude people from social life and the workforce just because they were chronically ill, 'disabled', or 'incurable'. Karl Heinrich Bauer, co-founder and first director of the Deutsches Krebsforschungszentrum (German Cancer Research Centre) in Heidelberg, pithily captured this view in a lecture held in Wiesbaden at the 1968 annual conference of the state of Hesse's cancer research society. He expressed doubt that post-treatment care or a stay at a health resort could increase cancer patients' chances of survival, but nevertheless pled for the expansion of rehabilitation services:

> Sure, the imported word 'rehabilitation' when used in connection with cancer sounds bad in us surgeons' ears, since the incurable cancer patient is so often not 'rehabilitable', but who can escape the subtle tyranny of such concepts when talking about legal claims in a welfare state![180]

The 'tyranny' to which Bauer was rhetorically capitulating was rooted in the social and political acceptance of a notion that had gained an international following during the Second World War and remained a permanent feature of public discourse in both German states after 1949. 'Rehabilitation' had affinities with some welfare programmes of the Weimar Republic, such as 'care for crippled persons', but most proponents sought to distance it from this history, and especially its fate under National Socialism.[181] New efforts at rehabilitation were focused on people with physical disabilities and, particularly in West Germany, 'combat wounded veterans', but the concept still had a broader scope.[182] The West German government convened a committee to reorganize social welfare services, which, in 1954, defined rehabilitation as a range of 'measures taken for the best possible recovery of the remaining abilities after illness or injury with the goal of optimal adaptation to living conditions through vocational training and occupational reintegration'.[183] In East Germany, the concept was understood even more expansively as the 'systematic and organized medical, psychological, social, and economic treatment of every sick, injured, or otherwise physically incapacitated person'.[184]

[180] Karl Heinrich Bauer, 'Wert der sogenannten "Krebsnachkur" für radikaloperierte Kranke', *Hessisches Ärzteblatt* 30 (1969): 215–18, 215.

[181] Wilfried Rudloff, 'Rehabilitation und Hilfen für Behinderte', in *1949–1957. Bundesrepublik Deutschland. Bewältigung der Kriegsfolgen, Rückkehr zur sozialpolitischen Normalität* (Baden-Baden: Nomos, 2005), 517–57, 517. For a survey, see Gabriele Lingelbach and Anne Kleinschmidt, 'Kontinuitäten, Zäsuren, Brüche in der deutschen Disability History nach 1945', in *Kontinuitäten, Zäsuren, Brüche? Lebenslagen von Menschen mit Behinderungen in der deutschen Zeitgeschichte*, ed. Gabriele Lingelbach and Anne Kleinschmidt (Frankfurt: Campus, 2016), 7–27.

[182] Rudloff, 'Rehabilitation und Hilfen für Behinderte', 524–5.

[183] Quoted in ibid., 518.

[184] Hans-Günther Häublein, 'Rehabilitation schafft Gesundheit und besseres Leben', *Arbeit und Sozialfürsorge* 13 (1958): 612–15, 612.

In both the GDR and the FRG, rehabilitation was first and foremost about restoring a person's ability to work. On the one hand, working was considered the foundation of a meaningful life in society. On the other, rehabilitation saved the welfare state the costs of early retirement.[185]

This reasoning defined rehabilitation programmes in both German states into the 1970s, perpetuating the exclusion of those seen as having little chance of re-entering the labour market.[186] Termed 'incurable' in the years before 1945, these persons simply fell out of sight. But when they were under discussion, it was with a new name. The German word '*unheilbar*' (incurable) was avoided on account of its negative association with Nazi euthanasia programmes. Preferred now was its Latinized form '*incurabel*', which had already been used in specialist publications and matched with its English counterpart.[187]

The new term 'the wretched' (*die Desolaten*) also entered into use.[188] It defined misery and bleakness as the essence of terminally ill cancer patients' experience while establishing a parallel between their physical and emotional state of being. But it was not just the words used to describe them that were new. The bodies of dying cancer patients had also changed. Improved radiotherapy techniques that more accurately targeted the body part to be irradiated as well as earlier diagnoses decreased the prevalence of visible 'deformities' caused by tumours. Moreover, the noxious smell given off by decaying tumours also became less common. The feeling of disgust that had so often determined others' comportment towards cancer patients diminished. As a perhaps paradoxical consequence, medical discourse more easily overlooked them and often unquestioningly grouped them together with all patients in need of intensive care.

During the 1950s, post-treatment care did not count among the prominent medical topics in the two Germanys. However, East Germany began building care centres early on, though not entirely out of humanitarian motivations: one reason was to relieve hospitals of having to care for 'incurable' cancer patients.[189] Soviet decree no. 92 from 22 April 1947 ordered that care centres be constructed in the Soviet Occupation Zone, which, in contrast to the Weimar Republic's cancer

[185] Rudloff, 'Rehabilitation und Hilfen für Behinderte', 556–7.

[186] Elsbeth Bösl, 'Die Geschichte der Behindertenpolitik in der Bundesrepublik aus der Sicht der Disability History', *Aus Politik und Zeitgeschichte* 23 (2010): 6–12; Dr Rautenberger, Letter to the District Health Official Responsible for Tumorous Diseases, Berlin, 23 April 1957, BArch DQ 1 6341.

[187] Prof. Dr Wilhelm Flaskamp, Oberhausen, Welche Forderungen stellt der DZA an die Krebsbekämpfung (presentation held at a conference of the Commission for the Economic Security of Cancer Patients, 3 and 4 March 1960 in Düsseldorf), BArch B 142/2027, 75–6.

[188] Linde, 'Krebsfürsorge im Rahmen der Krankenhausfürsorge', 638; H.-D. Jung, 'Das Waldkrankenhaus Lychen—ein neuartiges Rehabilitationszentrum für Geschwulstrekonvaleszenten', *Internationale Arbeitstagung über Fragen der Rehabilitation, Dispensairebetreuung und Prämorbidität* (Leipzig, 1958), 267–78, 274.

[189] Filing from the Head Doctor of the Municipal Women's Clinic of Leipzig, Dr Hirschberg, and the Clinic's Administrative Head Starge, to the Administrative Councilor for Labour and Welfare of Leipzig, 26 November 1953, BArch DQ1 6120.

treatment centres, were to be centrally administered by the state and taken out of the hands of religious organizations.[190] At the end of the war, there were roughly 20,000 care centre beds in the territory of what would become the German Democratic Republic—by 1961, the number had mushroomed to 37,000.[191] West Germany's Federal Social Assistance Act (Bundessozialhilfegesetz) gave legal priority to domestic care by paying 100 Deutschmarks a month to family members or loved ones to attend to the patient and by covering expenses they incurred in doing so.[192]

And while the principles guiding rehabilitation were similar in both states, their translation of these principles into practice diverged. Because of the dire situation of East Germany's economy into the mid-1950s, its local counselling centres for cancer patients focused on distributing coal vouchers and nutritional assistance to clients.[193] Beginning in the mid-1950s, the Ministry of Health instituted a programme for cancer patients with good chances of soon returning to work. It involved sending them to convalescence resorts without bureaucratic red tape immediately after they completed medical treatment. In order to facilitate this, all care centres for cancer patients were given a certain number of vouchers that allowed cancer patients to take the waters for a few weeks without having to submit a special application.[194]

Many doctors thought it pressing that the state construct convalescence centres for 'tumour patients', a word chosen to refer to cancer patients in the GDR in order to reduce fears, as tumours can be benign, too. Such institutions, they argued, could meet the particular needs of recovering cancer patients. Providing specialized rehabilitation services seemed more important than the old, still widespread concern that housing cancer patients together could negatively impact their mood and thus inhibit their betterment.

A 1955 draft from the Ministry of Health's archives records the specifications for such convalescence centres. They were supposed to be small buildings with a maximum of thirty beds in two-bed rooms, secluded in nature, and, 'in order to avoid visits, as far away from a train station as possible'. Equipped with a lawn, recreation rooms, and a library, they were supposed to offer cancer patients six weeks of peace, where they could recover their strength with a protein-rich diet and not have to worry about their families, who were taken care of by employees

[190] Matthias Willing, *'Sozialistische Wohlfahrt'. Die staatliche Sozialfürsorge in der Sowjetischen Besatzungszone und der DDR (1945–1990)* (Tübingen: Mohr Siebeck, 2008), 52–71.

[191] Jürgen Wasem, Doris Mill, and Jürgen Wilhelm, 'Gesundheitswesen und Sicherung bei Krankheit und Pflegefall', in *1961–1971 Deutsche Demokratische Republik. Politische Stabilisierung und wirtschaftliche Mobilisierung*, ed. Christoph Kleßmann (Baden-Baden: Nomos, 2006), 377–428, 383.

[192] Gerhard Igl, 'Sicherung im Pflegefall—Rechtsentwicklung', in *1957–1966 Bundesrepublik Deutschland. Sozialpolitik im Zeichen des erreichten Wohlstandes*, ed. Michael Ruck and Marcel Boldorf (Baden-Baden: Nomos, 2007), 426–32, 426–9.

[193] Meeting of the District Officials for Fighting Cancer, 19 April 1955, Berlin, BArch DQ1 6120.

[194] Preprint of a Letter from the Common Illness Division of the Magdeburg Health Department, 30–43, to the District Councillors and the Care Centres for Cancer Patients, 20 November 1956, BArch DQ1 6120.

of the counselling centres for cancer patients.[195] However, not everyone experienced this compulsory separation from family as a relief. A complaint about rules against phoning home or receiving phone calls exemplifies this. Its author, a civil servant employed with the Interior Ministry, wrote it in the name of his wife and a woman she met during her stay at the retreat. He detailed how the inability to know about the well-being of their families created a sense of insecurity harmful to the women, giving them the feeling that they were isolated from the world and 'locked up' on account of the severity of their illness.[196]

In 1956 and 1957, the state found three properties that fit its criteria. Until the GDR's demise in 1990, thousands of cancer patients would visit them for post-treatment care. All of their buildings had been constructed in the first half of the twentieth century and were retrofitted for the convalescence centres. Only one of the buildings had been originally built as a medical institution: the Waldkrankenhaus (Forest Hospital) in Lychen (Fig. 27), situated amongst lakes and woods, which had served as a sanatorium for tuberculosis patients. Without much new construction, the Waldkrankenhaus opened on 1 September 1957 as one of East Germany's first Geschwulstrehabilitationszentren (Tumour Rehabilitation Centres).[197] Equipped with forty beds, it was supposed to primarily serve women with cervical cancer and breast cancer from the Neubrandenburg district, the Greifswald University Hospital, and the Berlin Friedrichshain district hospital.

Two months earlier, the official at the Ministry of Health overseeing the rehabilitation centres toured the Georgi Dimitroff Rehabilitation Centre. Established in early 1957, it had capacity for eighty-four patients. Most of its rooms were larger than its counterpart in Lychen, since it was a veritable mansion that textile magnate Ernst C. Lehmann had constructed in 1928/29 in the village of Bärenklau in Lower Lusatia. In 1945, the Soviet Military Administration had seized the building and used it for a few years as a school for the Free German Trade Union Federation.[198] Like in Lychen, the resort had a library, a number of recreation rooms, a park, and access to the nearby woods. Its old fireplaces and stately furniture, which had remained after it was expropriated, impressed its visitors (Fig. 28).

In 1956, a rehabilitation centre was set up in Ziegenhals just southeast of Berlin. It was housed in an old building that was, however, a bit less grand. Built in 1906 on a peninsula in Lake Crossin, it had originally served as a restaurant and residence. Furnished in the style of the 1950s, the clinic began serving patients

[195] Copy of a Proposal for Establishing a Rehabilitation Centre for Post-Treatment Care of Women Who Have Undergone Operations for Genital Carcinoma, signed Hanke, BArch DQ1 6120.

[196] Complaint from Günther F. to the Ministry of Health, Division for the Organization of Prophylaxis, Berlin, 2 March 1967, 4 and 6–8; Statement from Dr Herold to the Filings from Günther F. and Ursula B., undated, BArch DQ1 2277.

[197] Jung, 'Das Waldkrankenhaus Lychen', 270.

[198] File Memo, signed Dr Rautenberg, Berlin, 29 June 1957, BArch DQ1 6341.

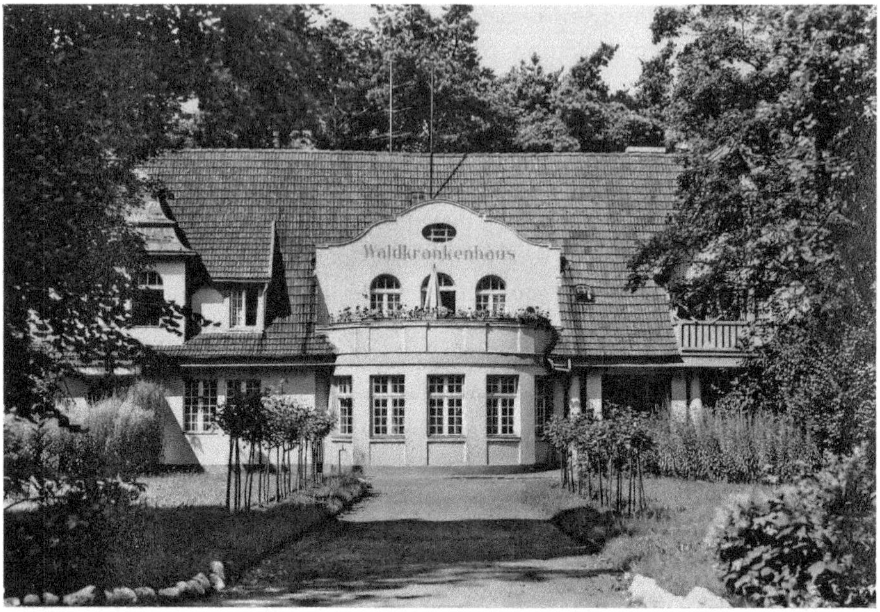

Fig. 27 Postcard of the Waldkrankenhaus in Lychen (before 1970).

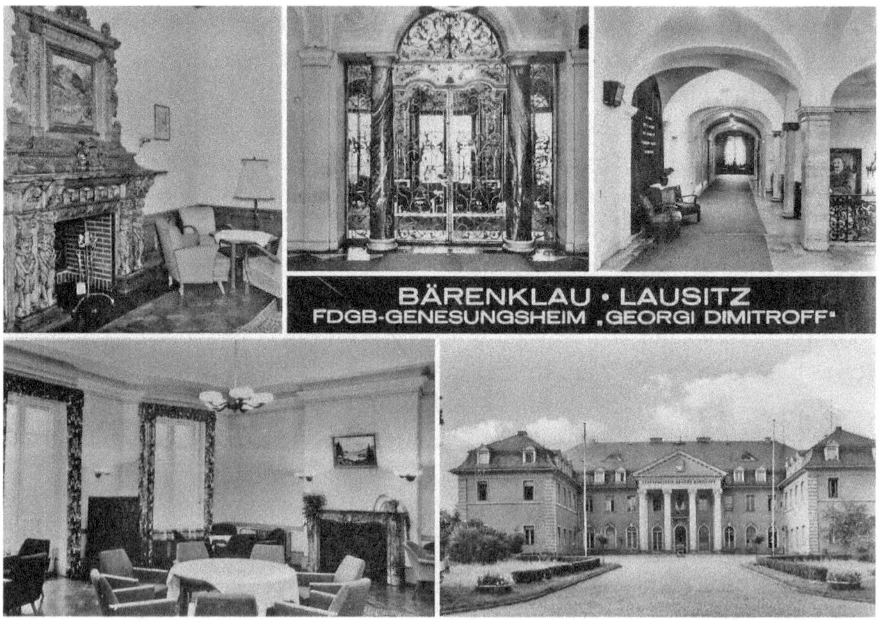

Fig. 28 Postcard of the Georgi Dimitroff Rehabilitation Centre in Bärenklau (before 1971).

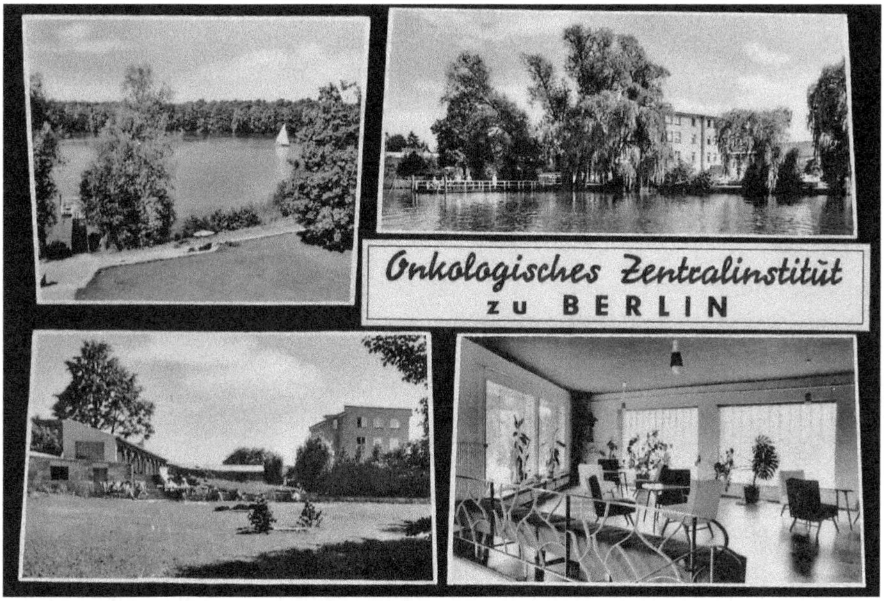

Fig. 29 Postcard of the Berlin Central Oncology Institute in Ziegenhals (*c.*1970).

from the counselling centres in the Berlin region in 1960. In January 1965, it became part of the new Onkologisches Zentralinstitut zu Berlin (Berlin Central Oncology Institute), which coordinated the work of rehabilitation centres for cancer patients in the GDR (Fig. 29).

The new name was used publicly and even appeared on postcards that patients could send to friends and family. However, this was not an expression of a new approach to cancer diagnoses, which were still being hidden from patients. Rather, the name 'Central Oncology Institute' was supposed to signal competence, scientificity, and the power and resources of state administration. That medical laypersons would know that oncology referred to the treatment of cancer was considered unlikely, since the word was new among doctors, too.

In contrast, the broadly familiar word 'cancer' was strictly avoided. Winfried Herberger, head doctor of Wittenberg's Hufeland Clinic, which specialized in treating cancer patients through a special diet, exercise, and other therapeutic methods, emphasized this in an unpublished annual report.[199] The clinic's house rules explicitly discouraged patients from 'talking with fellow patients about their own suffering'.[200] The proscription was motivated by the concern not only that the taboo word 'cancer' might be uttered, but also that patients talking about their

[199] Winfried Herberger, Annual Report 1961, 25 March 1961, 1, BArch DF 4/53231.

[200] Winfried Herberger, Behandlung und Pflege inoperabler Geschwulstkranker einschließlich Nachbehandlung von Krebsoperierten und Bestrahlten (Dresden: Steinkopff, 1960), 307.

illness could propel them into a spiral of fear and hopelessness. Thus, house rule number two asserted:

> While privacy and quiet calm is the goal, joy and cheerfulness should reign in the sick rooms. We prefer friendly patients more than constantly discontented, complaining, gloomy patients. Do not forget that a cheerful mood is more important for recovery than tablets and injections![201]

Similarly, nurses were told to bring 'sun' to the 'often morbid and unfriendly' patients and to avoid saying anything that might draw patients' attention to their potentially worsening state of health. Forbidden were expressions like: 'Can you STILL stand, walk? Are you STILL alright? Have you ALREADY started having back pain, received morphine? Hey, you are STILL alright! You look pale, weak! Did you lose weight AGAIN?'[202]

Nevertheless, these rules stopped short of commands that nurses and doctors be optimistic and deny concerns. They were limited to banning discussion of the sick and dying body and of emotions like sadness, fear, and despair. The clinic's leadership trivialized patients' problems as 'troubles and worries' and wanted them to talk about their issues not with fellow patients, but only with their doctor or nurse. As further evidence of its strictly pragmatic approach to patients' problems, the clinic sought to soothe patients' worries by offering them 'easy labour', handicapped passes, and help with daily affairs and diet after their release.[203]

In the 1960s, the GDR added a new technique to its toolbox of cancer therapy and rehabilitation called 'teaching solidarity and mutual aid', which saw doctors establishing 'clubs of former patients' and leading group therapy sessions.[204] The aim was to make (former) cancer patients into 'a positive collective of active persons with a shared fate who are full of hope and a desire to lead a reflected life'.[205]

But producing the feeling of being part of a 'collective' was not so easy, as exemplified by a letter written by Lotte B., who spent about six weeks at the Waldkrankenhaus in Lychen in early 1970. Towards the end of her stay, she wrote to the family of her nephew: 'We are 36 tumour patients, of them 14 men, and even 1 professor from Berlin.... I have... yet to find a sense of community and

[201] Ibid., 307. [202] Principles for Care Staff: ibid., 306 (emphasis in original).

[203] Marcel Boldorf, 'Rehabilitation und Hilfen für Behinderte', in Kleßmann, *1961–1971 Deutsche Demokratische Republik*, 451–69, 471–2.

[204] H. Berndt, H. Gummel, and G. P. Wildner, 'Zur Problematik und weiteren Entwicklung der Krebsbekämpfung in der Deutschen Demokratischen Republik', *Das deutsche Gesundheitswesen* 18 (1965): 786–97, 794, BArch B 142/3435, 50–61.

[205] Winfried Herberger, 'Die Rolle psychosozialer Faktoren im Rahmen der Rehabilitation Geschwulstkranker', *Zeitschrift für die gesamte Hygiene und ihre Grenzgebiete* 15 (1969): 67–72, 70.

have thus gone to church.'[206] In contrast, a young woman who resided at Bärenklau in 1965 wrote to her father: 'Already in Guben [the larger town nearby], the waiting room was full of "Bärenklauer". We had to wait there until the evening and all sat together at tables.... There are a bunch of young women here, some of whom are nice and intelligent.'[207]

Regardless of how well the patients got along, the East German Genesungsheime für Geschwulstrekonvaleszenten (Rehabilitation Centres for Tumour Convalescents) were the first dedicated treatment centres in Germany where cancer patients lived with one another for multiple weeks. In the decades before, cancer patients indeed had contact with others in the same situation at the clinics where they were housed, but it was at a time when pain, weakness, and other physical difficulties determined their experience to a great degree and placed serious constraints on socializing. The specialized rehabilitation centres changed all this. And even if all of their residents did not know that they had cancer, all of them had just completed similar treatments and were facing similar problems, among them the rigid rules of the resorts themselves.[208] Thus, despite all of the taboos, the centres provided the first spaces where cancer patients could consort with others who were passing through comparable times. This significantly shifted how cancer was experienced.

In West Germany, too, doctors and health policymakers pled for the establishment of special recovery centres. Spearheading this movement was a key project of the Deutscher Zentralausschuss für Krebsbekämpfung und Krebsforschung, the predecessor organization of the German Cancer Society.[209] In contrast to East Germany's convalescence resorts, which were run by a centrally organized health system with clearly defined regional subdivisions, post-treatment care in the Federal Republic of Germany remained in the hands of individual doctors, who had to refer patients to rehabilitation centres, and in the hands of the public health insurance corporations and regional anti-cancer associations, which ran the resorts. Some of these groups were able to reappropriate post-treatment centres that had been constructed in the 1920s and then used as military hospitals during the war.

One such site was Deisterhort in the town of Bad Münder in the Weser River Uplands (Fig. 30). Deisterhort was built as a tuberculosis sanatorium in 1920. In the 1950s, the stately four-storey building was converted into the first—and, for many years, only—post-treatment hospital in the state of Lower Saxony; it was administered by the federal state's Landesarbeitsgemeinschaft für Krebsbekämpfung (State Working Group for Fighting Cancer) and its public health insurance corporations.

206 Postcard from Lotte B. to the Family of Otto R., Lychen, 9 February 1970, private holding of Bettina Hitzer.

207 Postcard to Werner R., undated [around 1965], private holding of Bettina Hitzer.

208 Complaint from Günther F. and Reply from Dr Herold, BArch DQ1 2277.

209 Transcription of the Main Conference of the German Central Committee for Fighting Cancer and Cancer Research on 9 June 1956 in Göttingen, BArch B 142/411, 373–85, 381.

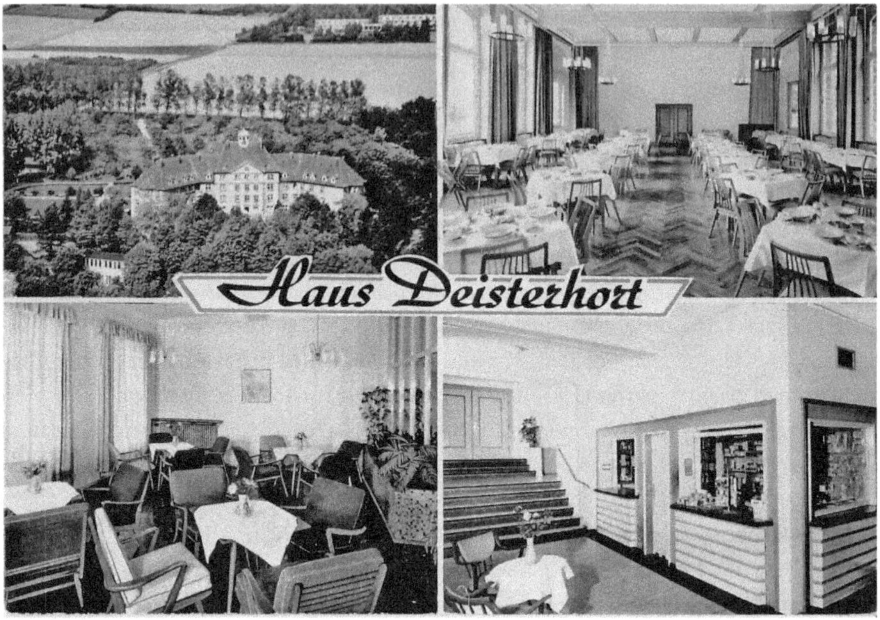

Fig. 30 Postcard of Deisterhort Convalescence Centre in Lower Saxony (before 1971).

In 1967, the government of Lower Saxony funded the construction of an annex, expanding its capacity to about 200 patients.[210]

Analogous recovery centres were set up in other West German states. In North Rhine-Westphalia, one of the first regional cancer associations of the post-war era was established in 1951. The first director of the Gesellschaft zur Bekämpfung der Krebskrankheiten Nordrhein-Westfalen (North Rhine-Westphalia Society for Fighting Cancer) was Wilhelm Flaskamp, who since 1935 had been working as the lead doctor of the women's clinic and as director of the radiology clinic at the Lutheran Hospital in Oberhausen and had close ties to the Ministry of Social Welfare in Düsseldorf.[211] In 1954, the public health insurance corporations and the retirement insurance administration in North Rhine-Westphalia founded the Arbeitsgemeinschaft für Krebsbekämpfung der Träger der gesetzlichen Kranken- und Rentenversicherung im Lande Nordrhein-Westfalen (Working Group for Fighting Cancer of the Statutory Health and Retirement Insurance Administrations of the State of North Rhine-Westphalia). By the mid-1970s, it was managing twenty post-treatment centres throughout West Germany.[212]

[210] K. Windstosser, 'Die nachsorgende Behandlung des Krebskranken. Begründung, Wesen und Wirksamkeit derselben. Gutachten in Sachen Bauer/Dr. Pauli' (Bad Salzuflen, 1976), 13, http://windstosser-museum.info/museum/veroeffentlichungen/1976.pdf. The number of 200 beds is referenced in Uta König, 'Ein Haus, das Mut macht', 37 (1980): 256.

[211] Windstosser, 'Die nachsorgende Behandlung des Krebskranken', 16.

[212] Ibid., 16.

Yet despite the early blossoming of recovery centres, the predecessor organization of the German Cancer Society published a critique of the lapidary state of post-treatment cancer care in West Germany in 1958.[213] They cited not only the inadequate number of beds, but also the fact that the public health insurers did not cover post-treatment care for unemployed women, which they underscored as particularly unjust for mothers and (soldiers') widows.[214] The only convalescence centre that offered rehabilitation to a limited number of women was the Müttergenesungswerk (Mothers' Rehabilitation Works), which was established in 1950 by Elly Heuss-Knapp, wife of West German president Theodor Heuss.[215] Moreover, the predecessor of the German Cancer Society charged that a single four-to-six-week stay was insufficient, demanding that it be supplemented with another round of post-treatment care after a few months of rest at home. This 'confirmation care' was supposed to comprise a special diet, fresh air, and exercise, as well as professionally supervised treatment with vitamins, hormones, and other medicines.[216]

The parliamentary Kommission für die wirtschaftliche Sicherung der Krebskranken (Commission for the Economic Security of Cancer Patients) took up these demands and ultimately helped translate them into a law that guaranteed convalescent care for cancer patients.[217] While resort stays in the 1950s had revolved around protecting and strengthening recovering patients through exercise, rest, and the like, the law ushered in a period of medicalization. Patients' vitals were constantly being measured and the body parts affected by cancer were regularly examined with x-rays. This was one reason why West German convalescence centres focused much more on the emotions and mental health of their patients than their East German counterparts. Another reason was German psychosomatics' interest in fear and anxiety, as discussed above, and the civil society movements of the 1970s.

For instance, in the early 1960s, North Rhine-Westphalia's cancer association conducted an evaluation of post-treatment care in which it explicitly studied the 'psychological effects of post-treatment care for tumour patients'. It concluded that 'the psychological trauma of the manifestation of the malignant tumour . . . causes

[213] Memorandum of the German Central Committee for Fighting Cancer and Cancer Research on the Care and Economic Security of Cancer Patients.

[214] Alfred Diller, Hamburg, 'Krebsbekämpfungswünsche zur Neugestaltung der Krankenversicherung', *Die Ersatzkasse H.* 5 (May 1959), BArch B 142/410, 496–7.

[215] Dr Nopitsch, 'Disskussionsbeitrag, im Anschluss an Karl Gemsjäger, Die Krebsbekämpfung in Hamburg', *Strahlentherapie* 96 (1955): 325–44, 341.

[216] Memorandum of the German Central Committee for Fighting Cancer and Cancer Research on the Care and Economic Security of Cancer Patients.

[217] Wilhelm Flaskamp, Oberhausen, 'Welche Forderungen stellt der DZA an die Krebsbekämpfung' (presentation held at a conference of the Commission for the Economic Security of Cancer Patients, 3 and 4 March 1960 in Düsseldorf), BArch B 142/2027, 75–6; Discussion Paper for a 'Comprehensive Program to Fight Cancer' as a Collective Task for the Federal and State Governments, Public Insurance Corporations, Doctors, Hospitals, German Cancer Aid, Research Associations, Research Funding Institutions, and Everyone Who Can Make a Direct Contribution to Fighting Cancer (for the 'Grand Cancer Conference' on 27 September 1979 in Bonn), 16, BArch B 138/25846.

serious mental stress, which is expressed in depression, increased affective sensitivity, decreased self-esteem and which is made noticeable—even to other tumour patients—by symptoms like inferiority complexes, distrustfulness, mental inhibitions.'[218]

The forms that doctors had to fill out after patients had completed post-treatment care also inquired into the patient's 'mood' during their stay. Their choices are indicative of what medical professionals saw as concerning behaviour: 'withdrawn, restless, anxious, depressive, exhausted, distrustful, resistant'.[219] Techniques like small group discussions moderated by doctors were supposed to result in a 'change of mood'. Thus, the head doctor of Deisterhort stated in an interview with *Stern* magazine:

> Here everyone can speak about their fears. Of course everyone who arrives here is downtrodden. But when they see how confident and joyful others are who had the same operation not a long time ago, they immediately feel better.[220]

Doctors thought that other patients whose recovery was further along could provide a powerful example for new arrivals. Perhaps already on their second or third stay at the 'house that makes courageous', as Deisterhort was called in the *Stern* article, their cooperation was deemed essential to the success of its post-treatment care.

And even if nobody in West Germany described such patient groups as 'collectives of active persons with a shared fate', as was the stated goal of their East German counterparts, in the end, both countries' rehabilitation centres served as places where cancer patients experienced a feeling of belonging to a group of people with similar experiences for the first time. This cultivation of a sense of community stood in stark distinction to the historically older feeling of exclusion and isolation experienced by many cancer patients.

The 'Radiology Bunker'

But it was not just practices, spaces, and conceptions of post-treatment care that changed after the war. Radiotherapy technology progressed by leaps and bounds,

[218] Carl Ludwig Paul Trüb and Carl Humperdinck, 'Ergebnisse einer Repräsentativstatistik über die Nachkuren bei Geschwulstkrankheiten vom 1. April 1960 bis 30. Juni 1961 in den Nachkurkliniken, Nachkursanatorien und Nachkurheimen der Arbeitsgemeinschaft für Krebsbekämpfung im Lande Nordrhein-Westfalen', in *7 Jahre Kampf dem Krebs 1956–1962*, ed. Arbeitsgemeinschaft für Krebsbekämpfung im Lande Nordrhein-Westfalen (Arbeitsgemeinschaft der Träger der gesetzlichen Kranken- und Rentenversicherung im Lande Nordrhein-Westfalen), Bochum 1964, BArch B 142/3436, 412–51, 430–1.

[219] State of the Art of Post-Treatment Care, Form published by the Arbeitsgemeinschaft für Krebsbekämpfung Nordrhein-Westfalen [undated, 1967], BArch B 142/3436, 328.

[220] König, 'Ein Haus, das Mut macht'.

which necessitated redesigning irradiation rooms. This shift had wide-ranging consequences.

The way was paved by technological innovations that physicists had been working on since the 1920s but that only entered into medical use in Europe, the United States, and the Soviet Union in the 1950s. The puzzle was to figure out how to increase the dosage of radiation to more effectively treat internal tumours without causing permanent or potentially fatal skin damage. Researchers believed the key to striking the right balance was in the percentage depth dose curve. This physical principle states that, because secondary electrons flow in the same direction as the primary beam that emits them, their effect is added to that of the primary beam and thus increases the dose of radiation absorbed by cells beneath the surface. Thus, the higher the quantum energy is, the lower the maximum dose bearable by living cells. The effect is more dramatic with electrons than with x-rays, as research in the early 1940s demonstrated.[221] In order to effectively irradiate internal tumours, beams produced with at least 1 million volts were required, which came to be called megavoltage therapy.

In the early 1920s, a patent for producing megavoltage x-rays by accelerating electrons in a magnetic field was filed. The construction of a betatron in 1935 at a lab of the Siemens-Schuckertwerke in Berlin represented the first successful realization of this concept. Military researchers in both Nazi Germany and the United States were interested in ultra-high energy radiation, too. Fascinated by its potential military utility, they poured considerable resources into studying it, which came to strongly influence the technological development of the betatron.[222] Military researchers were also interested in the cyclotron, a different type of particle accelerator invented around the same time.[223]

In the 1950s, oncological medicine began using gammatrons, another type of megavoltage radiation therapy unit that generated radiation with the radioisotope cobalt-60. In contrast to radium, cobalt-60 is not a naturally occurring element, but is produced synthetically by adding a neutron to the natural element cobalt-59. Manufacturing cobalt-60 first became possible after the discovery of the nuclear reactor by the Manhattan Project, an American military research programme that also provided the technology for the first atomic bomb. Like radium, cobalt-60 emits gamma rays, but they are much stronger and thus more effective

[221] Burghard Weiss, 'Von der Hochvolt- zur Megavolttherapie. Strahlentherapie und Großtechnologie in Deutschland und den USA, 1925–1955', in Eckart, *100 Years of Organized Cancer Research*, 137–41, 141; Josef Becker and K. E. Scheer, Introduction to *Betatron und Telekobalttherapie. Internationales Symposion am Czerny-Krankenhaus für Strahlenbehandlung der Universität Heidelberg vom 1.–3. Juli 1957* (Berlin: Springer, 1958), 1–4, 2.

[222] Weiss, 'Von der Hochvolt- zur Megavolttherapie', 140; Alexander von Schwerin, *Strahlenforschung: Bio- und Risikopolitik der DFG, 1920 bis 1970* (Stuttgart: Steiner, 2015); Bruce Cameron Reed, *The History and Science of the Manhattan Project* (Berlin: Springer, 2014), 315.

[223] Ellen Leopold, *Under the Radar: Cancer and the Cold War* (New Brunswick, NJ: Rutgers University Press, 2009), 105–6.

in therapy.[224] Moreover, the artificial synthesis of cobalt-60 was considerably cheaper than purchasing radium. The first doctor to seize on this new opportunity for cancer treatment was Harold E. Johns of the University of Saskatchewan, who conducted the first cobalt-60 therapy on a patient in 1951.[225]

The close connection between military and medical research and applications of the new radiation technologies had a number of consequences. First, there was no shortage of money for research and development, so that the first megavoltage machines with an intensity of 15 MV were soon supplanted by stronger ones. Second, military interest in the short- and long-term effects of these new types of irradiation influenced the speed at which the new devices, and in particular the gammatron, entered into clinical use. It also influenced decisions about which patients were treated with which kind of radiation. This was particularly apparent in the United States, where megavoltage therapy arrived at select clinics in the early 1950s. Cancer patients were irradiated with betatrons, cyclotrons, and gammatrons, even though scientists did not yet know which dosage would achieve the desired therapeutic result without causing devastating side effects. After all, the key advantage of megavoltage therapy—the ability to irradiate internal tumours with a high dosage of radiation—posed a serious conundrum for radiation dosimetry. The measurement unit used for x-ray treatment, the skin erythema dose, was not applicable to the new technologies, because visible reddening of the skin only occurred after the radiation had already caused serious internal damage. Despite this lack of knowledge about the proper dose, the new machines were used in normal clinical settings. Irradiated patients thus unknowingly became part of a medical experiment, even though the doctors treating them did not necessarily view it as such.

In 1955, Irma Natanson, a 35-year-old housewife and mother from Kansas, became one of the first patients in the Plains state to be treated with a gammatron. She suffered first-hand the consequences of the hasty, largely untested 'adaptation' of military technology for medical use.[226] During the first radiation series, she felt severe pain in her ribs and a tumour developed beneath her arm. Doctors soon confirmed that her ribs and the skin on her chest had been so damaged that the skin necrotized and her ribs were destroyed. More than twenty skin transplants were unable to close the large 'hole' in her ribcage. Her left lung collapsed, she could no longer lift her left arm, and she experienced terrible pain during her months-long hospital stay despite receiving high doses of painkillers.

[224] Ibid., 240; Angela N. H. Creager, 'Atomic Transfiguration', *Lancet* 372, no. 9651 (2008): 1726–27, https://doi.org/10.1016/S0140-6736(08)61721%963.

[225] Leopold, *Under the Radar*, 46.

[226] Ibid., 36–58. Many details can be gleaned from the files from the 1960 appeal, which are available online: Natanson v. Kline, Irma Natanson, Appellant, v. John R. Kline and St. Francis Hospital and School of Nursing, Inc., Appellees. No. 41, 476. Supreme Court of Kansas. Opinion Filed April 9, 1960, in *Justia US Law*, http://law.justia.com/cases/kansas/supreme-court/1960/41-476-2.html and Justia US Law, Opinion denying a rehearing filed August 5, 1960, in *Justia US Law*, http://law.justia.com/cases/kansas/supreme-court/1960/41-476-1.html.

In June 1957, she sued radiologist John R. Kline for medical malpractice for treating her with radiation even though a biopsy revealed that her tumour was contained and had not spread to lymph nodes, thus making the radiotherapy superfluous. In order to show the jury the damage that the treatment had done to her, her lawyers asked her to bare her upper body after sending the public out of the courtroom. One of the lawyers present later described what he saw: 'the ribs had been destroyed by the radiation and the best that [reconstructive surgery] had been able to accomplish, was to have a layer of skin over the opening. I recall seeing the beat of the heart reflected in movements of this skin flap.'[227]

However, the complicated nature of proving that the injuries had been caused by negligent use of a new technology made things difficult for Natanson's lawyers and the jury refused to award damages for malpractice. But she appealed and the Kansas Supreme Court overturned the ruling on the grounds that the jury had not sufficiently been allowed to consider how the doctor had failed to inform Natanson of the potential damage that cobalt treatment could have caused. The decision in *Natanson v. Kline* forced the doctor's lawyers to settle and became a milestone in the history of informed consent.

The military's role in pressing for rapid clinical use of gammatrons in order to study their effects is often overlooked.[228] The extent to which the American military influenced radiotherapy started coming to light in 1971, when American newspapers reported on experiments conducted by a team led by Eugene L. Saenger at the University of Cincinnati School of Medicine. Financed by the Department of Defence, Saenger irradiated eighty-eight cancer patients—most of whom were terminally ill—over their entire bodies, promising them that this represented the final hope at curing them or that it would have a palliative effect. He published the findings of this research in medical journals without mentioning who was funding it. In fact, Saenger and his team did not believe that irradiating patients' entire bodies would have any positive therapeutic effect. Like a series of tests that had been carried out on terminally ill cancer patients at the M. D. Anderson hospital in Houston a few years earlier, their true motive was to analyse the physical and mental effects of irradiating the entire body with different intensities of radiation—a question of considerable interest for generals thinking of deploying soldiers after dropping an atomic bomb.[229]

At first glance, this specifically American history (it is unclear if it had a Soviet complement) seems like it might have had little significance for radiotherapy in the two Germanys. The first gammatrons were installed in the GDR in 1957/8, and shortly thereafter West Germany acquired its own. Around this time, the first sets

[227] Quoted in Leopold, *Under the Radar*, 44.
[228] American historian Ellen Leopold has done excellent work analyzing this relationship. See Leopold, *Under the Radar*.
[229] Ibid., 80–98.

of verifiable data about the short- and long-term effects of local cobalt radiation were being published, making it possible to avoid the kind of horrific side effects endured by Irma Natanson.[230]

But the dual military and medical applications of the new machines helped define how they were perceived by Germans East and West. They shaped the images patients associated with the treatment. And they influenced the emotions felt by cancer patients as they waited on treatment, as they lie beneath the humming arm of the gigantic machine that 'shot' them with radiation that they could neither see nor feel. The media in West Germany in particular, but also in East Germany, dedicated much ink to the new methods of radiotherapy.

Newspapers, magazines, and radio and TV broadcasts employed the machines' military use as a metaphor to illustrate their incredibly destructive power in the fight against cancer. This followed earlier media discourse on atomic bombs, which held up the mushroom cloud 'as a clean symbol of political power and technological progress' and made it into a familiar everyday image.[231] In a 1948 article in *Der Spiegel*, the cyclotron was described as the 'strongest cannon of atomic physics'. In a 1951 article in *Das Ufer*, the author wrote how a brain tumour had been destroyed in the United States with an 'atomic explosion in [the patient's] head'. In short, the media depicted the image of radiation as a weapon in the fight against cancer more as a symbol of hope than as an object of dread.[232]

An unsettling image printed in the *Ufer* article rendered a procedure conducted at the Brookhaven National Laboratory, a research centre that was founded in 1947 at Camp Upton and run by the United States Atomic Energy Commission. It was one of four such cancer research centres where new forms of radiotherapy were experimented with on terminally ill cancer patients. The illustration shows a tiny patient strapped to a bed and isolated inside a brick depression at the top of a tower. It was intended to demonstrate the monstrous power of the therapeutic 'atomic explosion' while offering readers a look at the dangerous experiment that the patient heroically consented to. It was also touted as evidence that 'man has begun to tame the terrible violence of the atomic explosion'.[233]

In order to counter fears of nuclear winter, politicians, media, and radiologists all vigorously promoted the notion that atomic power could be 'tamed' and used for peaceful ends. Examples include the East German 'Atomic Power for Peace'

[230] T. A. Watson, 'Co60 Telecurietherapy—After Five Years', *Journal of the Canadian Association of Radiologists* 8 (1957): 22–6. See also Leopold, *Under the Radar*, 76.

[231] Gerhard Paul, '"Mushroom Clouds". Bilder des atomaren Holocaust', in *Das Jahrhundert der Bilder*, Vol. 1: *1900 bis 1949*, ed. Gerhard Paul (Bonn: Vandenhoeck & Ruprecht, 2009), 723–9, 725; Philipp Gassert, 'Popularität der Apokalypse: Zur Nuklearangst seit 1945', *Aus Politik und Zeitgeschichte* 46/7 (2011): 48–54, 50.

[232] 'Stoßkeile gegen den Krebs', *Der Spiegel* 51 (1948): 27; 'Krebs endgültig heilbar!', *Das Ufer* 13 (1951): 1–4.

[233] Leopold, *Under the Radar*, 75 and 245. Quote from 'Erste Atomexplosion im Innern des Menschen', *Das Ufer* 13 (1951): 25.

campaign and West German atomic physicist Otto Hahn's lecture on 'Atomic Energy for Peace'. But around the same time, it was becoming common knowledge that atomic energy was not as easy to control as its proponents claimed. The test of the first hydrogen bomb at Bikini Atoll in 1954 produced nuclear fallout well beyond expectations and contaminated many people on surrounding islands as well as Japanese fishermen on the boat 'Lucky Dragon No. 5'. In 1956, the American National Academy of Science released its first report on the biological effects of the fallout. Congressional hearings in 1957 engaged with the possibility that those exposed might get cancer.[234] Thus, the dangers of radioactivity were neither wholly known nor entirely calculable. New knowledge about the risks of atomic energy was thematized in film, literature, philosophy, and pop culture of the second half of the 1950s. Still, media representations of its peaceful potential remained largely unchanged until the mid-1960s.[235] The press greeted the first gammatrons that went online in East Germany in 1957/8 as the 'peaceful atom', as if peacefulness were one of their inherent attributes.[236] First and foremost, though, media reporting on the gammatron in both East and West Germany depicted it as a technological wonder, complete with detailed elucidations of how it functioned.[237] Questionable is whether cancer patients shared this hope in technology and faith in the possibility of harnessing the dangerous potential of atomic power.

After all, the spaces where radiotherapy was conducted underscored its dangers. Gammatrons, betatrons, and cyclotrons were housed behind concrete walls and thick, heavy doors. In order to effectively and economically protect others from radiation, they were almost always located in basements or bunkers.

The first gammatron used in Germany was a Canadian model set up in 1957 at the Klinik für Geschwulstkrankheiten (Clinic for Tumorous Diseases) in the Buch section of East Berlin, which later became the Robert Rössle Clinic.[238] In contrast to most machines that followed it, it was placed in a space above ground. Because of its relatively low voltage of 1.3 MV, a lead glass window was installed in the irradiation room so that patients did not have to lie in complete isolation behind concrete walls during the roughly thirteen-minute sessions. The company that manufactured it included a picture of a Canadian landscape with every order that the patient could look at during irradiation. Besides that, though, the space was empty and barren.[239]

[234] Leopold, *Under the Radar*, 23. [235] Gassert, 'Popularität der Apokalypse', 51–3.

[236] Heinrich Fritz, 'Die Kobaltkanone gegen Geschwulstkrankheiten', *Frau von heute* 13, no. 42 (1958): 24–5.

[237] Ibid.; 'Programmhinweis zur Sendung Strahlenmedizin auf neuen Wegen', *HörZu* 14 (1961): 19.

[238] Fritz, 'Die Kobaltkanone gegen Geschwulstkrankheiten', 25; author's conversation with Roland Jacob (4 November 2016); Bielka, *Geschichte der Medizinisch-Biologischen Institute Berlin-Buch*, 77 and 84.

[239] Fritz, 'Die Kobaltkanone gegen Geschwulstkrankheiten', 25; author's conversation with Roland Jacob (4 November 2016).

Throughout the late 1950s and 1960s, the rooms for gammatrons and betatrons in both East and West Germany had a similar design. For example, a radiotherapy clinic that opened in Düsseldorf in 1957 did not have a gammatron, but a powerful Siemens betatron. Its radiation rooms were partially underground, and the walls of the betatron room were twice as thick as those of the other treatment rooms. For additional protection, the architects constructed the betatron space as an annex that was essentially separated from the rest of the building and was only accessible through a door at the end of a hallway in the main building. The leaden door was so heavy that it could not be opened by hand.

After passing through the door, the patient was brought into a brightly painted space in the middle of which stood the huge betatron. Like most of the era's betatrons and gammatrons, it had a rotating head that could be moved around the patient, who would lie on the platform covered in a white cloth up to their neck. The Düsseldorf clinic had a window between the betatron room and the control room. The more powerful machines that quickly superseded it made such windows impossible. Now, clinics had to install cameras for radiologists to observe their patients, which of course did not allow patients to see the doctor treating them.

Like the gammatron, the betatron had a rotating head that emitted the radiation and lightly hummed as it moved during the session. The patient would not feel the radiation, nor would they have to tolerate the rank smell given off by the x-ray machines of the pre-war era. The inconspicuousness of the machines was praised by media as progress. In 1961, *Bunte* columnist Dr Fabian wrote: 'The primary advantages of the new machines are: no radiation hangover, no destruction of bones, no skin damage, significant effect on internal tumours.'[240] Sharing the same sentiment, if a bit more cautiously, a radiologist expounded on the gammatron's positives in a 1958 article in the East German women's magazine *Für Dich*, lauding the gammatrons purchased by the Soviet Union that year for how they 'protect the skin and the underlying tissue'.[241]

Even leaving aside the fact that gammatron irradiation did not always leave skin and bones unscathed, the new machines and the spaces that housed them were characterized by a new, singular unity of danger and safety, powerful efficacy and sensory invisibility. Just a few minutes of imperceptible radiation and four to six weeks of recovery were supposed to make the potentially fatal tumour disappear. In other contexts, the new technology seemed hardly controllable, threatening many healthy people with sudden death or torturous disease. But in proper doses, atomic power was now touted as destroying cancer and saving lives. However, even in its medical application, it was so dangerous that patients had

[240] Fabian, 'Neue Waffe gegen den Krebs'.
[241] See Fritz, 'Die Kobaltkanone gegen Geschwulstkrankheiten', 25.

to lie in a specially designed concrete room sequestered in a basement as if it were a bomb shelter.

Writers in the 1950s were themselves making the comparison, turning the word 'bunker' on its head.[242] While in wartime, bunkers protect people inside them from an external danger, 'radiology bunkers' were constructed to protect people outside the bunker from the dangerous radiation aimed at the patient alone inside of it. The dangerous instrument not only irradiated the tumour, but also affected the rest of the patient's body. Awareness of this double-sided nature of radiotherapy determined the language of discourse about it. The word 'gammatron' was rarely used in both mainstream media and specialist journals. Instead, two words that clearly identified the machine as a weapon predominated: in East Germany, it was the 'cobalt cannon', while in West Germany it was the 'cobalt bomb'.

However, did cancer patients in the late 1950s themselves experience these spaces, technologies, and the militarized language used to describe them as frightening? Did they feel emotionally isolated in facing both cancer and the dangerous machines that were supposed to cure it? Or is this just an anachronistic distortion of a perspective informed by the 1970s, when many came to perceive gammatrons and the like as symbols of the threatening, uncontrollable, 'cold' faith in technology and its dehumanizing effects? Might it perhaps have been true that up through the mid-1960s, cancer patients largely embraced the media's depiction of atomic power as peaceful and promising? Did they lie under the betatron or gammatron full of hope that it would relieve them of their illness? Did they see in the machine the only 'weapon' that was a match for their illness? Did they trust that the doctors knew how to properly measure the dosage and 'elegantly' employ the 'modern machines', as the staff of East Berlin's Robert Rössle Clinic told author Maxie Wander in 1976?[243]

The relative dearth of contemporaneous writings from first-hand experience makes it difficult to answer these questions. The bare white and grey walls and the tiling reminiscent of operating theatres suggest that doctors did not pay much mind to the emotions patients felt during radiotherapy sessions. Radiology journals seldom discussed how patients might perceive the radiation rooms and their gargantuan machines.

Patient files offer some clues, though. A few held in the archives of Heidelberg's Czerny Clinic, for instance, reveal how patients rejected operations that their doctors recommended with dire urgency. In at least two cases, the patients seem to have opted against surgery because they had seen the side effects that their parents had to endure and the futility of the entire ordeal, as those parents

[242] Heinz Vieten, 'Die neuerrichtete "Strahlen-Klinik" in Düsseldorf; zugleich ein Beitrag zur Stellung der Radiologie an der Medizinischen Akademie', *Strahlentherapie* 109 (1959): 161–8, 164.

[243] Wander, *Leben wär' eine prima Alternative*, 61.

succumbed to their cancer.[244] They requested radiotherapy with a gammatron instead, even though their doctors did not believe this to be the best option. Implied in this preference is that they did not fear the murkier dangers of the new technology as much as the familiar dangers of surgery. During the same period, patient files at the Czerny Clinic do not contain a single reference to a patient who turned down radiotherapy when it was recommended. This might be read as another sign that the hope of a cure overshadowed fears of megavolt therapy in the gammatron and betatron's initial years.

And one of the first personal accounts of radiotherapy written in German—Elisabeth Keller's diary, which was published in 1969—cast it in a generally positive light, too. Keller recounted her impressions and feelings during her treatment with cobalt-60:

> Like during an x-ray, I lie down again on a slightly mobile bed, which is then fixed into place. It can be set precisely with small adjustments. I observe the small, short nurse, who irradiates up to eighty women and men every day, various body parts.... Her responsibility is great, because everyone getting exactly the prescribed dose of radiation depends on her diligence. Any mistake would be a catastrophe that could lead to death. I observe this nurse's work with admiration.[245]

Offering a positive spin on the procedure by focusing on the nurse's great responsibility, the passage nevertheless testifies to an awareness that radiation could be dangerous and even fatal. By noting the large number of radiation sessions that the nurse had to prep every day, Keller highlighted the potential for exhaustion and with it, distraction, while measuring the dosage and aiming the beam. The discomfort in this situation derived less from the technology than from the fallibility of the human being operating it. A few months after radiotherapy, as Keller was recovering in a sanatorium, her scepticism towards it grew when side effects began appearing. Upon reading Johannes Kuhl's book on alternative medicine, *Schach dem Krebs* (*Putting Cancer in Check*), she wrote in her diary that she was 'very downtrodden': 'it shows the harmfulness so starkly that it almost makes you afraid. But it seems there is no choice in a case like mine: invasive formations of squamous cell carcinoma.'[246]

[244] The patients were Elise v. R., who was treated for breast cancer in 1961/2 in Heidelberg, and the retiree Karl Th., who was treated for bronchial cancer in 1965 at the radiology clinic and whose father died of laryngeal cancer: Patient Files of Elise v. R., UAH, preliminary signature: Acc. 14/02 (Radiology Clinic), 1961, no. 23176 and Patient Files of Karl Th., UAH, preliminary signature: Acc. 14/02 (Radiology Clinic), 1965, no. 9013.

[245] Keller, *Ich habe den Krebs überwunden*, 52.

[246] Ibid., 96; Johannes Kuhl, *Schach dem Krebs. Verhütung und erfolgreiche Behandlung der Krebserkrankung durch das Kuhlsche Kostsystem* (Zurich: Humata, 1954) (the most recent reprint was in 2014).

Her brush with fear was not directly linked to the radiation room and the foreboding technology. Rather, it evolved out of her first-hand knowledge of the painful, dangerous side effects of treatment that had, by all standards, proceeded normally and without issue. She was not alone with this fear in the second half of the 1960s. Support for this claim is provided by the film *Jeder Fünfte . . . Ein Bericht über den Stand der Krebsforschung in der Bundesrepublik* (*Every Fifth Person: A Report on the State of Cancer Research in the Federal Republic of Germany*), which was broadcast on West German television in August 1965. Director Marianne von Arnim wanted to document the state of oncological research in order to promote early detection. Towards the end of the film, she asks Werner Lorenz, professor of radiology and head of the Clinic for Radiotherapy and Nuclear Medicine at the University of Frankfurt, how his patients usually react when he tells them they should undergo radiotherapy. Lorenz responds:

> Most of our patients and their family members are very concerned about this radiation treatment. After all, they see in the choice of treatment confirmation that they have cancer. But this is not true. The population's anxiety complex about the use of invisible, powerful beams being dangerous is also totally unfounded. The most modern methods of treatment using the most modern sources of radiation allow us to avert the risks of earlier decades.[247]

This statement, which came from a doctor who encountered radiotherapy patients every day, indicates that popular fears about radiation treatment and its dangers were more widespread around 1965 than the patient files of the Czerny Clinic and Elisabeth Keller's diary suggest. But its normative content also offers a clue as to why there was so little discussion of these fears elsewhere. By giving them a voice, one ran the risk of being censured as irrational and uninformed, as a person whose emotions were not the expression of a legitimate, understandable premonition of danger, but the result of a pathological 'anxiety complex'.

Thus, it is likely that going back to the late 1950s, many cancer patients felt fear the moment that their doctors recommended they undergo radiotherapy. There is much to suggest that they were unsettled and anxious lying beneath the gammatron, thinking of atomic explosions that, in contrast to the intended message of the drawing of the Brookhaven experiment, were not lifesaving, but dangerous and destructive. Thus, the widespread view among historians of cancer and historians of atomic power that fears of 'peaceful' atomic energy only came about in the late 1960s should be relativized.[248]

[247] Script of the film *Jeder Fünfte: A Report on the State of Cancer Research in the Federal Republic of Germany*, Marianne von Arnim, BArch B 145/4719, 25.

[248] Marion Moamai, *Krebs schreiben. Deutschsprachige Literatur der siebziger und achtziger Jahre* (St. Ingbert: Röhrig Universitätsverlag, 1997), 112; Christa Karpenstein-Eßbach, 'Krebs—Literatur—

This periodization might hold for atomic fission for the purposes of electricity production. But it does not maintain for radiological cancer treatment, which was more associated with atomic energy's military uses in the metaphors employed to describe both it ('cannon', 'bomb', 'combat', 'crossfire irradiation') and the spaces where it was conducted ('bunker', 'radiation protection'). These terms from the 1950s speak to the specific fears attached to the new technologies of radiation treatment. Indeed, these fears might have contributed to a more general shift in perceptions of technology. However, they were not (and hardly could be) expressed publicly and were only 'utterable' in snippets. The late 1960s changed this, as critiques of technology and progress developed into a regular feature of public discourse. A growing number of autobiographical writings and fictional texts grappled with the 'radiology bunker' and 'cobalt cannon' in order to thematize the dehumanizing, isolating force of technology. In this matter, there were only slight differences between the numerous books and diaries published in West Germany and the few published in East Germany.

For example, author Brigitte Reimann, who received treatment for breast cancer in 1968 at East Berlin's Robert Rössle Clinic, confided in her diary in 1970:

> During the first sessions, I had terrible fear beneath this cobalt cannon. It was as comfortable as an inquisition dungeon, all kinds of strange and threateningly humming machines, and doctors and physicists with lead vests, while I was naked, exposed to the bombardment.[249]

Maxie Wander, who spent time in the same clinic six years later, reflected in her diary about why she was faring so poorly. She surmised: 'Maybe they are the symptoms—I have been unable to eat for a week—of the fear of the coming radiation from the cobalt cannon.'[250] Both authors foregrounded fear and pain. However, Reimann explained them by depicting the radiation machine as an instrument of torture and describing her feeling of being reduced to her naked, exposed body.

West German writings generally painted the spaces and machines in greater detail. In *Der Schattenfotograf* (*The Shadow Photographer*), Wolfdietrich Schnurre recounted his perception of the spaces where his wife Marina received radiotherapy treatment in 1978:

> The cobalt bunker. Steep stairs. Dampness, coolness. Banished beneath the earth. Mould spots. Crumbling plaster from the walls. Heating and ventilation room

Wissen. Von der Krebspersönlichkeit zur totalen Kommunikation', in *Epochen/Krankheiten*, ed. Frank Degler and Christian Kohlroß (St. Ingbert: Röhrig Universitätsverlag, 2006), 233–64, 239. On fear of atomic energy see Gassert, 'Popularität der Apokalypse', 52.

[249] Entry from 9 May 1970, in Reimann, *Alles schmeckt nach Abschied*, 316–17.

[250] Entry from 12 November 1976, Wander, *Leben wär' eine prima Alternative*, 77.

> repurposed into a waiting room. Scuffed chairs, water pipes, iron door. Yellowed newsprint: hummingbirds, exotic flowers . . . . The personnel runs out of the room where the patient lies beneath the cobalt beamer. The isolation and inner forlornness of the patient could not be more clearly represented. Additionally: 'cobalt bunker', 'cobalt bomb'. How powerful must the illness that I have be if it has to be treated with such warlike methods. Conceivably unpsychological, such words, conceivably logical: either way, we are on the frontlines where most of the fallen lie.[251]

Decay, paradise lost, the underworld, and lifeless grey were what Schnurre saw in the radiology department. Author Ilse van Heyst utilized similar imagery in her vehement rejection of the 'death rays' before she had even seen the machines that produce them:[252]

> I dreamed dreadful dreams. Every night I went through long subterranean passages in the middle of a stream of people. Right and left, doors led into dark chambers. They opened themselves. As if they were drawn by a magical power, one person after the other disappeared into the chambers. The door shut silently behind each one. And I knew—as one knows such things while dreaming—that none of them would ever come out. Or I experienced explosions, devastations, desert landscapes with entrances to bunker-like caves from which thick smoke seethed. No, I did not want to be irradiated. I felt that it would be my demise.[253]

Her dream connected radiotherapy with a loss of control and visions of a post-apocalyptic world. But the images leaned on descriptions of typical radiotherapy departments that she must have been familiar with, such as those of Schnurre or of Hildegard Knef in her 1975 *Stern* report. The anxious expectations churned up by her dream determined how she experienced her first real visit to a radiology clinic: 'What I found in K.—near busy streets—was exactly what I saw in my dream: long, grey, sad subterranean passages.'[254] During the actual irradiation, she feared that the machine would spin out of control and vaporize her:

> I was supposed to get oscillating cobalt radiation treatment. But the machine did not oscillate, not like one imagines when thinking of the pendulum of a clock; rather, the radiation lamp slowly moved over me and disappeared in the depth at the side of an exam table upon which I lied. Meanwhile, on the other side, a

[251] Wolfdietrich Schnurre, *Der Schattenfotograf* (Munich: List, 1978), 32–3.
[252] Ilse van Heyst, *Das Schlimmste war die Angst. Geschichte einer Krebserkrankung und ihrer Heilung* (Frankfurt am Main: Fischer, 1982), 31.
[253] Ibid., 36. [254] Ibid., 50.

> 'millstone' rose slowly and threateningly and for my feelings much too close to my body; the big leaden radiation guard. That was uncanny and I feared being grazed or even crushed. I breathed a sigh of relief every time the millstone returned to the depth and the radiation lamp returned.[255]

Similar accounts are contained in autobiographical writings, diaries, and letters published in West Germany between 1970 and the end of the 1990s. As the passage from Ilse van Heyst's work underscores, these texts did more than create a public voice for long existing fears. They also shaped expectations about what a radiology clinic should look and feel like. In some cases, they might have intensified fears by associating radiotherapy with foreboding images prominent in the criticisms of technology that were becoming popular at the time.

Once public opinion began to shift, some doctors began taking these fears seriously, and not just in West Germany, but also in the East. For example, when the hospital in Berlin's Buch section was first able to acquire a gammatron in the late 1970s, lead doctor Roland Jacob criticized the space intended for it—a former bomb shelter—even though it was well suited to the task. He rejected the idea of tiling the concrete walls, because it would have made the 'radiology bunker' look like a 'slaughterhouse'. Instead, he had green wood panelling installed and convinced the GDR's minister of culture to appropriate 100,000 marks so that he could furnish the radiology wing in a way that emanated what he thought was a vivid atmosphere of hope. Jacob realized that patients' perspectives could diverge from his own after he had the ceiling decorated with paintings of flowers, because staring at it for minutes gave some patients the feeling of already lying six feet underground. When Jacob learned of this, he had the flowers removed and commissioned an artist to paint abstract figures on the ceiling so that patients could speculate about their meaning while lying on the radiation table.[256]

Many radiology clinics of the 1980s, however, still looked just like they did in the writings of Wolfdietrich Schnurre, Ilse van Heyst, and others. The 'radiology bunker' was, for many patients, a place of emotional isolation, a dark place beneath the earth where the individual was exposed to foreboding machines and radiation that promised a cure while simultaneously posing a potentially fatal threat. In the 1960s, a new, third type of therapy gave rise to its own spaces of experience.

What Is a Day Worth? The Emotional Logic of Chemotherapy

Chemotherapy was not a post-war discovery. At the beginning of the twentieth century, Paul Ehrlich called his treatment for syphilis 'chemotherapy', by which he

[255] Ibid., 106. [256] Author's conversation with Roland Jacob (4 November 2016).

meant medicine that directly attacked the germ causing the illness. The idea garnered interest among oncologists. In Ferdinand Blumenthal's laboratory in Berlin, haematologist Hans Hirschfeld researched chemical substances effective against cancer cells, just as Ehrlich's Institut für experimentelle Therapie (Institute for Experimental Therapy) did in Frankfurt.

Beginning in the 1960s, though, the original, broad meaning of chemotherapy fell out of everyday language. The common usage of the word came to refer to medicine intended for one specific illness: cancer. The shift in language lines up with the amount of attention anti-cancer chemotherapy has received since then. Hopes were invested in it as a therapy that promised to not just locally treat the tumour, but also individual cancer cells detached from the primary tumour. Envisioned as a 'wonder drug', its severe side effects led it to become a symbol of the unbearable, unfeeling side of modern medicine.

The first chemotherapeutic agents effective in cancer treatment were nitrogen mustards, which are closely related to so-called mustard gas (sulphur mustard). During the First World War, scientists learned that mustard gas could alter a person's blood levels. In 1941, a team of pharmacologists led by Alfred Gilman and Louis Goodman at Yale University began systematically researching the biological effects of mustard gas and other alkylating agents.[257] Their studies were funded by the Office of Scientific Research and Development (OSRD), which was established in June 1941 by the United States government to coordinate scientific research in the service of the military. Gilman and Goodman's study was motivated by the fear that one of the belligerent states in the Second World War might deploy mustard gas.[258] After initial successful experiments on lab mice with malignant lymphoma, the two scientists tested nitrogen mustard on a human with lymphoma in 1942. For a short time, the lymphoma abated, only to reappear a short time later, after which the man died. The experiment was not made public during the war because it was considered a military secret, but it was discussed at medical conferences.[259]

A coincidence also fed hopes that nitrogen mustards could cure cancer. A German air raid on the port of Bari, Italy on 2 December 1943 hit an American freighter that was carrying mustard gas bombs. The mustard gas leaked

[257] Ilana Löwy, *Between Bench and Bedside: Science, Healing, and Interleukin-2 in a Cancer Ward* (Cambridge, MA: Harvard University Press, 1996), 40.

[258] Stacey L. Hail and Daniel C. Keyes, 'Vesicating Agents Including Mustard and Lewisite', in *Medical Response to Terrorism: Preparedness and Clinical Practice*, ed. Daniel C. Keyes, Jonathan L. Burstein, Richard B. Schwartz, and Raymond E. Swienton (Philadelphia: Lippincott Williams & Wilkins, 2005), 16–25, 16.

[259] Louis S. Goodman, Maxwell W. Wintrobe, William Dameshek, Morton J. Goodman, Alfred Gilman, and Margaret T. McLennan, 'Nitrogen Mustard Therapy: Use of Methyl-Bis(Beta-Chloroethyl)amine Hydrochloride and Tris(Beta-Chloroethyl)amine Hydrochloride for Hodgkin's Disease, Lymphosarcoma, Leukemia and Certain Allied and Miscellaneous Disorders', *Journal of the American Medical Association* 132, no. 3 (1946): 126–32, https://doi.org/10.1001/jama.1946.02870380008004.

into the water and caused severe chemical burns to the ships' crews. But it also caused a stark reduction in their white blood cell count.[260]

Nazi Germany also invested considerable resources in studying chemical weapons and, indirectly, on the effects of mustard gas on humans. After 1933, close cooperation developed between the military, the seven branches of the Kaiser Wilhelm Institute that were working on weapons research, industrial enterprises like the Auergesellschaft, and the Institut für wehrwissenschaftliche Zwecke (Institute for Military Science), a division of the SS's Forschungsgemeinschaft Deutsches Ahnenerbe (Research Association on German Ancestral Heritage), which was run by Heinrich Himmler.[261] In contrast to American research, there seems to have been little overlap between chemical weapon research and cancer research in Nazi Germany.[262] It is hard to say why Germany did not explore the connection between the two. One reason may have been that German cancer research during this period was concentrated on analyzing the effects of vitamins, hormones, and workplace carcinogens and on how blood tests might offer a way to detect cancer early on. Second, Nazi chemical weapons research was primarily interested in nerve agents. Its work on mustards was mostly concerned with their ability to cure exposure and less with their effects on humans' metabolism and blood levels. Third, cancer patients were probably rarely used as test subjects by German chemical weapons research because researchers conducted their experiments on concentration camp prisoners.[263] In short, most of the earliest research on cytostatic cancer treatment came from the United States.

American scientists were commissioned by the military to study not only chemical weapons, but also methods to prevent and treat infected wounds, which often killed soldiers in the field. This spurred the mass production of penicillin, which had already been discovered but was not seeing the sort of broadscale application that it would soon be known for. Meanwhile, researchers conducted expansive tests in the search for new antibiotics. Their successes raised hopes that similar largescale studies conducted by the pharmaceutical industry could discover chemotherapeutic agents for cancer treatment.[264] The American government thus initiated two research programmes that tested the ability of

[260] Löwy, *Between Bench and Bedside*, 40; Carsten Timmermann, '"Just Give Me the Best Quality of Life Questionnaire": The Karnofsky Scale and the History of Quality of Life Measurements in Cancer Trials', *Chronic Illness* 9, no. 3 (2013): 179–90, 181, https://doi.org/10.1177/1742395312466903.

[261] Florian Schmaltz, *Kampfstoff-Forschung im Nationalsozialismus. Zur Kooperation von Kaiser-Wilhelm-Instituten, Militär und Industrie* (Göttingen: Wallenstein Verlag, 2005); Julien Reitzenstein, *Himmlers Forscher. Wehrwissenschaft und Medizinverbrechen im 'Ahnenerbe' der SS* (Paderborn: Schöningh, 2014).

[262] Moser, *Deutsche Forschungsgemeinschaft und Krebsforschung 1920–1970*, 153–4, 203–4 and 231.

[263] Schmaltz, *Kampfstoff-Forschung im Nationalsozialismus*, 521–62; Reitzenstein, *Himmlers Forscher*, 129–47.

[264] On this and the following, see Ilana Löwy, 'Cancer: The Century of the Transformed Cell', in *Science in the Twentieth Century*, ed. John Krige and Dominique Pestre (Amsterdam: Routledge, 1997), 461–77, 467.

thousands of natural and synthetic substances to destroy cancer cells. They were carried out between 1945 and 1954 at two of the country's most renowned centres for cancer treatment: the Sloan Kettering Institute in New York and the National Cancer Institute in Bethesda, near Washington, DC. The industrial-sized programmes were expanded after 1955, receiving millions of dollars of funding as they were brought under the helm of the Cancer Chemotherapy National Service Centre (CCNSC). With that, the United States ascended to become the capital of international oncological research.[265]

The main focus was on substances that could hinder the growth and spread of cancer cells, substances that had been given the name 'cytotoxic agents' by Freiburg-based internist Ludwig Heilmeyer in 1947.[266] Like radiotherapy before it, chemotherapy was based on the assumption that cancer was a disease of rapid cell division.[267] Still today, alkylating agents, which include nitrogen mustard and its derivatives, remain one of the most important types of anti-proliferative substances in chemotherapy. In the 1950s, another group of chemicals entered the scene: antimetabolites, which disrupt cell division. A third group of chemotherapeutics called mitotic inhibitors also interrupt the process of cell division; their cytostatic properties began being studied after the war. The last group of cytostatic agents that drew the attention of researchers in the post-war period were antibiotics that attack not illness-causing germs, but human cells.[268]

Initial medical experiments with these substances primarily tested their efficacy on patients with different types of leukaemia and lymphoma, such as Hodgkin's lymphoma. Two factors informed this choice. First, in contrast to tumorous carcinomas and sarcomas, these forms of cancer could not be treated locally. This made treatment with chemotherapy, which worked throughout the entire body, particularly attractive. Second, at the time, there was no cure for leukaemia, which always ended in death. This was also true for most types of lymphoma. Chemotherapy thus seemed to finally offer hope for diseases that generally led to death within weeks of diagnosis if they were not treated. In contradistinction to other types of cancer, leukaemia afflicts a considerable number of children. In the face of the negative prognosis, many doctors, patients, and family members were willing to accept the risks associated with these largely untested drugs and their severe side effects.

However, the yet-new chemotherapeutic methods also could not entirely rid patients of cancer. Sidney Farber, a pathologist at the Boston Children's Medical Centre and one of the pioneers in using chemotherapy to treat children with cancer, described the best-case scenario in a 1949 article. An 8-year-old boy who

[265] Ibid., 471.

[266] Peter Voswinckel, *50 Jahre Deutsche Gesellschaft für Hämatologie und Onkologie*, 116.

[267] Löwy, 'Cancer: The Century of the Transformed Cell', 466–7.

[268] Hormones are among the chemotherapy agents that were used to treat cancer after the late 1940s. However, they do not have a cytostatic effect and are thus not part of this analysis.

entered the clinic with acute leukaemia in February 1947 had continued to take various antifolates after his initial treatment. Farber wrote: 'Leukemia is still present and there have been many complications, but he is still alive twenty-three months after the onset of his disease.' At the time, the maximum life expectancy for a child with leukaemia was six months. Still, Farber knew that 'no evidence has been presented which would justify the use of the word "cure" of acute leukaemia'.[269]

Fourteen years later, little had changed. Thus, paediatrician Johannes Oehme began his article on leukaemia therapy for children with the categorical qualification: 'A treatment that achieves a true cure does not exist.'[270] In 1966, a gynaecologist from Regensburg stated that while chemotherapy was becoming a preferred form of treatment for advanced or metastasizing solid tumours, it could still only have 'temporary' success.[271]

In the 1970s, the life expectancy of children with leukaemia increased dramatically. Some survived years after their diagnosis. Leading paediatric oncologists cautiously expressed hope that some of these children might indeed be cured.[272] But similar breakthroughs in the treatment of adults with solid tumours were lacking.[273] Thus, during these first decades, curing cancer with chemotherapy remained outside the realm of possibility. Remission, the temporary disappearance of symptoms, was the goal. Chemotherapy staved off death but could not ultimately prevent it. In this respect, it represented a wholly new type of cancer treatment. Even though surgery and radiotherapy often did not deliver a cure, doctors and patients embarked upon these paths in the hope that they would. In the first years of chemotherapy's existence, doctors knew that it could 'only' defer death for a certain period of time. This confronted doctors with a conundrum. In their attempts to solve it, they searched for new procedures and treatments, while at the same time changing their view of cancer as well as their approach to the doctor-patient relationship.

Experiments with chemotherapy in the United States had already demonstrated that the difference between the dosage effective for treating cancer and the dosage fatal for the individual patient was minute, making it necessary to test new substances in extensive clinical studies.[274] The end result was an unprecedentedly tight integration of pharmaceutical laboratory research, preclinical research, and clinical research. In order to arrive at and compare findings, though, researchers

[269] Sydney Farber, 'Some Observations on the Effect of Folic Acid Antagonists on Acute Leukemia and Other Forms of Incurable Cancer', *Blood* 4, no. 2 (1949): 160–7, 165–6.

[270] Johannes Oehme, 'Die Therapie der Leukämien im Kindesalter', *Blut* 9 (1963): 471–80, 471.

[271] W. Schärtl, 'Interne Karzinombehandlung mit dem Zytostatikum Proresid®. Vorläufige Mitteilung', *Münchener Medizinische Wochenschrift* 108, no. 2 (1966): 112–14, 112.

[272] Krueger, *Hope and Suffering*, 138–9.

[273] W. E. Berdel and U. Fink, 'Internistische Tumortherapie. Stand, Probleme, Perspektiven der Chemotherapie', *Münchener Medizinische Wochenschrift* 126, no. 41 (1984): 1166–71, 1171.

[274] Löwy, 'Cancer: The Century of the Transformed Cell', 467.

had to try to control their experiments' variables as much as possible. A key variable was the tumour itself. Unlike in animal experiments, it could not be artificially induced, but had always grown 'uncontrolled'. Thus, scientists needed to derive categories to ensure comparability. Unfit for the task were the concept of inoperability, the old assumption that some tumours were just incurable, and the simple distinction between local tumour and cancer that encompassed the entire body. Doctors and medical scientists had been trying to classify some types of cancer since the early twentieth century, such as the aforementioned Steinthal classification system for breast cancer. Ultimately, a classification system for comparing different cases of cancer gained footing. Created by French pathologist Pierre Denoix in 1943, the TNM staging system laid out three key criteria for judging the severity of tumours and comparing them with one another: the expansion of the tumour (T), whether and the extent to which lymph nodes were affected (N), and the presence of metastases (M).[275] In 1953, a research committee of the Union for International Cancer Control began working on fleshing out the TNM classification system for every known type of cancer.[276] It divided cancers into stages, which could assist in making prognoses and deciding which form of treatment to take.

Defining the stages through which cancer 'naturally'—i.e. without therapeutic intervention—progressed was supposed to enable doctors to assess how effective chemotherapy might be in a specific case, since entirely eliminating cancer from the body no longer counted as the exclusive measure of success.[277] At first glance, it seemed easy to determine whether chemotherapy had been effective: Did the tumour involute? Was there remission? But what if the tumour indeed got smaller, but then grew rapidly and the patient died? Did the chemotherapy extend their life? How long would they have lived without it? And if the tumour continued to grow, did that mean that the chemotherapy was not working? Perhaps it would have grown faster without cytostatic agents. Could it be counted as a success if symptoms like ascites subsided and breathing became easier, even though the tumour remained the same size? What if the tumour shrank but the patient felt just as sick and immobile as before, but also lived longer?

Finding answers to these questions demanded that clinics reflect on what constituted 'successful' treatment. In the West and East German clinics that had been offering chemotherapy since the 1950s, doctors were guided by criteria developed in the United States. One was the visible and palpable shrinkage of tumours and metastases. Doctors then confirmed their observations with x-rays

[275] Patrice Pinell, *The Fight against Cancer: France 1890–1940*, trans. David Madell (London: Routledge, 2002), 683.

[276] Timmermann, *A History of Lung Cancer*, 140–1.

[277] Elizabeth Toon, 'Measured Responses: British Clinical Researchers and Therapies for Advanced Breast Cancer in the 1960s and 1970s', in Timmermann and Toon, *Cancer Patients, Cancer Pathways*, 130–60, particularly 138–47.

and checked on the diminution of other symptoms like ascites. If they determined that the tumour had involuted, they wrote that the case was in remission.[278] It might be full remission—the complete disappearance of symptoms for at least four weeks—or partial remission—a 50 per cent reduction in symptoms over a period of four weeks.[279] They deemed treatment a partial failure when symptoms remained the same or when some lessened while others worsened. A total failure was when the tumour continued to grow and additional symptoms or metastases appeared. These definitions clearly show that chemotherapy's success was defined using a fairly narrow window of time, as a mere month was sufficient to register the statistically relevant result 'full remission'.

Alongside these 'objective' criteria, doctors also drew on subjective criteria. They might interview the patient about how they felt, though their responses never made their way into statistics. Still, some doctors did work with manuals that combined objective and subjective criteria and coded them for statistical evaluation.[280] These manuals were based on an evaluation table devised in 1948 by American doctor David Karnofsky when he was holding a presentation on the first chemotherapy experiments at the Sloan Kettering Institute.[281] Karnofsky offered patients three responses to assess their improvement: G = good, F = fair, O = none. A further criterion was what he called the 'performance status', which denoted the patient's ability to work and take care of themselves. His system of evaluation struck a chord with German doctors between the 1950s and early 1970s. However, the use of subjective factors to determine the effectiveness of chemotherapy for a particular patient remained a topic of heated international debate.[282]

In fact, questions about whether chemotherapy was justified at all revolved around this nexus. When it worked, it could beat back primary tumours and metastases and thus reduce pain and other symptoms. It could sometimes improve the patient's general state of health to such a degree that they could

[278] Stephan Tanneberger and Giovanni Bacigalupo, 'Einige Erfahrungen mit der individuellen zytostatischen Behandlung maligner Tumoren nach prätherapeutischer Zytostatika-Sensibilitätsprüfung in vitro (Onkobiogramm)', *Archiv für Geschwulstforschung* 35, no. 1 (1970): 44–53, 48; H. Martin and J. C. F. Schubert (1967), 'Behandlung der Lymphgranulomatose mit Vincaleukoblastin', *Blut* 16 (1967): 157–60, 159.

[279] P. Drings, R. Allner, N. Brock, H. Burkert, M. Fischer, E. Fölsch, H. Gerhartz, P. Götzky, I. Hoppe, G. Kanzler, H. O. Klein, K. Mainzer, H. Martin, P. Obrecht, G. Palme, H. Paulisch, H. Riegg, J. C. F. Schubert, U. Treske, W. Weise, D. Willems, H. Wilmanns, S. Witte, and H. Wohlenberg (1970), 'Erfahrungen mit neuartigen N-Lost-Phosphamidestern', *Deutsche Medizinische Wochenschrift* 95, no. 10 (1970): 491–7, 494, https://doi.org/10.1055/s-002%9614389.

[280] Hans Ehrhardt, 'Chemotherapie maligner Geschwülste', *Münchener Medizinische Wochenschrift* 115, no. 18 (1973): 814–32, 816.

[281] D. A. Karnofsky, W. H. Abelmann, L. F. Craver, and Joseph H. Burchenal, 'The Use of the Nitrogen Mustards in the Palliative Treatment of Carcinoma: With Particular Reference to Bronchogenic Carcinoma', *Cancer* 1, no. 4 (1948): 634–56, 634, https://doi.org/10.1002/1097%960142(194811)1:4%3C634::AID-CNCR2820010410%3E3.0.CO;2-L.

[282] Toon, 'Measured Responses', 146–50.

again care for themselves and work, and sometimes it extended their life expectancy. But at the same time, chemotherapy could cause serious, sometimes life-threatening side effects.[283]

Thus, a pressing goal of research was to identify dosages, intervals between sessions, and chemical combinations that would not have such intense side effects. Medical scientists were only able to accomplish this in clinical studies that precisely prescribed, for patients with a particular type of cancer at a particular stage, how many milligrams of which substance per kilogram of body weight should be administered over a therapy cycle, whether the cytostatic agent should be given daily or weekly, whether it should be administered through transfusion or tablet, whether it should start with a single high dose and then step down to low doses, and whether cytostatic agents should be given in the interval between two therapy cycles. Although only a few substances were in widespread use in the early 1960s, there were a multitude of variables to consider, which only expanded as more cytostatic agents were discovered over the following years. Thus, the difference between experimental clinical protocols and the so-called standard protocol was often slim.[284]

Drawing a line between experimental chemotherapy and clinical applications was further complicated by the observation that patients with seemingly identical cancers at a similar stage on the TNM scale reacted differently to chemotherapy administered according to the established protocols. In many cases, the tumour did not involute or the patient's health declined dramatically, necessitating a change in dosage or drug. One reason was simply that patients' bodies escaped total classification. But that did not explain everything. Different reactions of seemingly similar tumours to the same chemical substance led doctors to the realization that there must be differences between the tumours that research simply did not yet understand. In effect, this meant that the medicine simultaneously functioned as a diagnostic instrument. This new form of 'diagnostic therapy' was extremely burdensome for patients. They not only had to fear they were among the so-called non-responders, which would reduce their prospects for remission, at least in the near-term. In some cases, they also had to shoulder the side effects of chemotherapy without any benefit. According to a study of the most common cytostatic agents in the early 1970s, this affected different groups of patients differently according to tumour type, stage, and cytostatic agent: in the best-case scenario, it was only 10 per cent; for other groups, it was 70 per cent.[285] In order to avoid this problem, some cancer researchers tested the efficacy of a cytostatic agent on a patient's cells or tissue samples before therapy began, a

[283] See, for example, the list of general side effects in Ehrhardt, 'Chemotherapie maligner Geschwülste', 827–8.

[284] Peter Keating and Alberto Cambrosio, 'Cancer Clinical Trials: The Emergence and Development of a New Style of Practice', in Cantor, *Cancer in the Twentieth Century*, 197–223, 216.

[285] Ehrhardt, 'Chemotherapie maligner Geschwülste', 817–20, 822–3 and 826–7.

method that had proven useful with antibiotics in the past.[286] Growing tumorous tissue cultures was exceptionally difficult with some patients, though. For others, tests were developed that reliably showed which tumours would not react to a specific agent, while doctors only had limited success in predicting whether a tumour would respond. Still, the experience gave rise to the idea that an individualized course of therapy had to be designed on the basis of lab tests *before* treatment began. This further contributed to an unprecedented melding of laboratory and clinic, experiment and standard clinical practice. For both doctors and patients, the differences between therapy that accorded with standard protocol and therapies in pharmaceutical tests in Phase II (dosage determination) and Phase III (verification of efficacy) seemed minimal.

In the GDR, at least forty-four studies in oncological medicine commissioned by West German pharmaceutical corporations were conducted between 1961 and 1990.[287] The overwhelming majority were Phase II or Phase III studies.[288] However, Phase I studies on humans were also conducted after the obligatory testing of the substance on animals. Dr Helgard Lenk conducted one such study at the Robert Rössle Clinic in East Berlin between February 1986 and March 1987.[289] She was testing the recombinant human tumour necrosis factor rhTNF PAC-4D, which was developed by Japanese pharmaceutical corporation Asahi Chemical Company. The substance was supposed to trigger the immune system to fight or cure cancerous tumours. Lenk selected seventeen cancer patients who could not be treated with clinically permitted drugs or who had already tried all existing methods without success. All patients confirmed that they had been informed about the run of the study and possible complications and that they still wanted to participate.[290]

The patients received regularly increasing doses of the tumour necrosis factor so that researchers could determine the maximum dosage tolerable without severe side effects. They suffered from nausea, vomiting, fever, chills, serious pain in the tumours, drowsiness, and light-headedness. After the metastases in one patient's intestines necrotized—the desired effect—the necrotized tissue leaked into her abdomen, causing a fatal case of peritonitis. All the other subjects survived. Most

[286] Tanneberger and Bacigalupo, 'Einige Erfahrungen mit der individuellen zytostatischen Behandlung maligner Tumoren'; Stephan Tanneberger and A. Mohr, 'Biological Characterization of Human Tumours by Means of Organ Culture and Individualized Cytostatic Cancer Treatment', *Archiv für Geschwulstforschung* 42, no. 4 (1973): 307–15; K. Ebeling and H. Spitzbart, 'Zur Erfassung zytostatischer Effekte an Zellkulturen in vitro und deren gegenwärtige Bedeutung für eine individualisierte Tumortherapie des fortgeschrittenen Ovarialkarzinoms', *Zentralblatt für Gynäkologie* 99 (1977): 1041–54.

[287] Volker Hess, Laura Hottenrott, and Peter Steinkamp, *Testen im Osten. DDR-Arzneimittelstudien im Auftrag westlicher Pharmaindustrie, 1964–1990* (Berlin: Be.bra Wissenschaft, 2016), 194–243 and 255.

[288] Ibid., 179.

[289] Helgard Lenk, 'Tumornekrosefaktor in der Behandlung maligner Tumoren—Stand und Perspektiven aus klinischer Sicht' (PhD diss., Akademie der Wissenschaften der DDR, 1990).

[290] Ibid., 79.

complications subsided forty-eight to seventy-two hours after intake. Because the tumour necrosis factor seemed to effectively target the tumour in some cases, Lenk conducted a Phase II study.

This study stood at the centre of a February 1991 report in *Der Spiegel* that criticized how the 'pharmaceutical hustle' in the GDR was exploited by 'pimps from the West' who wanted to carry out medical tests that would be impermissible elsewhere.[291] In fact, if the published findings and information on the study's design are a reliable source, the study conformed with East Germany's testing standards, which were not much different from those in West Germany and other Western countries.[292] A study conducted around the same time in the United States with a tumour necrosis factor produced by biotech company Genentech followed a nearly identical study design. All thirty-nine test subjects suffered serious complications similar to those in the East German study; one patient was blinded, but nobody died.[293] Thus, the outrage over the scandal in the GDR may have been more of a sign of how little the public knew about the proximity between clinic and laboratory in the world of chemotherapy.

There are other explanations as to why the West German pharmaceutical industry sought to recruit East German clinics for its studies. The GDR had a highly centralized health system that accelerated both the administration and evaluation of the studies—an advantage that translated directly into increased revenue for the pharmaceutical companies.[294] For its part, the East German government could get sorely needed foreign currency from the studies, since it, and not the participants, received the remunerations for test subjects.[295] Doctors benefitted from invitations to conferences in the West and the chance to publish in West German medical journals.[296] Moreover, the host clinics received experimental drugs from West Germany free of charge in order to compare their effectiveness with established cytostatic agents. In a handful of cases, the remuneration was paid in medical technology unavailable in the GDR, which the clinic could use during the duration of the study and sometimes even retain afterwards.[297]

291 '"Das ist russisches Roulett". Schmutzige Geschäfte mit westlichen Pharmakonzernen brachten dem SED-Regime Millionen', *Der Spiegel* 6 (1991): 80–90, 80.

292 On drug trials in East Germany commissioned by West German pharmaceutical companies, see Hess, Hottenrott, and Steinkamp, *Testen im Osten*, 180.

293 B. Feinberg, R. Kurzrock, M. Talpaz, M. Blick, S. Saks, and J. U. Gutterman, 'A Phase I Trial of Intravenously-Administered Recombinant Tumor Necrosis Factor-Alpha in Cancer Patients', *Journal of Clinical Oncology* 6, no. 8 (1988): 1328–34, https://doi.org/10.1200/JCO.1988.6.8.1328.

294 Hess, Hottenrott, and Steinkamp, *Testen im Osten*, 118–23.

295 For a detailed analysis, see ibid., 54–9.

296 Ibid., 132–6.

297 For instance, as compensation for participating in a Phase III study of the cytostatic agent Ifosfamid, Frankfurt-based pharmaceutical corporation ASTA offered East Berlin's Robert Rössle Clinic a high-performance liquid chromatography machine manufactured by Hewlett-Packard. See Beratervertrag zwischen dem Beratungsbüro beim Ministerium für Gesundheitswesen für Arzneimittel und medizinisch-technische Erzeugnisse, Herrn Prof. Dr St. Tanneberger, Robert-Rössle-Institut, Zentralinstitut für Krebsforschung und der Firma Asta-Werke AG, 7 February 1985, BArch DQ 105/34, 4.

Last but not least, the studies gave the clinics access to new chemotherapeutic drugs unattainable in East Germany. There were quite a few of them, as evidenced by a list compiled in 1980 by Stephan Tanneberger and his colleagues at the chemotherapy division of East Berlin's Institute for Cancer Research, which enumerated known cytostatic agents, where they were produced, and whether they could be obtained in the GDR.[298] Doctors saw in this a potential boon for their patients. The hope that a newly discovered substance could provide a breakthrough led many patients to consent to participate in such studies.[299] Things were not much different in West Germany. There, too, patients with late-stage tumours who had already tried out all other forms of treatment hoped that they would be helped by participation in medical studies, some of which had designs similar to those conducted in the East.[300]

Almost all chemotherapy patients in the 1960s and 1970s, whether treated with experimental drugs or according to established protocol, had already been operated on and irradiated, because few doctors were willing to risk employing cytostatic agents to treat early-stage cancers.[301] These patients were already familiar with the hospital. But what they experienced during chemotherapy was significantly different from everything else they had gone through. Before it began, doctors performed extensive tests to ensure that their health and, above all, their blood levels were relatively stable. Most cytostatic agents were first administered intravenously in high doses. In order to avoid having to repeatedly reinsert the infusion needle, some patients got a long-term catheter, a foreign body that regularly reminded them of chemotherapy that also had to be carefully cleaned because it posed an acute danger of infection.

In most cases, infusions were supplemented with a drip that intermittently dosed the patient with drugs that mitigated side effects like nausea and vomiting; they were often combined with anti-anxiety meds that could make the patient drowsy. Infusions usually lasted roughly an hour. But the cytostatic agents used to

[298] Stephan Tanneberger, R. Gürtler, B. Tschiersch, and B. Heise, 'Klinisch gebräuchliche antineoplastische Pharmaka und deren Charakteristika', in *Experimentelle und klinische Tumorchemotherapie. Spezielle Tumorchemotherapie*, ed. Stephan Tanneberger (Stuttgart: Fischer, 1980), 317–43.

[299] In contrast to the legally defined parameters in the FRG, GDR law only required oral assent. However, it had to be documented with a signature or at least confirmed on paper by the lead doctor. Before assenting to participate, patients had to be informed about the 'type, extent, and risks' of the treatment, which a witness had to confirm had actually occurred. It is not possible to reconstruct what exactly this information consisted in. See the form Nachweis der Einwilligung, BArch DQ 105/34. In 2013 and 2014, Volker Hess, Laura Hottenrott, and Peter Steinkamp conducted interviews with study participants and doctors who had taken part in the studies. According to the interviewees, participants voluntarily participated. See Hess, Hottenrott, and Steinkamp, *Testen im Osten*, 145–7.

[300] G. P. Breitbach and N. Marschner, 'Droloxifen beim metastasierenden Mammakarzinom: Dosierung und Pharmakokinetik', *Archives of Gynecology and Obstetrics* 254, no. 1 (1993): 903–5, https://doi.org/10.1007/BF02266228. There is an entire volume of files on Lenk's study in the GDR: BArch DQ 105/43, vol. 1.

[301] C. G. Schmid and S. Seeber, 'Neue Perspektiven für eine adjuvante Chemotherapie bei soliden Tumoren', *Deutsche Medizinische Wochenschrift* 100, no. 45 (1975): 2342–8, https://doi.org/10.1055/s-0028-1106547.

treat some types of cancer were infused over a span of a few hours. During the infusion, patients generally lied down, though some could and wanted to remain sitting. If the procedure was conducted during a stay at the hospital, patients were often together in a single room with others who were also undergoing chemotherapy or had just completed an infusion. Outpatient chemotherapy allowed family or friends to accompany the patient and speak with them during the infusion, something that had been impossible during operations and radiotherapy.

The first side effects suffered by many chemotherapy patients set in shortly after or, if the infusion lasted a long time, during the process. Almost all cytostatic agents caused nausea and vomiting, which persisted for hours and could be so intense that some patients could not even look at the infusion apparatus without feeling nauseous or throwing up.[302] Once the infusion began, many patients felt an unpleasant, metallic taste in their mouth, which often led to a loss of appetite. A recurring topic of accounts on chemotherapy was the struggle to eat something in order to withstand the process. Friends and family developed strategies to get patients to eat, nudging them with small portions and offering them their favourite foods.[303] But nausea and loss of appetite were not the only barriers to eating. Chemotherapy patients often developed infections in their mouth that made consuming food painful. Diarrhoea and constipation were also problems that some patients had to contend with.

Another common side effect only set in a week or more after the infusion, at a point when the first treatment cycle, which often lasted three to six weeks, was not yet finished.[304] The patient's hair began to fall out in clumps. Many autobiographical accounts, especially those written by women, recount this experience as one of shock. In 1984, a teacher with breast cancer writing under the pseudonym Christiane Lenker described the event:

> But after the first night that I could finally spend at home, I woke up to find a fine network of blonde hair on my pillow. Appalled, I grasped at my head and held a whole bunch in my hand.[305]

Hair lends beauty and vitality and its loss completely altered the appearance of the person's face, particularly for people who had long hair. But that was not the only reason hair loss was a shock. The balding head, dry skin, and edema in the face were external markers of cancer that were difficult to cover up and drew stares

[302] Christiane Lenker, *Krebs kann auch eine Chance sein. Zwischenbilanz oder Antwort an Fritz Zorn* (Frankfurt am Main: Fischer, 1984), 54; Judith McKay and Nancee Hirano, *The Chemotherapy Survival Guide* (Oakland: New Harbinger Publications, 1993), 68–9.

[303] Dieter Wellershoff, *Blick auf einen fernen Berg* (Gütersloh: Kiepenheuer and Witsch, 1991), 132.

[304] Ehrhardt, 'Chemotherapie maligner Geschwülste', 822–3 and 826–31; Tanneberger et al., 'Klinisch gebräuchliche antineoplastische Pharmaka'.

[305] Lenker, *Krebs kann auch eine Chance sein*, 57.

from other people.[306] In order to hide their baldness, women in both the GDR and FRG could be prescribed wigs, though the public health insurers did not always cover the entire cost.[307] However, many were uncomfortable with wearing a wig and preferred to wear a headscarf, even though its rarity as an accessory in both countries during the 1970s and 1980s also made it into a symbol of chemotherapy.[308]

From the doctor's perspective, other side effects were more concerning, among them altered blood levels and the potential for the cytostatic agents to affect other organs, particularly the kidneys, heart, and nervous system. Thus, everyday life as a chemotherapy patient involved not only infusions, but also weekly—and sometimes daily—blood tests. Additionally, manual examinations, x-rays, and, beginning in the mid-1970s, computer tomography were used to check if and to what extent tumours and metastases were responding to the chemotherapy. If something was not right, then the therapy might be ended. Such exams determined whether patients could sustain their hope for more time. Thus, some jotted down their platelet and white blood cell levels in their diaries as a daily judgement of fate.[309]

However, blood levels and the like did not have any necessary correlation with a patient's feeling of wellness. Surely, poor blood levels often found expression in exhaustion, weakness, and headaches, but having blood levels good enough to set forth chemotherapy did not necessarily mean the patient felt healthy. Many patients thus fluctuated in a limbo state between their quantified state of health and their own feeling of sickness or well-being. On the one hand, they hoped for good 'objective' levels that would enable the therapy to continue. But on the other, the weakness, disgust, and pain many felt was caused by the very chemotherapy that they hoped could proceed.[310]

Chemotherapy patients thus experienced a dramatic decline in their feeling of wellness *during* the treatment itself. This stood in contrast to the experiences of cancer patients in the previous decades, as surgery and radiotherapy generally worsened the patient's feeling of health only *after* the procedure, when their decision to undergo treatment could no longer be reversed. For this reason, the side effects of chemotherapy could pose a medical problem, even though doctors did not consider them in and of themselves dangerous. For instance, an article on the state of chemotherapy published in a 1984 issue of the *Münchner Medizinische Wochenschrift* (*Munich Medical Weekly*) stated: 'The partially very uncomfortable side effects of the cytostatic agents as well as an insufficient doctor-patient relationship often lead to the *abandonment* of an *in principle promising*

[306] Schnurre, *Der Schattenfotograf*, 33; Helmut Ulrich, *Verknotet. Tagebuch einer Krebstherapie* (Kiel: Rake, 2000), 175.

[307] Letter to the District Leadership of FDGB, Health Insurance Administration, Welfare and Health Services Division, Frankfurt an der Oder, 28 June 1983, BArch DY 34/15383; McKay and Hirano, *The Chemotherapy Survival Guide*, 117–19.

[308] Lenker (1984), *Krebs kann auch eine Chance sein*, 52–3; McKay and Hirano, *The Chemotherapy Survival Guide*, 119.

[309] Ulrich, *Verknotet.* [310] Lenker, *Krebs kann auch eine Chance sein*, 54.

treatment.'[311] Thus, the authors concluded that 'the treatment of acute leukaemias, but also chemotherapy for solid tumours [is] today no longer conceivable without supportive measures', which had to have as their goal the improvement of the patient's 'quality of life'.[312]

Almost always, though, doctors' definition of 'quality of life' was purely physical. Accordingly, they thought it could be achieved through purely medical means, such as prescribing painkillers, developing better antiemetics, and identifying and addressing infections early on. But the concept of 'quality of life' had other connotations. Fields like social medicine and stress research had begun integrating it into their work, while patients' rights movements also championed it as a primary value of ethical medical treatment.[313] In oncology in West Germany, 'quality of life' supplanted the notion of 'performance' on the Karnofsky Scale. Oncologists continued to understand 'quality of life' on the basis of measurable parameters and sought to quantify it in statistics.[314] But because it acknowledged the patient's subjective feeling of health as significant, it empowered patients to define for themselves what constituted well-being and the acceptable limits of treatment and its side effects.

More and more patients in West Germany were demanding that a reasonably good quality of life be placed on equal footing with prolongation of life expectancy. They were bolstered by critiques of cold, anonymous, technologized medicine. Looking back on her experience with chemotherapy, the aforementioned 32-year-old teacher writing under the pseudonym Christiane Lenker reflected:

> I would never again put myself through it, because chemotherapy, at least for breast cancer patients, is an inhumane form of treatment. Successful experiments with lab rats do not provide legitimation for the application of the same treatment on humans.[315]

Although she might have been cured, and although the chemotherapy might have achieved not only remission, but long-term elimination of the cancer, she felt as if it had reduced her to a laboratory animal. As she wrote elsewhere, it transformed her into a 'frightened bunny rabbit' by robbing her of her human dignity.[316] Her perception was echoed by Dora Hauri, a Swiss woman not quite 30 years of age who felt that chemotherapy had made her life unliveable. She lambasted her doctors: 'The doctors seemed to me to be like goblins who were playing an evil game with me. They poison me, they deceive me. They try to convince me that a

311 Italics in original, see Berdel and Fink, 'Internistische Tumortherapie', 1167.

312 Ibid., 1168.

313 Patrick Kury, 'Vom physiologischen Stress zum Prinzip "Lebensqualität": Lennart Levi und der Wandel des Stresskonzepts um 1970', *Body Politics* 1, no. 1 (2013): 119–37; Stoff, 'Franz Klose', 186–8.

314 Timmermann, '"Just Give Me the Best Quality of Life Questionnaire"', 184–97.

315 Lenker, *Krebs kann auch eine Chance sein*, 54.

316 Ibid., 55.

life without hair is still worth living.'[317] In a book published in 1991, author Dieter Wellershoff metaphorized the very aggressive chemotherapy regimen that his brother went through as 'chemical warfare':

> This method of treatment was comparable to the most brutal military strategy, the 'scorched-earth' policy.... Of course, such a general attack on life is not the goal of chemotherapy, but it is its unavoidable consequence.... Its end result is not seldom just as catastrophic as the scorched-earth policy: one has only defeated the cancer by destroying its host. Mocked by gradually disappearing hope, the patient has passed through the valley of tears only in order to die at the end.[318]

The military metaphor was also used by his brother's doctors. But the author engaged it for another purpose: to question the utility of a form of treatment that declares 'war' on the patient's body, even though he himself ultimately refused to give a definitive opinion.

The few autobiographical accounts of chemotherapy published by East German writers do not contain analogous critiques of the treatment and its detrimental effects on 'quality of life'. Maxie Wander, the aforementioned author treated for breast cancer at East Berlin's Robert Rössle Clinic in the mid-1970s, frequently mentioned chemotherapy in her posthumously published diaries and letters. But usually, she simply stated that she had to return to the clinic for an infusion; though like Wellershoff, she called chemotherapy 'poison': 'Afterwards I feel awful, but the poisonous stuff in me goes away and I feel better again.'[319] Nowhere did she cast doubt on its potential benefits, even if she knew that 'the poisonous stuff will cause some damage, to the heart, bones, stomach. But in the end, one does not need to live to be 120 years old.'[320] Shortly before her death, she wrote a letter to her sister in which she remarked in passing and without complaint that she was about to undergo another session of chemotherapy.[321]

But some West German chemotherapy patients also endured its side effects while maintaining faith in the notion that only radical treatment that pushed their body to its limits could effectively repel their cancer.[322] According to Wellershoff, his brother assented to this 'strategy' out of hope:

> At any rate, it is certain that the head doctor told him when making his rounds the day before the chemotherapy began: 'Tomorrow you are going into the deepest basement that I have. And then we will carry you out step by step.'...

[317] Dora Hauri, *Ich habe den Herbst gesehen*, ed. Walter Graber and Ruedi Passavant (Basel: Passavant, 1982), 47.

[318] Wellershoff, *Blick auf einen fernen Berg*, 130–1.

[319] Wander, *Leben wär' eine prima Alternative*, 241.

[320] Ibid., 259.

[321] Letter from October 1977: ibid., 278.

[322] See, for instance, Ulrich, *Verknotet.*

> Surrounded by his staff, the doctor had approached the patient's bed and bent towards him. He uttered the two sentences while lightly grasping the hand resting on the blanket. It was a gesture of solidarity intended to give the patient courage, and a distinction, and, I believe, an unconscious act of consecration. Because without having explicitly thought it, he said to the patient: You are now the chosen hero who must descend into the realm of the dead for seven days and seven nights. And then you can try to return to life from there.... At any rate, my brother seems to have been more encouraged than terrified by these words.[323]

Canadian medical sociologist Arthur W. Frank detailed the 'spiritual experience' of his own fight with cancer in a book translated into German shortly after its original publication in 1991. He describes his own 'personal mythology of illness as adventure' and concludes:

> My body was a toxic waste dump, but it was also a living miracle. Twenty years before, maybe even ten, I would have been dying instead of getting chemotherapy. Now the ultimate slo-mo of the CAT scan cameras showed the tumors shrinking. My existence was a wonder, living it an adventure. I could believe in prevailing until the sun rose. The blessing was that I was seeing life, face to face.[324]

Frank's account partook in a development in the 1990s that saw the two tendencies described here converge: the radical critique of chemotherapy on the basis of subjective feelings of quality of life, and the hope that chemotherapy could cure cancer, however unbearable its side effects might be. After all, only a handful of cancer patients categorically refused chemotherapy from the outset.[325] Instead, doctors began taking more consideration of quality of life when treating their patients. As a result, techniques that originated from 'alternative medicine' ended up entering the mainstream, viewed as helpful for reducing the patient's stress and their feelings of being isolated in a dangerous situation. Advice manuals funded by the Deutsche Krebshilfe and recommended by self-help groups advised patients on how to relax and visualize positive outcomes in order to make chemotherapy more bearable and facilitate healing.[326]

Thus, chemotherapy played a much more significant role than radiotherapy or surgery in spurring doctors to be more open towards such 'alternative' methods. One reason was that doctors wanted to keep patients from choosing to end treatment before its completion and showing more sensitivity towards their subjective experience seemed like the best method for doing so. At the same

[323] Wellershoff, *Blick auf einen fernen Berg*, 167–8.
[324] Frank, *At the Will of the Body*, 81–2.
[325] Peter Noll, *Diktate über Sterben und Tod* (Zurich: Pendo, 1984).
[326] McKay and Hirano, *The Chemotherapy Survival Guide.*

time, public discussion regularly thematized concepts like quality of life and psychosomatic reflections on the necessity of heeding the patient's emotions and mental health. Another contributing factor was the time that patients had to spend during their infusions and between chemotherapy sessions at the hospital, as well as the weeks and months claimed by chemotherapy, in contrast to the more punctual duration of radiotherapy and surgery.

During these weeks and months, patients were forced to confront the vicissitudes of their own embodiment. Their lives were dominated by medical routines that measured their body as an object. The integrity of their body was incessantly taken from them by the pokes of infusion needles and blood sample extractions, the injection of medicine, the installation of catheter tubes. Pain, nausea, weakness, exhaustion, digestive problems, loss of appetite, skin changes, and hair loss all absorbed the patient's energy and turned their body into the focal point of their everyday life. Some patients' accounts painted chemotherapy as an experience that constantly drew their attention to their own sick bodies, draining them so much that they became apathetic and burnt out.[327] During the afternoons, days, or weeks that could pass between two infusions, many were too weak to really do anything; but at the same time, they were, to an extent, able to take a break from the constant focus on their bodies. Many autobiographical accounts discuss this free time that had to somehow be filled. Many complained about their situation or their fellow patients—the sight of whom often reminded them of their own finitude and the possibility that the treatment might not work; whose everyday conversations they often overheard; with whom they themselves talked.[328]

A number of autobiographical writings depicted this time as an opportunity to reflect and practice living in the present. Similar arguments appeared in advice guides for patients, which began being published in ever greater number in the 1990s by German Cancer Aid, the German Cancer Society, self-help groups, and public health insurers. For instance, a booklet for men with testicular cancer stated: 'You face the challenge of actively grappling with the effects of your illness. This generally means developing a new sense of your body and perhaps a new approach to life.'[329] One of Germany's largest public health insurance corporations recommended that patients enjoy the present and fill it with laughter so that they might activate the body's power to heal itself and regain a good quality of life.[330] Thus, these advice texts drew on ideas that had originated in psychotherapy and psychosomatics and had grown popular in the 1970s. Psychotherapy and psychosomatics had emphasized the importance of mental health for overcoming

[327] Lenker, *Krebs kann auch eine Chance sein*, 52; Frank, *At the Will of the Body*, 167.

[328] Wander, *Leben wär' eine prima Alternative* (1994), 247–8; Lenker, *Krebs kann auch eine Chance sein*, 55–6; Frank, *At the Will of the Body*, 133–4.

[329] Deutsche Krebsgesellschaft e.V., *Diagnose Prostata-Karzinom. Das geht den Mann an. Patientenratgeber*, undated [before 2001], DHMD 2001/228, 43.

[330] AOK, *Mit neuem Lebensmut. Nachsorge bei Krebs*, undated [before 2001], DHMD 2001/1652, 21.

physical illness and the significance of activating the immune system through various bodily techniques. Now, these notions were rounded out with the cultivation of positive images and emotions, not as counterpoints to mainstream medical methods, but as their necessary counterpart. Autobiographical texts, advice guides for patients, and self-help books all began regularly framing cancer as an opportunity to make a change in one's life.

Visualization, relaxation, and stress reduction were supposed to make chemotherapy more bearable. But patients were also encouraged to continue these practices after treatment was over. Chemotherapy led both doctors and patients to a new understanding of cure and remission. Curing cancer was still the goal. But when it was not possible, something more remained than giving up or dying. Doctors no longer viewed remission as the result of a failed attempt at curing, but as gained time. Moreover, during the 1990s in particular, remission started promising more time for a greater number of patients with a range of different cancers. Now it was a question not of weeks or months, but years.

Hope: Promise or Burden?

Remission became a new state of being between sickness and health. Operations and radiotherapy had always been depicted to patients as episodes: either the treatment failed and the patient died or the treatment worked and the patient was cured. Doctors knew that in many cases, the cure would not last, that relapses or metastases would occur that ruled out further treatment once and for all. But they rarely passed this knowledge on to patients. Since the 1950s, regular post-treatment examinations in intervals of six months or a year that could continue for a span of five years—and for breast cancer patients considerably longer—had become a standard feature of cancer treatment, even if it was not always adhered to. Thus, a practice that suggested to patients that the elimination of their cancer was not necessarily permanent did predate chemotherapy. However, they were considered cured until the relapse actually happened, and indeed, many patients seem to have viewed themselves as such.[331]

'Remission' was not a new experience for cancer patients in every respect. But it still marked a notable departure from the past. Cancer treatment had once lasted seldom more than a week. For many, it now involved a series of treatment cycles that could take months and, in some cases, a year or longer. Whether the cancer had been cured or the patient had entered into remission often remained unclear for a long time—and sometimes an entire lifetime. Feeling healthy while not definitively knowing the state of one's treatment became, in the eyes of Arthur

[331] Baines, 'Three Stories: Generations of Breast Cancer', 22.

W. Frank, a state of existence. Those living through it like himself became citizens in a 'remission society'. Unlike Susan Sontag's 1978 analysis, they are not temporary citizens in the kingdom of the sick who then return to that of the healthy. Instead, they perpetually travel between the two, relying on a visa that regularly has to be renewed.[332]

Whether it is renewed depends, on the one hand, upon the cancer's development and regular check-ups. But on the other hand, many see its renewal as the result of a personal decision. Should I be mindful of my life as someone in remission, or should I be indifferent about it?[333] Should I choose to be done with cancer and dispense with check-ups? This was the path travelled by Gerda A.: 20 years old when she was diagnosed in 1969, she did not miss a check-up for ten years and regularly complained of pains and concerns that she had metastases. But then she stopped going to check-ups, informed the clinic she was pregnant, and wrote them a Christmas card three years later.[334]

Did this young woman and mother remain cured and completely return to the realm of the healthy? Many oscillate between the lands of sickness and health or even lose their visa, because the tumour starts to grow again or metastases are detected. But because chemotherapy always straddles the line between standard procedure and experimental therapy, it repeatedly delays the moment at which doctors can definitively say that the patient is 'incurable' or untreatable. While in the nineteenth century, doctors often made this determination right after settling on a diagnosis, chemotherapy has consistently fed hope over the past decades. The large number of available cytostatic agents has enabled patients to try again if the first or second treatment cycle fails, even if they and their doctors know that the chances of success will be slimmer with each round. Surgery and radiotherapy placed firm limits on the quantity of treatment a patient could undergo. But with the advent of chemotherapy, ending treatment has often been a conscious decision of doctors and patients who do not want to endure the remaining, yet less promising possibilities of treatment.

Among them was (and still is) the choice to participate in a pharmaceutical study. But doing so is generally limited to a small group of patients who meet certain criteria. Self-help groups around the world have worked to allow certain patients who have already tried all extant medicines access to these not-yet approved drugs outside the framework of studies. In 2005, Germany passed a law permitting such 'compassionate use' under certain conditions.[335] This might

[332] Frank, *The Wounded Storyteller*, 9.

[333] Angelika Mechtel, *Jeden Tag will ich leben. Ein Krebstagebuch* (Frankfurt am Main: Fischer, 1990), 142 and 145.

[334] Patient's file of Gerda A. UAH, preliminary signature: Acc. 14/02 (radiology clinic), 1968/9, no. 22630/69.

[335] 'Compassionate use' was first legally codified in Germany in § 21, no. 6 of the 14th Änderungsgesetz zum Arzneimittelgesetz (Modification of the Pharmaceutical Drug Code). The law entered into effect on 6 September 2005. See Gesetz über den Verkehr mit Arzneimitteln

perhaps open the door to remission or a cure for a few patients. At the same time, it fuels hope that there is always one more treatment that can be tried.[336]

American author Rafael Yglesias captured the complexities of this internal compulsion to hope in a scene from his 2009 novel *A Happy Marriage*. After undergoing chemotherapy for over three years and fighting hard to be allowed to try new forms of treatment, the protagonist, Margaret, decides that she no longer wants to try another. Her oncologist, a specialist at the internationally renowned Sloan Kettering Institute, pleads with her to take one last shot at it. Her husband Enrique observes him and notes:

> The handsome, dictatorial, and—Enrique could now see—softhearted man argued passionately, and against all the evidence.... 'There are new drugs all the time', he said. 'You don't know how long you can live on TPN. I have patients who have lived for years with metastasized cancers worse than yours. The scans show your tumors aren't growing. We can find you a drug trial—.'
>
> Enrique knew that these statements were nonsense.... And yet. And yet Enrique found himself engaged by the specialist's irrational invocation of what had certainly died for Margaret, namely the belief that further struggle was worthwhile. Enrique kept his pace, but the [doctor's] words filled him with shame and doubt. In September Enrique had supported Margaret's search for a miracle cure....
>
> Trying desperate measures had also reassured all who knew her, especially her sons, her parents, and her siblings, that everything had been done to save her life. But for Enrique there had been the cost of time, robbed from her farewell....
>
> Margaret answered the pleading doctor in utter despair. Tears flowed and her voice quaked while she curled up into a fetal position. She shrank from his words of optimism, wincing as if they were lashes of a whip. She pleaded 'I can't do this.... Please, please let me go....'[337]

Hope for a new, effective medicine is depicted here as an exceptionally powerful emotion that drove everyone involved—the patient, her husband, her doctor—to search for over three years, even though they knew that the chances were diminishing with every attempt. The medicine that tortured Margaret also represented hope, both for her and the others. But even though she was firm in her decision and her husband supported it, the power of this hope was so great that he

(Arzneimittelgesetz—AMG) (24 August 1976), Bundesministerium für Justiz und für Verbraucherschutz, *Gesetze im Internet*, https://www.gesetze-im-internet.de/bundesrecht/amg_1976/gesamt.pdf, 32–3.

[336] Ilana Löwy, 'La standardisation de l'inconnu: les protocoles thérapeutiques en cancérologie', *Techniques and Culture* 25/6 (1996): 73–108, 77, https://doi.org/10.4000/tc.507.

[337] Rafael Yglesias, *A Happy Marriage* (New York: Scribner, 2009), 61–4.

could hardly resist the promise uttered in the doctor's words. For Margaret, hope mutated into an almost corporeal pain that she fought against with her last bit of strength. The price that she and her husband had to pay for having held out hope for so long was the lost time that they could have spent with one another—not struggling to save Margaret's dying body, but talking with one another and saying goodbye.

6

Cancer and Emotions in the Twentieth Century

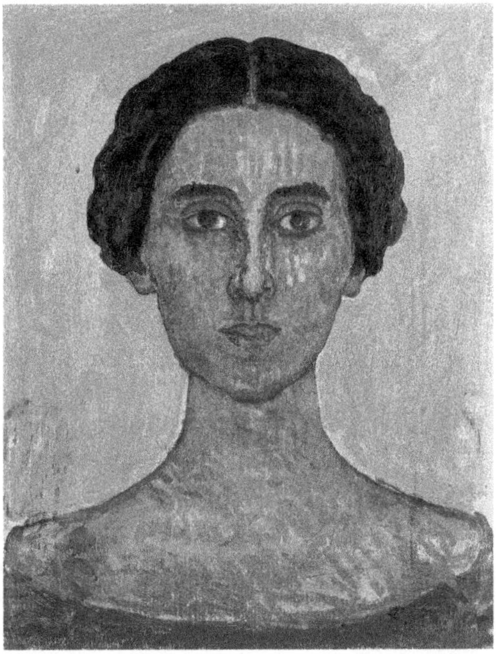

Fig. 31 Ferdinand Hodler, *Portrait of Valentine Godé-Darel* (*c.*1910).

Valentine Godé-Darel's gaze is still fixed on us (Fig. 31). We still do not know what she was feeling when Ferdinand Hodler painted her portrait over a century ago. When we look at her portrait, we fill her eyes with our thoughts, our knowledge of her fate, our emotions that flow out of this extinguished future. Her gaze captures our gaze. It seems as if it demands that we reflect on Godé-Darel as well as on her experiences and those of other cancer patients, that we try to comprehend them and grasp all of the labour, challenges, treatment, and research that have shaped them.

This is why the book travelled through the history of cancer in the twentieth century four times. Emotions were the common thread that tied together its diverse narratives. In some places, emotions were almost imperceptible, almost faded into other story lines. But they were never absent. The four main chapters illuminated why the texture of the history of emotions always has to draw on a range of sources and engage with multifarious topics in order to piece together its analysis. The history of emotions cannot be understood in and of itself, nor can its effects be reduced to practices, knowledge, spaces, and things that exclusively have to do with emotions. The book's four main chapters traced these complexities of the history of emotions and cancer. This conclusion ties up loose ends with the common thread of the history of emotions in each of those four chapters. It then reflects on the historically relative nature of which emotions qualify as significant and which do not; which emotions could be expressed openly and which could not; which emotions were valued as moral or healthy and which were not valued or even discouraged. It wraps up with a discussion of how emotions—and particularly fear, hope, and disgust—gained new significance through scientificization, rationalization, and therapeutization, while medical, social, ethical, and personal approaches to emotions underwent profound shifts.

Emotions in Science and History

Encyclopaedia entries from the late nineteenth century suggest that contemporaneous medical research rarely explored whether emotions might be a cause of cancer. This aligns with the conclusion drawn by most scholarship that has been conducted on the history of medicine: late nineteenth-century medicine was dominated by the rise of cellular pathology and bacteriology. But in fact, long-standing notions about how long-term negative emotional states could contribute to cancer continued to influence medical practice and discourse.

The new discipline of psychoanalysis engaged with how psychological factors influence health, but its model of the body, emotions, and psyche differed from those of the past. The still young concept of the psychogenesis of organic illnesses claimed that unresolved psychic conflicts could be converted into bodily ailments via the vegetative nervous system. Its proponents believed that this conversion of psychological forces—among them emotional conflicts—evoked reversible dysfunctions that could transmute into irreversible corporeal damage over the long-term. Debates on the psychogenesis of illness focused on the feeling of fear, leading one of the pioneers of psychosomatic medicine, Felix Deutsch, to postulate in the 1920s that every illness was, in essence, an illness of fear.

But they generally ruled out the possibility that cancer could have psychogenetic origins, since it seemed implausible for illnesses that began at a specific part of the body. In the words of neurologist Viktor von Weizsäcker, cancer was considered to be so deeply corporeal that a psychological influence was inconceivable. Contributing to this assessment was that cancer was, at the time, almost always fatal. Most doctors thus held it preposterous to think that such a disease could have some kind of deeper psychological meaning, as doctors influenced by psychoanalysis believed was true of other illnesses. At the same time, doctors wondered what the point of psychoanalytic research on cancer could possibly be if nobody thought it could be cured with psychotherapeutic methods.

There was, however, one exception to this general viewpoint: the unorthodox psychoanalyst Georg Groddeck, who theorized that cancerous tumours were a bodily reaction to an unfulfilled wish to have a child. However, the hypothesis that cancer was caused by psychological factors seemed to him too simple. Instead, he asserted that body and mind interacted in an indeterminate manner in the 'id'. Groddeck modelled his theory of the pathological relationship between body, mind, and emotions on the female body, a gendered analysis that drew on historical stereotypes and was perpetuated by other thinkers throughout the twentieth century.

Initially, nobody seemed interested in Groddeck's psychoanalytic theory of cancer. However, in the 1920s, a different school on the margins of conventional medicine thematized the possible significance of emotions as a cause of cancer: the Neue Deutsche Heilkunde, or New German Medicine. The politically right-wing movement latched onto holism and natural medicine in its diatribes against what it saw as 'materialistic' mainstream medicine. It trumpeted the special status of humans, which its proponents believed was being diminished by laboratory experiments on animals. They included doctors like Erwin Liek, who asserted that diseases are generally not started by *one single* cause or germ and that the body's constitution and disposition play just as significant of a role in the aetiology of illness. He and his counterparts viewed specifically human approaches to emotions as constitutional factors in the causation of illness, including cancer. The school's ideals were productivity and increased individual performance, which it shared with the National-Socialist Deutsche Seelenheilkunde (German Psychotherapy). Accordingly, its representatives defined as 'false' those emotions that weakened the body's constitution or the person's capacity to work. In contrast to Groddeck's theory, the New German Medicine interpreted emotions as a matter of will power and attitude, while asserting that they could be influenced by adopting the 'correct' disposition and by therapeutic interventions like autogenic training.

Among the ranks of the Deutsche Seelenheilkunde were prominent members of the Heidelberg School, which, in the post-war era, continued to develop theories of biographical and anthropological medicine under the leadership of Viktor von Weizsäcker. Wilhelm Kütemeyer, a student of Weizsäcker who had conducted most of his research on psychosis, claimed that there was a complementary relationship between psychosis and cancer. He reasoned that both were rooted in similar patterns of pathology that were simply situated in different spheres, namely mind and body. Mirroring contemporary discourse on schizophrenia, Kütemeyer traced cancer back to emotional disturbances in childhood. He concluded that cancer was the end result of an inner emptiness and emotional anaesthesia that followed out of an inability to reckon with and express one's own emotions. In his model, the cause of this emotional disturbance was a person's choice to subordinate themselves to the brutal authority of the father, thus sacrificing their own feelings of love and affection. This linked up with discussions of other intellectuals like Margret Boveri, who inquired into Germans' culpability for the crimes of National Socialism. Kütemeyer thought that the same pathological structure of self-betrayal and emotional anaesthesia was responsible for both guilt and illness.

Kütemeyer's theory remained contentious and was considered methodologically unsound, because he did not develop a generalizable model of the relation between mind and body and almost exclusively relied on case studies. This could not be reconciled with calls for causal hypotheses and verifiable, reproducible experiments. The new scientific standard in medicine also altered researchers' and clinicians' approach to and definition of emotions.

German medical science adopted tests from American personality psychology that were designed to explain with objective measures the role of psychological factors in the aetiology of illness. This approach focused not on autobiographical accounts and case studies, but on standardized responses to standardized questions or stimuli. Findings were compiled in statistics in order to determine whether the personality profile of patients with a certain disease diverged from those of other groups to a significant degree. Researchers defined the personality types of people with various types of cancer not as pathological in and of themselves, but as potentially being conducive to cancer.

Media simplified the various psychosocial factors contributing to cancer by inventing the concept of a 'cancer personality' applicable to all cancer patients. The 'type C' personality was characterized by the inability to articulate negative, conflictual emotions. In turn, researchers asserted that this inability derived from either too much or too little motherly love. They thought that the resulting inner compulsion to 'be nice' was particularly pronounced in women who later got cancer, as it encumbered them in acknowledging their own emotional needs.

In the GDR, research in psychotherapy and psychosomatics only began slowly gaining ground in the 1960s, after psychotherapy had spent the 1950s being forced by the ruling party to stick to Pavlovian psychology. As these dictates were gradually lifted, psychotherapists in East Germany could work with Western European and American methods like personality tests, but their resources remained limited and the pressure to justify their work high. Because of this, psychosomatic cancer research—the methods of which were heatedly debated even in the country where it was pioneered, the United States—never blossomed in East Germany. At the same time, civil society movements in West Germany held up the 'cancer personality' as the prototype of the inauthenticity of bourgeois life and oppressive social norms, which was then translated into political critique in works like Fritz Zorn's autobiography *Mars* (1977). This politicized form of cancer psychosomatics contradicted the social ideals of the GDR's ruling party; moreover, it found little resonance in East German literature and autobiography.

The second pillar of post-war psychosomatics, on the other hand, enjoyed undivided acclaim in both East and West: stress research. 'Stress' defined emotions as *one* endocrinologically significant factor among *many* others. The concept was so vague that both human and animal emotions could be studied in the lab without drawing any distinction between them. Stress research interpreted emotions as an evolutionary response to environmental challenges. It discarded the division between 'positive' and 'negative' emotions and asserted that emotions like fear had, at least in principle, a purpose. The decisive question was how humans and animals dealt with such emotions and which behaviours were forced on them by external circumstances. This moved researchers' attention towards the ways in which people processed 'emotional stress' in particular situations. They realized that people can learn 'salutogenetic' techniques of grappling with stress and can 'work' on their emotions without having to undergo years-long therapy. This insight fostered a budding shift in psychosomatics, which was tending away from the aporias of causal analysis and towards studying how doctors and nurses could better provide treatment. In West Germany, this trend was picked up by advice literature during the 1970s, and 'working on emotions' became a core component of self-help groups. In East Germany, this shift was limited to the engagement of a handful of doctors, psychologists, and psychotherapists who organized group therapy for (former) cancer patients in clinics, rehabilitation centres, and patients' clubs. In the 1970s and 1980s, therapy sessions revolved around expressing difficult, but 'authentic' emotions and making them bearable. Since the 1990s, the production of 'positive' emotions ascribed with a salubrious effect has become the primary concern of many psychotherapists. The field has moved from 'talking against fear' (Anne-Marie Tausch) towards the call to 'have some illusions, no big deal!' (*Psychologie Heute*).

Corporeal Emotions—Prevention and History

At the beginning of this history was the hope that cancer could be cured. It was fuelled by the advent of full anaesthesia and anti-septic standards in the second half of the nineteenth century, which made it possible to operate on patients without causing unbearable pain and significantly reduced the danger of potentially fatal infections. Only at this juncture did the early detection of cancer seem to make sense. After all, the smaller the tumour was, the less risky was operating on it. Moreover, because cellular pathology defined cancer as an illness with local origins, early surgery promised increased chances of curing it.

One of the first early detection campaigns was organized by gynaecologist Georg Winter in the late nineteenth century. His goal was to inform women that painless, seemingly harmless symptoms like intermenstrual bleeding might be early signs of cervical cancer and needed to be checked by a doctor. These campaigns provided a model for many others in the first third of the twentieth century.

But the point was not just to determine how to best communicate knowledge about early symptoms. Public health campaigners and officials were similarly concerned with how to get people to care for their bodies and identifying emotions that would encourage self-care. Winter and his colleagues at the newly established Committee for General Cancer Research did not want laypersons to rely on their intuitive sense that the absence of pain equalled health. Additionally, they did not want people to take their bodies for granted as a tool of labour that needed no attention so long as it was properly functioning. In order to awaken people out of their 'indolence' towards their own bodies, producers of early detection campaigns liberally employed frightening images and wax models of tumours. They were convinced that fear could occasion deliberate self-care.

The more expansive early detection campaigns became, the more doctors and health officials realized that the 'obtuse' behaviour of many people was not the only threat to their initiatives. They identified three 'adversaries'. First on the list were doctors who did not share their hope that cancer could be cured. As a result, these doctors often did not send their patients to clinics, believing that this refusal at least spared them the pain and suffering of surgery or radiotherapy. Second, campaigners thought that women's 'false shame' inhibited them from attending the 'embarrassing' appointment with their gynaecologist. In order to overcome this feeling, campaigns tried to cultivate a more matter-of-fact approach to female genitalia through schematic representations. Third, they sought to counter a different type of shame: the shame of potentially suffering from an illness that many believed was contagious and that could cause physical disfiguration, which led some people to prefer suppressing possible symptoms over revealing them to their doctor.

In the late 1920s and early 1930s, they bucked these emotional 'adversaries' with exhibitions, publications, lectures, and stage plays that sought to evoke both fear and hope. They shocked people with moulages and images of tumours, mobilizing a kind of fascination with fright. These images were juxtaposed with images of hope, of cured cancer. In order not to relativize hope, organizers concealed the fact that in many cases, such cures were only temporary.

'Before-and-after' images and stories told of protagonists who made the right decision at the right time, went to the doctor, and were cured, and of protagonists who passed up the brief window of hope and died because they had missed their one and only chance. Parallel narratives about a 'rational' character and a 'foolish' one almost always had a woman play the latter. 'Rational' concern and 'foolish' fear were thus imbued with moral, gendered meanings.

The moralizing strategy reached its apex in the 1930s. The exhibition 'Kampf dem Krebs', produced by Dresden's Hygiene Museum in 1931, expanded its scope. In the stories from the 1920s, the 'foolish' person had to bear the consequences of their 'false' decision as an individual. But the exhibition framed it as part of a cavalier attitude that posed a burden to family, society, and the '*Volk*'. Because a mother or father waited too long to go to the doctor, their children were left orphaned and destitute. Because cancer patients failed to respond to their early symptoms in time, society had to shell out lots of money to treat them in vain, money that could have been used for sorely needed housing. Listening to one's fears and avoiding early detection was explicitly condemned as cowardice. Overcoming fear through courage, in contrast, was depicted as a one-way street to being cured, as if courage in itself was sufficient for successful treatment. This narrative coupled courage with detached observation of the body, even without symptoms: monthly breast self-examinations and menstrual calendars were promoted as methods to frequently check the body for 'irregularities'.

The moralization of emotions was propelled by the depiction of health as a matter of will power, which had been catching hold since the late 1920s. National-Socialist health policy embraced this notion and placed considerable weight on prevention through lifestyle changes. At the same time, the world's first epidemiological studies on the relation between tobacco consumption and lung cancer were published. Exhibitions about cancer seized on this research and placed quitting smoking alongside more general health advice about exercising, taking cold showers, and avoiding processed foods. Conversely, many took this advice to mean that people who got cancer had failed to do their 'duty' to maintain their own health.

The use of 'cancer' as slander for political opponents and as an antisemitic slur exacerbated the moral and ideological stigmatization of cancer patients. But their exclusion from society went beyond language. Those considered 'incurable' fell into the same category as others whose lives were considered 'not worth living' by Nazi health policy. It was no coincidence that seriously ill cancer patients counted among them. The call to kill cancer patients had already been made in the 1920s by proponents of euthanasia like the racist author Gerhard Hoffmann, who published under the pseudonym Ernst Mann. There is evidence that towards the end of the Second World War, cancer patients were killed through starvation. The emotional strategies of the era's early detection campaigns certainly played some role in facilitating acceptance of such brutality.

In the immediate post-war period, attention shifted away from early detection and prophylaxis in both the eastern and western parts of Germany. However, it did not take long for the newly formed East German state's health officials to declare 'prophylaxis' as one of its fundamental values. Early detection was considered part of it, even though it was not really identical with prophylaxis in the sense of illness prevention. East Germany's health policy cast early detection examinations as the natural continuation of prophylactic measures undertaken during childhood. Weighing, measuring, and vaccinating children habituated them for routine check-ups and procedures, making them ready to undergo cancer screenings as adults without thinking twice. The strategy shifted the focus away from the illness itself, images of tumours disappeared from films and posters, publications no longer showed treatments in detail. In short, GDR health policy sought to supplant frightening images with optimistic images of socialist joy.

In the Federal Republic of Germany, early detection of cancer first became prominent in the run of the 1960s. In contrast to socialist 'prophylaxis', West German 'prevention' was defined as the responsibility of the individual, while informing people about it was not in the hands of the state, but of doctors and public health insurance corporations. This approach gave rise to strategies that adopted aspects of the moralization widespread in the first half of the twentieth century. However, West German moralization was increasingly paternalistic, and the doctor's wagging finger became its symbol. Like in East Germany, images of disease gradually fell out of use in West German early detection campaigns. They were substituted with images of familial happiness rather than optimistic solidarity. Fear remained in the background, but images and language avoided it. However, simply swapping out the emotional surface of campaigns was not the only thing at stake. Early detection was supposed to be redefined from a technique of *averting* health risks into a technique of *producing* health and happiness. This shift was helped along by other trends of caring for the symptomless body.

Prevention—in the strict sense of avoiding the risk of ever getting cancer in the first place—occupied more space, and both West and East German campaigns promoted the avoidance of health risks. These campaigns, which exhorted consumers to change their lifestyles, continued to work with fear and frightening images all the way into the 1970s. However, a gradual shift was beginning to take hold here, too. Instead of fuelling fear and harping on morality, more campaigns sought to associate not smoking with a 'positive' image. The turn of the twenty-first century brought with it yet a new paradigm.

Knowledge and Ignorance—Ethics and History

In the late nineteenth century, doctors adhered to the principle that patients should not be told they have cancer. The practice of concealing diagnoses was informed by both medical paternalism and by specific assumptions about emotions and their power.

In the late nineteenth century, the chances that someone could be cured of cancer were slim to none. Many cancer patients faced a future of pain and other symptoms that were often impossible to ameliorate. Thus, a cancer diagnosis seemed not only to be an almost certain death sentence, but also an omen of a miserable death. Doctors were convinced that if their patients knew they had cancer, they would fall into despair and hopelessness. Additionally, the overwhelming majority of doctors believed that fear and hopelessness would be detrimental to their patients' health and would shorten what little bearable time they had left.

Still, the taboo of speaking about diagnoses did not reign everywhere. Especially when male patients had occupational or familial responsibilities, some doctors thought it best to inform them of their diagnosis. This set in motion a complex linguistic machinery that at once concealed and revealed the diagnosis. The goal was to get patients to take necessary measures while also leaving room for doubt. The latter part was essential, as doctors believed that hope was so vital that doubt could preserve it and let it grow anew.

Around 1900, the practice of silence came under fire more and more. Jurists pointed out how it conflicted with ideals of individual self-determination and remonstrated that patients must consent to all medical procedures. Some doctors, like psychiatrist and medical ethicist Albert Moll, thought that concealing a diagnosis was only acceptable in a few exceptional cases. Moll argued that hope was nearly indestructible and would always return anyways, even if the patient was clearly told that they were suffering from a potentially fatal disease.

In the 1920s, though, most doctors continued to insist that cancer diagnoses should not be communicated. Advice guides for doctors offered various explanations for why knowledge of their cancer diagnosis would rob patients of their hope and that without hope, life was impossible. They argued that the lack of hope not only destroyed the ability to enjoy life, but also weakened the body. However, patients' friends and family generally were informed that their loved one had cancer in order to allow them to organize the patient's domestic and occupational affairs—but also so that the doctor had a witness that they had properly conducted the diagnosis. The expectation was that relatives would play along and continue to deceive the patient about the state of their health. The price to be paid was, in some cases, emotional distance towards their relative, as if they were just a patient and not a loved one. Historical documents do not provide a clear answer as to how silence affected the emotional relationship between husband and wife, parents and children. However, there is evidence that it was not always experienced as emotional isolation. Instead, some seem to have perceived silence as an act that preserved their dignity. While it concealed a harsh truth, it made it possible to foster hope together; while that hope might have been superficial, it also opened space for intimacy.

But criticism continued unabated. In precedent-setting decisions from the 1930s, the Reichsgericht held that the right to self-determination superseded all else without exception and that knowing one's diagnosis was necessary for its actualization. The judges offered an interpretation of the emotional effects of knowledge that diverged from earlier judgements. They thought it would cause not hopelessness or despair, but just a temporary dip in the patient's mood. After all, they asserted, strong people would know how to come to terms with losing hope for survival. This reasoning drew on discussions influenced by German Psychotherapy, which promoted a dispassionate approach to fear and dying.

In the early post-war period, these conceptions of emotions fell out of favour. West Germany's Federal Court of Justice wrote decisions that characterized the emotional effects of knowing one had cancer as grave. These judgements positioned fear closer to panic and cast it as an irrational emotion that inhibited reason and decision-making processes. Early West German psychosomatics defined hopelessness as an extremely dangerous state that could break a person's will to live. Indeed, this was the conclusion drawn by internist Arthur Jores in his analysis of narratives told by concentration camp survivors and returned prisoners of war.

Thus, in the 1950s, doctors and others discussed hope a lot. East German officials, however, had ideological reservations about such discourse. Socialist health policy was geared towards curing people, and everything that might encumber that goal was treated as a secondary concern. East German medical law reflected this hierarchy. While doctors were required to obtain their patients' consent in order to ensure they actively participated in the process of betterment, they were permitted to dispense with informing patients or getting their consent if they believed that doing so might endanger the hope of curing them.

Beginning in the 1960s, East Germany witnessed objections to the practical impossibility of concealing diagnoses from patients undergoing multi-month therapies. And, medical professionals and ethicists noted, if the deception failed, then the patient's trust in their doctor would be enduringly damaged. Around the same time, American and British doctors, sociologists, and theologians were also raising concerns about harming the integrity of the doctor-patient relationship, and their counterparts in both West and East Germany adopted their arguments. While Hungarian-British doctor Michael Balint wrote that the doctor's unconscious emotions could influence their therapeutic decisions and be perceived by the patient as well, American sociologists Barney Glaser and Anselm Strauss demonstrated that doctors and nurses often intentionally avoided dying patients in order not to have to answer their questions, bear the burden of deceiving them, and confront their own fear of death. These theories all shared the basic assumption that fear could not be managed through deception and repression, but that these attempts only fed into it and that in the end, it was the patient who had to shoulder it.

These studies were published at a time when therapy was exploding in popularity, particularly in West Germany. Emotions appeared as a significant aspect of the doctor-patient relationship that could influence the course of therapy. But social views on the meaning of emotions in relationships between patients and their family and friends also shifted. Intimacy was no longer defined simply on the basis of intense feelings. Rather, definitive became whether patients and their loved ones spoke about intimate emotions and 'worked through' them together. From this perspective, discrepancies between the knowledge of family members and patients' knowledge or lack thereof appeared as a serious issue that stood in the way of intimacy. The concept of emotional labour entered into widespread use. While advice books and self-help groups in West Germany fleshed out this notion in countless ways, a more limited number of doctors and psychologists in East Germany organized group therapy sessions for (former) cancer patients where they could speak about everyday problems and anxieties related to their illness.

In the 1970s and 1980s, the perception of cancer as an 'illness of the psyche' grew popular in West Germany, which fundamentally altered the debate on communicating diagnoses to patients. After all, if particular character traits and a particular approach to emotions contributed to causing cancer, then curing cancer would require grappling with one's own emotional disposition. But cancer patients could only do so if they knew what illness they had. Knowing that one had been diagnosed with cancer thus took on a new meaning: it became the necessary condition for analysing the emotions that supposedly caused the disease, an act that in turn harboured the chance for a new beginning.

Since the 1990s, there has been broad consensus that cancer patients should be informed about their diagnosis in almost all cases. The debate now revolves around the 'how', not the 'whether'. Economic pressures and the new definition of the patient as an autonomous consumer of medical services have led some doctors to lay all the details of diagnosis and prognosis out on the table. Though strictly speaking, they fulfil their legally prescribed duty to inform the patient in doing so, the approach can come off as cold and detached. Other doctors have looked for better ways. Over the past years, medical professionals have made more and more attempts to develop communicative techniques that their colleagues can use to guide these sometimes life-changing conversations in a sensitive manner. Empathy often stands front and centre. The shift relegates to the background the doctor's emotions and moral authority, which long played an outsized role in the history of cancer, because it favours an emotional disposition primarily geared towards acknowledging and respecting the patient's feelings. At the same time, the new guides go beyond the old concept of 'emotional work' by asserting that communicative techniques can help shape the other's emotions. In a sense, 'work on one's own emotions' has given way to the management of other peoples' emotions.

Spatial Emotions—Experience and History

At the end of the nineteenth century, there was only one professionally recognized option for treating cancer: surgery. If a tumour could not be operated on, then it was considered incurable.

There was still hope for other patients. Surgeons who almost always operated when the entire tumour could still be excised were particularly driven by this hope. But operating on internal tumours was dangerous. On average, somewhere between 15 and 30 per cent of patients died during or shortly after such operations. Statistics let surgeons know that many patients would experience relapses. 'Cured' was generally defined as surviving three or five years after the operation, which could be said of only a handful of patients. Nevertheless, doctors continued to operate and fostered hope without relativizing it—the only condition was, of course, that the cancer be 'detected early'.

Thus, they did not tell patients about the risk of relapses and metastases, nor did they inform them about potential post-operation complications. The assumption was that if patients knew all of this, they would get scared and might opt against surgery. Moreover, anxious, frightened patients were more difficult to anaesthetize; this necessitated more anaesthesia, increasing the risk of the procedure. Finally, doctors were convinced that fear could weaken the body or disturb its equilibrium, thus creating suboptimal conditions for operating. Suppressing information seemed to be a way to manage fear. The price to be paid was shock and despair when patients realized after the operation what kind of pain and limitations they would have to suffer with. But placed on the scale with death, many doctors did not think this was a price too high to pay.

Cancer treatment was generally conceived of as an episode that ended when the wounds had healed and the patient learned how to deal with the physical disabilities that surgery caused in some cases. By the 1920s, doctors were indeed requiring patients to come in for regular post-operation check-ups. However, they placed little weight on it, since in their experience, relapses and metastases usually meant that only palliative measures were possible.

The first decade of the twentieth century ushered in a new reason to hope: x-rays could sometimes shrink tumours so much that they could be operated on. Radiologists and gynaecologists also had encouraging successes with radiotherapy by itself. Radium reduced tumour growth and infections, weakening the often noxious smell given off by open tumours.

But radium was expensive. Though a substitute was found in mesothorium, it was also costly and had to be regularly swapped out on account of its short half-life. This made hope into more of a financial issue than it had been before. Radiotherapy was covered for patients with public health insurance, but only if doctors believed they had strong chances of being cured. Many civil servants and self-employed people, who had neither statutory nor private insurance, could hardly afford it. Because only large university hospitals had sufficient stores of radioactive substances, the costs of radiotherapy were often compounded by expenses for travel and accommodation. Thus, families generally chose to pay for this 'luxury' only when the hope of a cure was very good; for some, it was entirely out of reach.

Radiotherapy isolated patients. Because of the high price of radioactive substances and the need to protect others from them, patients were sequestered in a separate room during their multi-day treatment. They were not allowed to leave it and nobody except nurses was allowed to enter it. They were not told that they would suffer from diarrhoea, drowsiness, and nausea for days after undergoing treatment. Because dosimetry was still in its fledgling stages, some patients' tissue necrotized, which was difficult to reverse and indeed sometimes never was.

In the 1920s, when a shortage of hospital beds became a widespread problem, hospital administrations insisted on only accepting or retaining patients whose chances at being cured were considered good. This policy affected patients with late-stage cancer particularly severely. Caring for them demanded considerable resources: they often required a special diet, their bandages had to be regularly changed, and they had little energy to help care for themselves. Their cries of pain bothered other patients. Moreover, their tumours sometimes exuded an odour that many described as unbearable. Some were visibly disfigured. Thus, fellow patients complained about them, nurses had to be forced to care for them as a punitive measure, and some doctors tried to be rid of them.

However, many patients could not be sent home, because their dwellings were too small and their families did not have enough time to provide the intensive care they needed. The last resort were the old infirmaries and hospitals for incurables, but they hardly had the staff to offer adequate care. Moreover, they were often located on city outskirts, far away from patients' families, and they had limited visiting hours, making them more of a place to house sick people than to give them a home.

Heidelberg and Berlin each had special clinics for cancer patients, though. They specialized in treating patients who had unsuccessfully tried all other available forms of treatment. Heidelberg's Samaritan House and the chronically underfunded cancer pavilions at Berlin's Charité hospital were intended to give patients one last hope. Their medical care kept up with the state of the art in cancer research. But this implied that patients could be turned into objects of experiment. The line between legally permissible attempts at treatment welcomed by the patient with hope and illegitimate human experiments was not always clearly drawn. This was not so much a problem at the clinics in Heidelberg and Berlin as it was at the clinics in the German Empire where doctors conducted experiments on dying patients. Archival sources underscore that some patients were aware of and feared this danger.

After 1933, the Berlin cancer pavilions and Heidelberg's Samaritan House increasingly fell into a precarious state. Antisemitic laws caused many doctors to lose their positions or forced them to resign. These institutes also suffered because their work did not align with National-Socialist politics. The Nazi state did fund cancer research and new clinics for curable cancer patients. But the clinics for severely ill patients began crumbling even before the war, not to speak of their abysmal situation after the war began.

Once the Second World War was over, the occupying powers focused on rebuilding hospitals and fighting rampant infectious diseases like typhus and tuberculosis. In the run of the 1950s, both German states funnelled resources into a new form of healthcare that would definitively alter cancer patients' experiences. Rehabilitation seemed to represent a marked rejection of the Nazis' euthanasia policies, while also offering combat-wounded veterans a chance at recovery.

Extending convalescent care services to cancer patients was a decision rooted in researchers' observation that, while cure rates had generally stagnated, wealthier patients who could afford to take time off of work and pay for home care ultimately had better chances of survival than those who could not. They reasoned that despite surgery or radiotherapy, some cancer cells would remain in the body, and that the only way the immune system could hold them in check was through rest and recuperation.

Convalescent care for cancer patients had special requirements, leading both states to establish special resorts that only or primarily admitted people who had just completed cancer treatment. The fear that bringing many cancer patients together might create an atmosphere of hopelessness seemed secondary in the face of the resorts' potential medical benefits. Still, this concern was not entirely relegated to the wayside. House rules admonished guests not to speak about their illness with the other convalescents. Employees were ordered never to use the word 'cancer' and to refrain from remarks that might remind guests about their physical disabilities or declining state of health. However, the resorts were indeed supposed to offer recovering cancer patients emotional support—not through speaking about their 'deepest' fears, but through advice on how to grapple with everyday 'needs and concerns'.

Despite these policies, patients lived at the resorts for multiple weeks with others who had gone through similar treatments and faced similar problems. And many surmised that the 'lump' that had been surgically removed or irradiated was in fact a cancerous tumour. Postcards, letters, and autobiographical writings suggest that during their stays, many patients felt for the first time like they were no longer alone with their illness. Post-treatment care centres offered (former) cancer patients a sense of belonging, which fostered feelings of solidarity and enabled concrete support measures. Thus, the post-treatment resorts were predecessors of the self-help groups that began proliferating in the 1970s in West Germany and, to a lesser extent, in East Germany, too.

A shift in treatment techniques was one factor that brought medical professionals to the realization that solidarity among patients was important. In the run of the 1950s, gigantic betatrons and gammatrons supplanted the pre-war x-ray machines. The new machines' incredible destructive power was perceived as a positive, adequate to the task of curing cancer. But the language of 'cobalt cannons' and 'cobalt bombs' was a regular reminder of these technologies' military origins. The spaces where radiotherapy took place underscored that these 'weapons' did not just pose a danger for cancer cells: thick concrete walls, leaden doors, and locations in basements or former bomb shelters all protected 'the healthy' from radiation. In contrast, cancer patients were left alone with the source of both danger and potential cure inside the 'radiation bunkers'. The rays could be neither seen nor felt, they emitted little sound beyond a ticking noise, they did not produce any smell, and they moved over patients like an 'animal'. All this evoked fear and a feeling of nakedness in many patients. As autobiographical texts began spreading such images and scepticism about atomic energy grew, gammatrons were turned into a symbol of the technologized, emotionless healthcare industry.

In the 1960s, chemotherapy rose in both Germanys. It, too, had origins in military research. However, the metaphor 'chemical warfare against the body' was much less prominent in discussions about chemotherapy than the atomic war rhetoric was in discussions about radiotherapy. Rather, since its beginnings in the late 1940s, chemotherapy was viewed as the most radical form of cancer treatment. Doctors involved in clinical research were convinced that the highest doses of cytostatic agents that patients could still bear would be the most successful. The line between effective and fatal dosage, though, was extraordinarily thin. Thus, during therapy cycles, the patient's vitals had to be closely monitored to ensure that the treatment did not slip into the grey zone of life-threatening poisoning. During and after treatment, patients often felt considerably worse than they did before. The meaning of this decline in subjective wellness was ambivalent: it could be a sign that the therapy was having its desired effect, but it could also mean that the treatment might have to be cancelled.

Over the first few decades of chemotherapy's existence, standard protocols were hardly distinguishable from experimental protocols. A combination of agents being studied one year might be standard protocol the next. The constant slight adjustments in dosage, the combinations of chemicals, the administration and duration of treatment, and the regular discovery of new cytostatic agents—the blazing pace of developments in chemotherapy made it into a practice of hope in a special sense. With the multiplication of different cytostatic agents came the possibility of trying a different combination if the first attempt was unsuccessful, which set it apart from operation and radiotherapy, where failure signalled the end of treatment.

Doctors and patients shared in the belief that new cytostatic agents could harbour new chances. The legalization of 'compassionate use' extended the horizon of hope. It offered a different promise of increased life expectancy and perhaps even of a cure. But when things did not get better despite advances in medical technology, patients confronted the burden of deciding whether to give up hope and focus on living a life different from the one imposed on them by chemotherapy, a life in which they, indeed, had to confront the difficulties of their dying body, but were no longer subject to the cycles of treatment and could thus more freely choose how to spend the time they had left.

But chemotherapy also altered the face of hope because it lent it the character of a kind of emotion on demand. In contrast to surgery and radiotherapy, chemotherapy was unable to eliminate cancer completely well into the 1960s. The cytostatic agents used at the time could significantly improve leukaemia patients' blood levels and shrink the size of some tumours, but these changes were always temporary 'remissions'. At some point, the tumour would begin to grow again and the white blood cell count would increase. Before children with leukaemia were cured with chemotherapy in the late 1960s, the purpose of the treatment was to extend life expectancy. But this served to shift focus to the side effects of treatment: What was the point of extending a patient's life for a few months if the gained time was spent suffering from the serious side effects of the treatment itself? While the old dichotomy of 'maybe surviving' or 'certainly dying' left little room for considerations of the patient's subjective sense of well-being, chemotherapy gave it new weight. Gained time had to be coupled with 'quality of life', a concept developed in the 1970s that quickly ascended to become a fundamental principle of health policy and medical ethics. The necessity of maintaining a certain quality of life opened doctors' minds to methods previously laughed at and maligned as alternative. Psycho-oncological care, group therapy, and visualization and relaxation techniques were recommended to patients and sometimes even offered by clinics themselves.

Today, the number of people who call themselves cancer survivors is swelling. There are also many cancer patients who live in a state of remission, whether it be because their tumour's growth has been brought to a halt for an indeterminate period of time, or because their symptoms have disappeared but they or their doctors are not certain that they are definitively cured. In such unclear cases, health can seem to be a question of one's own decision and subjective feeling. In early 2017, an article published by the *Süddeutsche Zeitung* quoted a woman who had leukaemia as a child who said of her current state: 'I *feel* healthy.'[1]

Fear, Hope, and Disgust in Historical Context

Do some emotions disappear while others are 'discovered'? Can an emotion define a period to such an extent that it justifies speaking of an 'age of fear'?

[1] Christiane Löll, 'Besser überleben', *Süddeutsche Zeitung* 47, 25/6 February 2017, 35.

This history of the relationship between cancer and emotions reveals the methodological deficiencies of the notion that emotions adhere to a logic of boom-bust cycles. After all, what constitutes the 'upvaluation' of an emotion? Perhaps that it is frequently thematized in public discourse? Would the reverse then follow that emotions seldom discussed in public are undergoing a 'decline'? But in some circumstances, unexpressed emotions can occupy more attention and influence decisions more than emotions that are constantly on everyone's lips. Indeed, the complicated practices surrounding the taboo of speaking about cancer and the emotions associated with it exemplify this point. And in other cases, intentionally suppressed emotions can be utilized to political ends, as was the case with disgust in the public awareness campaigns of the 1920s. Moreover, the notion that emotions undergo upswings and downturns is complicated by the fact that public perceptions of a specific emotion's 'function' change over time. For instance, the fear tapped by producers of early detection campaigns in the 1920s was a different emotion than the fear avoided by organizers in the 1950s and 1960s because of what they saw as its dangerous irrationality.

The meaning of an emotion in its historical context can only be accurately understood when the analysis of public discussions is tied to an analysis of how that emotion was defined at that moment, the extent to which talk about it was suppressed, and the extent to which it unfolded its power despite not always being explicitly named. The following provides a survey of the vicissitudes of three emotions that left an indelible mark on the history of cancer in the twentieth century: fear, hope, and disgust.

Fear

Fear was heatedly discussed in debates about the first early detection campaigns at the beginning of the twentieth century. Campaigners, doctors, and public health officials wondered if knowledge about health risks would incite fear and whether it was a good idea to use fear in order to motivate people to take better care of their bodies. Many believed that healthy people had few fears about their bodies and that instrumentalizing fear in public health campaigns would not pose a problem. The guiding assumption was that people with a good upbringing knew how to parry fear. Though they viewed it as a strong emotion, they also thought it could only have an effect when bound to a particular situation. The first early detection campaigns and exhibitions thus employed frightening images and moralistic narratives. As a remedy for fear, they proposed simply going in for an early detection check-up, while 'proving' the efficacy of this remedy with images and stories of cured cancer.

But in the context of surgical operations, fear was viewed as medically detrimental. A number of animal experiments demonstrated that fear could have a negative effect on organ functions, occasioning surgeons to take great pains to rid their patients of the emotion. The strategy of choice was to dampen fear before surgery by deceiving the patient.

Doctors also deceived patients about their diagnosis and prognosis. Most did not think that knowledge about one's imminent death had any positive value, while most did believe that it would trigger insurmountable fear that would permanently capture the patient's body and mind. In sum, in the early twentieth century, most doctors and medical scientists conceived of fear as a physiological emotion developed through evolutionary adaptation. As a consequence, they thought there was a biologically predetermined way to overcome it through action. Education and character development could be used to habituate people to deal with their fears, but they hit their limits when all treatment options were exhausted.

After the First World War, more people came to view fear's physical effects as serious and long-lasting; accordingly, they doubted that fear could be overcome so simply. Psychoanalysis focused on fear and its role in conversion neuroses. Some thought these 'illnesses of fear' were caused by unaddressed psychological conflicts that had initially had short-term physiological effects, which then became chronic, caused functional disturbances, and ultimately left irreversible scars. From this perspective, it seemed plausible that early detection campaigns themselves might cause irrational, uncontrollable fears about cancer among the population. Exhibitions and campaigns of the 1920s continued to play on fear, because organizers still believed it was a singularly powerful motivator to act and, moreover, because they thought that fear could elicit curiosity and excitement. However, they learned to exert more caution, using fear in moderation and never without counterbalancing it with hope.

Towards the end of the 1920s, fear was re-evaluated as a positive emotion. This viewpoint was embraced by the Nazis, who blamed the individual's cowardice for the aforementioned problematic aspects of fear. National Socialism touted the theory that courage developed out of an open confrontation with one's own fears. Like the New German Medicine and German Psychotherapy movements, the Nazis wanted people to 'toughen up'. While in their theory, 'cowardly' people avoided or repressed fear, self-certain 'German' people tackled their fears and cultivated strength and courage through action. Instilling the appropriate attitude demanded the right kind of upbringing, they thought, but they also asserted that people had to choose to identify with their 'true' will.

Conceptions of cancer replicated this fusion of inside and outside. As in the past, cancer was still considered to be a cellular illness located within the body. But at the same time, metaphors identified it with the state's political or 'racial' enemies. The fight against cancer was analogized with the fight against an external enemy, and 'defeating' it with the 'purification' of oneself. But what dying of cancer meant within this discursive framework remained an open question. Still, the National-Socialist approach maintained that nobody should be denied the chance to confront this question by being deceived about their approaching death. Here, too, a particular understanding of fear, courage, and cowardice dominated the conversation. Reckoning with the frightening knowledge of one's coming death was cast as the final test on the way to discovering one's true self, which counted for nothing outside the ethnically defined '*Volk*'. This shifted fear from being a biological emotion to a test of character. Courage and fear appeared as interrelated emotions, while cowardice was grasped as their true opposite and thus identified as the source of all the negative effects associated with fear.

In the post-war period, conceptions of fear diverged in the two German states. In East Germany, fear was stripped of its positive dimension, while optimism was crowned as the official emotion of the new socialist state. The ruling party thought that fear and the pessimism associated with it was unjustified, since socialism had been realized and the future was in the hands of the collective. Thus, East German early detection campaigns dispensed with fear. Instead, they focused on habituating prophylactic measures from the cradle to the grave while attaching positive emotions to them. Even though early detection was not the same as disease prevention, GDR health officials depicted it as just one part of the latter. Campaigns discussed fear of early detection screenings, while explaining that it was unnecessary because they were not painful and the chances of being cured in the case that something was detected were good. In short, they adopted strategies from the past. However, they were informed by a different understanding of why fear was dangerous, concerned less with its bodily effects than with its potential to fracture rosy images of the present and future.

In West Germany's early years, too, the strategy of intentionally inciting fear lost its backers. This shift was informed by a return to a conception of fear as an irrational emotion akin to panic. Multiple decisions handed down by the Federal Court of Justice emphasized the detrimental physical and mental effects that could follow out of frightening information and learning of one's cancer diagnosis. Thus, withholding knowledge from patients once again seemed legitimate.

As contemporaneous debates on the recent Nazi past suggested, fear could lead to a loss of control, both personally and politically. Thus, doctors and health policymakers were much warier about evoking it. Instead, West German early detection campaigns condemned in moralizing fashion the fear of people who refused to go to check-ups, while praising those who did as rational people. This trend pushed early detection to a new level, from a technique of dispelling fear to a technique of the rational, controlled production of security. Public representations of new radiotherapy technology, though, demonstrate that fear continued to be a factor. While the medical profession emphasized that they had control over the machines, the depiction of them as powerful anti-cancer 'weapons' only worked because it touched on the association of atomic power with massive death and destruction. This threatened to permanently derail the image of harnessed energy.

In the run of the 1960s, the 'repressed', 'unconscious' emotions of the Federal Republic of Germany became a central topic of both psychological and medical debate as well as more general public discourse. West German doctors, psychologists, sociologists, and theologians drew on psychoanalysis to analyse how repressed emotions—and particularly fear—could influence the body, therapeutic decisions, and doctor-patient relations. Their work was particularly influenced by American and British research. The shift expanded medical professionals' perspective on the significance of emotions to encompass those of doctors, rather than just those of patients. They reflected on which emotions led doctors to want to protect their patients from fear and what effects this might have on their relationship. They concluded that a doctor's fears—including that of death—could guide their medical decisions and mould their interactions with dying patients. These findings of sociological, psychiatric, and psychoanalytic research fundamentally altered future approaches to fear. At the same time, fear was politicized by the alternative left in the 1970s, which redefined it as a human, 'authentic' emotion that derived from the subject's sensitivity towards hidden dangers and had been 'sugar-coated' by bourgeois norms.

Doctors, therapists, and patients slowly recognized that fear had to be addressed, both for therapeutic and for social reasons. But in contrast to the model of open confrontation and heroic individualism that dominated the National-Socialist conception of fear, perspectives informed by psychoanalysis held that fear could not simply be overcome through action. Instead, they claimed that fear first had to be talked about. But they read the desire to overcome fear ambivalently, since articulating one's fears was viewed as an act of self-discovery and a critique of taboos. As a consequence, fear could never be banished once and for all, but had to be repeatedly spoken about in therapy. And an emotion that required so much energy in therapy was little suited to be used in public health campaigns. Accordingly, campaigns produced by West Germany's public health insurers and the Federal Centre for Health Education after 1971 sought to depict early detection as a way to be happy instead of being stuck in the cycle of feeling fear and searching for security.

In the 1970s, only anti-smoking campaigns still wielded fear as their tool of choice, in East and West Germany alike. Organizers thought that this 'strong' emotion was indispensable for moving people to make the kinds of lifestyle changes they were trying to spur. But psychological research and surveys cast doubt on the long-term efficacy of fear. Beginning in the 1980s, shocking images of decaying lungs gave way to attempts to give the choice not to smoke a positive image. Only recently have gruesome pictures found their way back onto cigarette packaging.

Thus, throughout the twentieth century, fear assumed a number of forms and was used in multifarious ways. In public health campaigns, it was employed, and then consciously avoided; in medical research and clinical treatment, it was attributed with various meanings and effects; it figured prominently in debates on whether and how to talk about cancer; and for many people, it fundamentally shaped the experience of the disease. But what fear was changed over time. Feelings of fear changed, as did moral evaluations of them. How people were expected to confront their fears, whether fear could be utilized for political ends—on these points, too, the twentieth century witnessed significant shifts. This history cannot be accurately captured by linear narratives that encompass the entire century; the notion that, for instance, fear was increasingly internalized over its course does not do justice to the manifold aspects of fear in the twentieth-century history of cancer. Certainly, the instrumentalization of fear is viewed much more critically today than it was during the turn to the twentieth century, because fear is now considered a complex emotion that has to be worked through. Early twentieth-century doctors withheld important information from their patients in order to avoid making them afraid, because they themselves worried about fear's negative physiological effects. Today, doctors and psychologists generally believe that this strategy is unjustified because repressed fears pose a danger to both physical and mental health. In short, contemporary discourse seems more sensitive to fear's pathological potential, rarely judges experiencing fear as a moral shortcoming, and prizes speaking about it. But this transformation was not a smooth-running, unidirectional development. Making these claims is only possible from a bird's-eye perspective, which fails to capture deviations and contemporary tendencies to once again label fear as irrational.

Hope

The temporality of hope is similar to that of fear. Hope is directed towards the future. But in contrast to fear, hope is geared towards inducing a particular vision of the future. Because it is impossible to know what the future will be, hope fills it with dreams and desires and motivates action to make them real. But despite these structural similarities, historians of emotions have conducted little research on hope. Perhaps the dismissal derives from views of hope as a passive disposition that exerts little influence on decisions and actions, as if it were more linked to political or religious visions than concrete objects and objectives, thus making it a better topic for historians of ideas than historians of emotions. However, hope played a significant role in the history of cancer in the twentieth century, one comparable to fear in its scope and impact, even if conceptions of hope changed more slowly and drew less on biology and medical science.

In the early twentieth century, two perspectives on the relation between hope and cancer were dominant. Early detection campaigns sought to appeal to the concrete hope for a cure. This hope was tightly bound up with a single action and end result. It could only be realized if people went to the doctor the moment they showed symptoms. Because this hope was entirely new and many doctors thought it was unfounded, campaigners believed that relativizing it in any way would undermine their campaigns' efficacy. Thus, the new slogan 'detected early, curable' suppressed any hint of the fact that this hope was, indeed, statistically improbable. By opting for this approach, campaign organizers tacitly accepted that patients might blame themselves for going to the doctor too late if their hope to be cured could not be realized.

The second variant of hope was also directed at being cured, or at least at surviving. The majority of doctors in the early twentieth century were convinced that hope was necessary for survival. The conviction was not limited to the belief that life without hope would be unbearable, because doctors thought hope had real effects on the body. However, they did not define these effects in physiological terms—it was not for nothing that, in contrast to fear, hope was never tested in laboratories and animal experiments. This version of hope was conceptualized in vitalist terms as an inner life force, as a necessary element of the desire to live without which the body would give up. In order to not run the risk of destroying this more fundamental hope, doctors thought it advisable to deceive patients about their cancer diagnosis. In the eyes of doctors, it seems, the hopes sown by early detection campaigns were not strong enough to withstand a cancer diagnosis. As a result, the period witnessed a paradoxical tension between open public discussion about cancer on the one hand and private silence about it on the other.

But the conviction that maintaining hope for survival was indispensable had another effect. There was no established approach for treating people who were dying and could not be deceived into believing they would be fine. Because doctors wanted to avoid inducing hopelessness at all costs, they had a difficult time dealing with terminally ill cancer patients. In the name of preserving other patients' hopes, they were hidden away—behind curtains, in asylums for incurables, and at special clinics like Berlin's cancer pavilions.

The exclusion of dying patients was the dark side of a hope propagated in absolute terms. And the practice continued well into the 1950s. But as early as the First World War, advocates wanted to wrest hope from the grip of the life/death dichotomy by giving it a new object. For instance, psychiatrist and medical ethicist Albert Moll argued that hope should be directed not primarily towards bodily survival, but towards being part of something greater, something indestructible, whether it be in religious transcendence or community belonging. National Socialism took this idea to its extreme. While it ruled out deception as a buoy of hope, it also devalued individual life. Because the dying, 'incurable' patient was just one small piece of the racially defined body of the nation, they had to come to terms with the hopelessness of their individual situation on their own. Institutions that had cared for dying cancer patients before 1933 were stripped of their funding and were increasingly unable to provide care, while some were likely shut down during the Second World War.

After the war, new discussions in both Germanys distinguished between the hope for bodily survival and a transcendental, but not necessarily religious hope that was only unfettered by the dissolution of the first type of hope. Debates questioned whether this was a process in which the hope for life almost automatically dissipated with the body's gradual weakening, or whether doctors and therapists had to cautiously unmask the first form of hope as an illusion in order to allow the second type of hope to break through.

But can people live without hope for their own future? Psycho-oncology, which arrived in West Germany in the 1970s but was also registered in East Germany, offered a different answer. Most people, its proponents claimed, needed hope throughout their entire lives. But their hope can be oriented towards small, attainable things, such as sailing on a boat again, seeing the springtime bloom again, not having to suffer unbearable pain, hugging their family tomorrow. Psycho-oncologists thought hope could best be preserved by chopping up the big hope for survival into a bunch of little hopes and drawing hope for the future closer to the present. This sort of hope management broke down the unattainable into a number of attainable hopes that made death almost invisible. As sociologist Zygmunt Bauman wrote about the fear of one's own mortality:

> The big carcass of mortality has been sliced from head to tail into thin rashers of fearful, yet curable (or potentially curable) afflictions; they can be now fit neatly into every nook and cranny of life.... Fighting death is meaningless. But fighting the causes of dying turns into the meaning of life.[2]

Chemotherapy fit well with this concept of small hopes. New cytostatic agents were regularly being discovered, thus helping sustain hope if one form of treatment did not work. Chemotherapy's goal was also different: remission and gaining life expectancy were sufficient; achieving a definitive cure was not necessary to call it a success. In the 1990s, positive psychology reassessed the salubrious effects of 'cultivating' hope through certain techniques. The assumption is that hopeful thoughts and images of healing can actually influence the body and benefit the immune system.

By the twenty-first century, hope had become an emotion closer to the present while becoming decoupled from grand visions of the future. At the same time, hope has gradually come to be seen as an act accomplished by the person doing the hoping.

[2] Zygmunt Bauman, *Mortality, Immortality and Other Life Strategies* (Cambridge: Polity Press, 1992), 140.

Disgust

In contrast to fear and hope, disgust had an identifiable highpoint in discussions about cancer in the twentieth century, after which it declined in prominence. Disgust was an emotion of the first half of the twentieth century's history of cancer, after which it abruptly dropped off the radar. The reasons lie in the history of cancer treatment: disgust was generally felt as a reaction to the unpleasant stench given off by decaying, infected tumours. Radiotherapy was often able to eliminate the causes of the smell, so that by the 1950s, it was seldom an issue. But this was not the only reason why disgust almost entirely disappeared from cancer history after the 1950s.

Before 1945, taboos regulated what could be said about disgust and what could not. A glance at health exhibitions and early detection campaigns reveals that publicly speaking about disgust was unwelcome then, too. With the aim of evoking a visceral reaction in visitors, they featured images that would have been considered disgusting by standards of the time. But exhibition producers had to be careful and balance out disgust with other emotions. Many perceived explicit descriptions of disgust as something scandalous, as the reaction to Gottfried Benn's 'Morgue' poems make clear. Still, people could certainly discuss lived feelings of disgust in partially public spaces. In letters of complaint, official communications, and expert journals, doctors, patients, and administrators did not shy away from writing about the disgust they felt towards patients with advanced tumours. Disgust with the smell, excretions, and sight of tumours was seen as a justified feeling: Charles Darwin and, later, philosopher Aurel Kolnai, defined disgust as an involuntary reaction to decay, secretions, and rotting food.

Disgust was ascribed with a life-preserving function, protecting the organism from danger. As such, biologists and philosophers alike thought it neither could nor should be overcome. This naturalistic concept of disgust was applied to cancer patients without qualification, since other factors seemed to justify it. Their hopelessness made them emotionally and morally reprehensible, and their 'incurable' state was viewed by eugenicists as proof of their 'inferiority'. Added to all that was the long debunked, yet widespread fear that cancer was contagious. These points not only seemed to legitimize feelings of disgust towards certain cancer patients. They also seemed to recommend a certain course of action, since people were supposed to avoid and discard disgusting things. Thus, many doctors, patients, and nurses demanded that cancer patients with advanced tumours be excluded from normal clinics. Feelings of disgust as well as convictions about others' moral and 'racial' inferiority reinforced one another. Only a handful of people spoke out against the exclusion of terminally ill cancer patients and sought ways to hem or overcome disgust.

After 1945, this complex of exclusion, morality, eugenics, and disgust was discredited. Descriptions of disgust generally disappeared from public forums, as did demands that people seen as 'disgusting' be hidden from view. Feelings of disgust continued to exist in silence, though. Despite advances in medical technology, some tumours broke through the skin and exuded a heavy odour. But discussions on how doctors, nurses, and pastors could dampen the smell were now held in private. In post-1945 writings on cancer treatment, disgust was hardly mentioned. However, interviews suggest that in the second half of the twentieth century, those who felt disgust took greater consideration of the shame felt by cancer patients for having a tumour perceived as disgusting. Contemporary palliative medicine places more weight on the patient's concerns that their tumour might evoke disgust in others. The primary goal is to ensure that disgust does not lead to exclusion or isolation, even if in some cases an animal can better provide compassion than a person can.[3]

When Emotions Became Rational

This history of cancer analysed three modes of the disease's relation to emotions: first, it studied the genesis of scientific, and above all medical and psychological concepts of what emotions are; second, it tracked the shifts in different types of knowledge about emotions and cancer; and third, it detailed the role that emotions played in clinical, preventive, palliative, and private approaches towards cancer and those diagnosed with it. This synthesis uncovered manifold insights into processes of rationalization, scientificization, and therapeutization.

Research literature seems to agree that it was during the 'long turn of the century', reaching from the 1890s to the 1930s, that the emotions were discovered as an object of scientific inquiry. In this first phase, they were studied as a physiological phenomenon, captured in the imagery of the 'hydraulic model' of control, restraint, and potential release. The history of the relation between cancer and emotions reveals a different, less clear-cut form of scientificization and rationalization, illustrating that two divergent conceptions of emotions coexisted in the early twentieth century: a scientific concept of emotions and a pragmatic, moral-philosophical concept, which were fitting for different situations and thus never came into conflict with each other. The scientific concept pigeonholed emotions as a bodily function devoid of intention and cognition. This idea was used to describe physiological reactions in medical contexts and surgery theatres, where doctors withheld information from patients in order to avoid evoking feelings of fear and the negative physiological effects they were thought to cause.

But when the issue was how emotions might spur people to act and make decisions, emotions in the physiological sense had secondary status as mere

[3] Christine Holch, 'Worauf es in der Palliativmedizin ankommt. Die Schrecken am Ende des Lebens. Interview mit Sven Gottschling', *Chrismon* 3 (2017): 12–18, 16.

arousers of attention and signals of urgency. After the initial sign was registered, it was believed, the person's character grabbed the reins, following the rules of action perceived to be adequate to the emotion. This shift was thought to have the potential to transform fear into courage.

The social expectation that people would manage their emotions demoted speaking about and showing strong emotions to undesirable choices. The external expression of a person conforming to this expectation might have given off the impression of 'coldness', but doctors' continued interest in and engagement with hope underscores that the appearance of an absence of emotions should not be equated with the genuine item. The sovereign mastery of one's emotions was viewed as the epitome of the educated character, an ideal that fell in line with other contemporaneous social norms about what constituted rational action.

Since the 1920s, though, a long process of change has been underway. The psychoanalytic acknowledgement of emotions entered into everyday discourse. Psychoanalysis elevated fear to a paradigmatic emotion, theorizing it as standing at the juncture between feeling and drive and evaluating it, for the first time, with the categories 'normal' and 'pathological'. This context saw the 'hydraulic model' of emotions turn into a pathological correlate to the pragmatic model. The new discipline postulated that emotional energies not discharged through action would be converted into psychological and physical symptoms. At the same time, emotions were recovered from the margins of academic medicine and turned into an object of science, particularly by the New German Medicine movement. Thus, on the whole, the medical, psychological, and biological sciences began considering emotions as a phenomenon worth researching. Still, 'bodily medicine' continued to bracket emotions because it attributed to them little capacity to influence somatic pathologies. Believing that they could only cause hormonal imbalances and similar disturbances expressed in symptoms such as ulcers, many doctors relegated their study to neurology, psychiatry, and psychology.

In the late 1920s and under National Socialism, psychology and psychotherapy became the authoritative sciences of the emotions. Dominated by the Nazi-sanctioned New German Psychotherapy, they redefined the psyche and expanded the moral implications of mastering one's emotions. Fighting against 'Jewish', 'mechanistic' psychology and psychotherapy, the school sought to bring Germans into touch with their 'German essence'. Its racist ideology encouraged patients to let feelings like fear flow and then overcome them in an act of will motivated by a consciously adapted moral certitude. This process became a key medium of subjectification in which the National-Socialist self had to reproduce and 'prove' itself again and again. Scholars have described this ideal as emotional dispassion. More accurate would be to describe it as a detached emotional style that justified itself through an arrogated attitude of heroism.

The year 1945 ushered in a caesura in the history of emotions, but not a full-scale break. On the one hand, emotions were repositioned as the clear opposite of rational thought, which temporarily put a freeze on earlier tendencies to rationalize them. Fear, for instance, was now perceived as being closely related to panic, which made questionable the notion that it could be rationally overcome through resolute action. On the other hand, emotions were placed in proximity to pathological disorders, which dangerously shrank the thin line between the normal and the pathological. This hard turn was new in Germany and, like the renewed assertion that emotions were irrational, represented a reaction to certain interpretations of the Nazi past. But at the same time, the pathologization of emotions set forth older developments that could be traced back to changes in American psychoanalysis and psychosomatics in the late 1930s as well as to discourses in the Weimar Republic.

Two contrary trends emanated out of this re-evaluation of emotions. Fields like psychiatry, clinical psychology, medicine, and law that explicitly dealt with illness researched emotional pathologies with more intensity than ever before. Other fields more interested in social structures like economics, sociology, and political science retreated from studying emotions, pushing them out of their models as best they could. Accordingly, emotions in public life seemed problematic and were, in the 1950s in particular, only expressed with extreme caution—and even then, they were always paired up with rational 'counterweights' like the promise of security and control.

Since the beginning of the 1960s, the emotions have increasingly been returned to the orbit of science and rationality. The trailblazers here were the psycho-sciences, which studied with new experimental methods how the emotions exert their effects. These sciences and their models fostered an ambivalent (de)pathologization of the emotions. What seemed to them dangerous and potentially causative of illness were not emotions as such, but 'false' approaches to them. This shift in accent helped blur the division between normal and pathological and shook up longstanding emotional topographies. Fear, anger, and rage were no longer the problems. Rather, the gravest pathology was seen as being the incapability of perceiving and adequately expressing one's own feelings.

This shift quickly proved to be political dynamite, because it implied a new ideal of emotional life: the emotionally authentic person able to withstand conflict. This ethic was cultivated by the alternative left in the 1960s and then entered into the mainstream, so that by the 1970s and 1980s, the psycho-sciences' concept of the emotions had asserted itself in society and contributed to the 'process of value change' observed by many at the time. The history of cancer, in short, had a considerable part in the scientific run-up to this more general social turn.

The new focus on the individual's ability to reckon with their feelings and experiences was open to a plurality of different psychotherapeutic methods. The 'proper' approach to one's emotions came to be grasped as a process, not something that could be finished once and for all, and character building now seemed inadequate for the task, too. Instead, the goal became the development of one's own individual emotional ethics in collaboration with one's therapist. As a consequence, perceiving emotions, speaking about them, and showing them became fundamental components of working on oneself in therapy. This positioned emotions as a key nexus between inner psychic life and the outside world, and as a primary medium of therapeutic, private, and even political relations.

While the therapeutic rationalization of emotions expanded, so too did the public visibility of emotions and their political and scientific reassessment. Thus, these developments should be read as the prehistory of the emotional turn, which most historians and sociologists date to the early 1990s. Emotions now attracted the attention of sciences that had previously neglected them and attributed to them little physiological significance and little importance for inter- and intrapersonal conflicts. The discovery of the emotions' rational aspects, their relevance for health and illness, and their proximity to cognition increased scientific interest in 'positive' emotions like hope, which sent a sonic boom through the history of cancer.

Alongside the therapeutic processing of already existing emotions, contemporary self-help guides promote the 'production' of salutiferous emotions through cognitive effort or consciously enacted bodily exercises. And certain communicative techniques have been designed to help doctors and therapists engage the emotions of cancer patients through rational, empathic conversation.

Ultimately, the rationalization of emotions has today reached a highpoint. Contemporary consensus is that emotions are rational because they play an important role in decision-making, can be intentionally evoked, and can be managed through communication and therapy. It is not for nothing that public debate today wonders whether robots can have feelings. But then what constitutes an emotion, and what distinguishes emotions from cognition? To what extent are my feelings mine? At our current juncture, emotions are enjoying more public and scientific interest than they have at any time over the past century. A renewed appreciation of emotions and the discrediting of their depreciation as irrational have made it possible to speak openly about them, get help in working on them, and to not just take them seriously in cases of grave illness.

After all, emotions have themselves undergone fundamental changes in the run of this century-long history, too. Thinking about how and why they have changed is important so as to not rest satisfied with the 'emancipation of the emotions'. Because analysing what has been lost and which new constraints have arisen is just as significant. This, ultimately, is what the history of emotions is all about.

Select Bibliography

Alexander, Franz. *Psychosomatic Medicine: Its Principles and Applications*. New York: W. W. Norton, 1939.

Arikha, Noga. *Passions and Tempers: A History of the Humours*. New York: HarperCollins, 2007.

Arnold-Forster, Agnes. *The Cancer Problem: Malignancy in Nineteenth-Century Britain*. Oxford: Oxford University Press, 2021.

Aronowitz, Robert A. 'The Rise and Fall of the Psychosomatic Hypothesis in Ulcerative Colitis'. In *Making Sense of Illness: Science, Society, and Disease*, edited by Robert A. Aronowitz, 39–56. Cambridge: Cambridge University Press, 1998.

Aronowitz, Robert A. *Unnatural History: Breast Cancer and American Society*. Cambridge: Cambridge University Press, 2007.

Atzl, Isabel, and Roland Helms. *Die Geschichte der Deutschen Krebsgesellschaft*. Germering: Zuckschwerdt, 2012.

Bahnson, Claus Bahne. 'Das Krebsproblem in psychosomatischer Dimension'. In *Lehrbuch der psychosomatischen Medizin*, edited by Thure von Uexküll, 685–98. Munich: Urban & Schwarzenberg, 1979.

Baines, Joanna. 'Three Stories: Generations of Breast Cancer'. In *Cancer Patients, Cancer Pathways: Historical and Sociological Perspectives*, edited by Carsten Timmermann and Elizabeth Toon, 13–35. New York: Palgrave Macmillan, 2012.

Balint, Michael. *The Doctor, His Patient and the Illness*. New York: International Universities Press, 1957.

Bauer, Karl Heinrich. *Mutationstheorie der Geschwulst-Entstehung. Übergang von Körperzellen in Geschwulstzellen durch Gen-Änderung*. Berlin: Springer, 1928.

Baumgart, Winfried, ed. *Kaiser Friedrich III. Tagebücher 1866–1888*. Paderborn: Schöningh, 2012.

Beddies, Thomas. *'Du hast die Pflicht, gesund zu sein!' Der Gesundheitsdienst der Hitler-Jugend 1933–1945*. Berlin: Be.bra, 2010.

Bielka, Heinz. *Geschichte der Medizinisch-Biologischen Institute Berlin-Buch*. 2nd edn. Berlin: Springer, 2002.

Biess, Frank. 'Feelings in the Aftermath: Toward a History of Postwar Emotions'. In *Histories of the Aftermath: The Legacies of the Second World War in Europe*, edited by Frank Biess and Robert Moeller, 30–48. New York: Berghahn, 2010.

Biess, Frank. *German Angst? Fear and Democracy in the Federal Republic Germany*. Oxford: Oxford University Press, 2020.

Biess, Frank, and Daniel M. Gross. 'Emotional Returns'. In *Science & Emotions after 1945: A Transatlantic Perspective*, edited by Frank Biess and Daniel M. Gross, 1–38. Chicago: University of Chicago Press, 2014.

Biro, David. *The Language of Pain: Finding Words, Compassion, and Relief*. New York: W. W. Norton, 2000.

Boddice, Rob. 'Introduction: Hurt Feelings'. In *Pain and Emotion in Modern History*, edited by Rob Boddice, 1–15. London: Palgrave Macmillan, 2014.

Boddice, Rob. *The History of Emotions*. Manchester: Manchester University Press, 2018.

Boddice, Rob. *A History of Feelings*. London: Reaktion Books, 2019.

Boddice, Rob, and Mark Smith. *Emotion, Sense, Experience*. Cambridge: Cambridge University Press, 2020.

Boddice, Rob, and Bettina Hitzer, eds. *Feeling Dis-Ease in Modern History: Experiencing Medicine and Illness*. London: Bloomsbury Academic, 2022.

Bösl, Elsbeth. 2010. 'Die Geschichte der Behindertenpolitik in der Bundesrepublik aus der Sicht der Disability History'. *Aus Politik und Zeitgeschichte* 23 (2010): 6–12.

Bothe, Detlef. *Neue Deutsche Heilkunde* 1933–1945. Husum: Matthiesen, 1991.

Bourke, Joanna. *Fear: A Cultural History*. London: Counterpoint, 2006.

Bourke, Joanna. *The Story of Pain: From Prayer to Painkillers*. Oxford: Oxford University Press, 2014.

Boveri, Margret. 'Körpergeschehen und Psychose. Eine Studie aus der Landschaft des Verrats'. *Merkur* 8, no. 74 (1954): 371–8.

Bowlby, John. *Maternal Care and Mental Health. A Report Prepared on Behalf of the World Health Organization as a Contribution to the United Nations Programme for the Welfare of Homeless Children* (Bulletin of the World Health Organization 3). Geneva: WHO, 1951.

Buchanan, Roderick D. *Playing with Fire: The Controversial Career of Hans J. Eysenck*. Oxford: Oxford University Press, 2010.

Cantor, David. 'Cancer'. In *Companion Encyclopedia of the History of Medicine*, vol. 1, edited by W. F. Bynum und Roy Porter, 537–61. New York: Taylor & Francis, 1993.

Cantor, David, ed. *Cancer in the Twentieth Century*. Baltimore: Johns Hopkins University Press, 2008.

Cantor, David. 'Choosing to Live: Cancer Education, Movies, and the Conversion Narrative in America, 1921–1960'. *Literature and Medicine* 28, no. 2 (2009): 278–332.

Cantor, David. 'Before Survivorship: The Moment of Recovery in Twentieth-Century American Cancer Campaigns'. *Social History of Medicine* 27, no. 3 (2014): 440–65. https://doi.org/10.1093/shm/hkt100.

Cantor, David, and Edmund Ramsden, eds. *Stress, Shock, and Adaptation in the Twentieth Century*. Rochester: University of Rochester Press, 2012.

Cocks, Geoffrey. *Psychotherapy in the Third Reich: The Göring Institute*. 2nd edn. Piscataway: Routledge, 1997.

Cocks, Geoffrey. *The State of Health: Illness in Nazi Germany*. Oxford: Oxford University Press, 2012.

Creager, Angela N. H. *Life Atomic: A History of Radioisotopes in Science and Medicine*, Chicago: University of Chicago Press, 2014.

Daston, Lorraine, and Peter Galison. *Objectivity*. New York: Zone Books, 2007.

Dehli, Martin. *Leben als Konflikt. Zur Biographie Alexander Mitscherlichs*. Göttingen: Wallstein, 2007.

Dixon, Thomas. *From Passions to Emotions: The Creation of a Secular Psychological Category*. Cambridge: Cambridge University Press, 2003.

Duttweiler, Stefanie. *Sein Glück machen. Arbeit am Glück als neoliberale Regierungstechnologie*. Konstanz: UVK, 2007.

Eckart, Wolfgang U., ed. *100 Years of Organized Cancer Research. 100 Jahre organisierte Krebsforschung*. Stuttgart: Georg Thieme, 2000.

Eckart, Wolfgang U. *Medizin in der NS-Diktatur. Ideologie, Praxis, Folgen*. Vienna: Böhlau, 2012.

Ehrenreich, Barbara. *Smile or Die: How Positive Thinking Fooled America & the World*. London: Granta, 2009.

Eitler, Pascal (2011), '"Selbstheilung". Zur Somatisierung und Sakralisierung von Selbstverhältnissen im New Age'. In *Das beratene Selbst. Zur Genealogie der Therapeutisierung in den 'langen' Siebzigern*, edited by Sabine Maasen, Jens Elberfeld, Pascal Eitler, and Maik Tändler, 161–81. Bielefeld: transcript, 2011.

Elias, Norbert. *The Loneliness of the Dying*. Translated by Edmund Jephcott. New York: Continuum, 2001.

Elkeles, Barbara. 'Die schweigsame Welt von Arzt und Patient. Einwilligung und Aufklärung in der Arzt-Patienten-Beziehung des 19. und 20. Jahrhunderts'. *Medizin, Gesellschaft und Geschichte* 8 (1989): 63–91.

Elkeles, Barbara. *Der moralische Diskurs über das medizinische Menschenexperiment im 19. Jahrhundert*. Stuttgart: Fischer, 1996.

Elkeles, Barbara. 'Wissenschaft, Medizinethik und gesellschaftliches Umfeld: Die Diskussion um den Heilversuch um 1900. In *Medizingeschichte und Medizinethik. Kontroversen und Begründungsansätze 1900–1950*, edited by Andreas Frewer and Josef N. Neumann, 21–43. Frankfurt: Campus Verlag, 2001.

Eysenck, Hans J. *Smoking, Health and Personality*. New York: Basic Books, 1965.

Eysenck, Hans J. *The Causes and Effects of Smoking*. Beverly Hills: Sage, 1980.

Eysenck, Hans J. 'Personality as a Predictor of Cancer and Cardiovascular Disease, and the Application of Behaviour Therapy in Prophylaxis'. *European Journal of Psychiatry* 1 (1987): 29–41.

Faden, Ruth R., and Tom L. Beauchamp. *A History and Theory of Informed Consent*. New York: Oxford University Press, 1986.

Frank, Arthur W. 'The Rhetoric of Self-Change: Illness Experience as Narrative'. *Sociological Quarterly* 34 (1993): 41–5.

Frank, Arthur W. *At the Will of the Body: Reflections on Illness*. New York: Houghton Mifflin, 2002.

Frank, Arthur W. *The Wounded Storyteller. Body, Illness & Ethics*. 2nd edn. Chicago: University of Chicago Press, 2013.

Freimüller, Tobias. *Alexander Mitscherlich. Gesellschaftsdiagnosen und Psychoanalyse nach Hitler*. Göttingen: Wallstein, 2007.

Freund, Michael. *Das Drama der 99 Tage. Krankheit und Tod Friedrichs III*. Cologne: Kiepenheuer & Witsch, 1966.

Frevert, Ute. 'Defining Emotions: Concepts and Debates over Three Centuries'. In *Emotional Lexicons: Continuity and Change in the Vocabulary of Feeling, 1700–2000*, edited by Ute Frevert, Monique Scheer, Anne Schmidt, Pascal Eitler, Bettina Hitzer, Nina Verheyen, Benno Gammerl, Christian Bailey, and Margrit Pernau, 1–31. Oxford: Oxford University Press, 2014.

Frevert, Ute. 'Rationalität und Emotionalität im Jahrhundert der Extreme'. In *Das 20. Jahrhundert vermessen. Signaturen eines vergangenen Zeitalters*, edited by Martin Sabrow and Peter Ulrich Weiß, 115–40. Göttingen: Vandenhoeck & Ruprecht, 2017.

Galison, Peter. 'Image of Self'. In *Things That Talk: Object Lessons from Art and Science*, edited by Lorraine Daston, 257–94. New York: Zone Books, 2004.

Gammerl, Benno. 'Emotional Styles: Concepts and Challenges'. *Rethinking History* 16, no. 2 (2012): 161–75. https://doi.org/10.1080/13642529.2012.681189.

Gardner, Kirsten E. *Early Detection: Women, Cancer, and Awareness Campaigns in the Twentieth-Century United States*. Chapel Hill, NC: University of North Carolina Press, 2006.

Gassert, Philipp. 'Popularität der Apokalypse: Zur Nuklearangst seit 1945'. *Aus Politik und Zeitgeschichte* 46/7 (2011): 48–54.

Gebhard, Bruno. *Kampf dem Krebs*. Dresden: Deutscher Verlag für Volkswohlfahrt, 1933.

Geisthövel, Alexa, and Bettina Hitzer, eds. *Auf der Suche nach einer anderen Medizin. Pychosomatik im 20. Jahrhundert*. Frankfurt: Suhrkamp, 2019.

Geyer, Michael, ed. *Psychotherapie in Ostdeutschland. Geschichte und Geschichten 1945–1995*. Göttingen: Vandenhoeck & Ruprecht, 2011.

Glaser, Barney C., and Anselm L. Strauss. *Awareness of Dying*. Chicago: Aldine Publishing Company, 1965.

Gleßmer-Junike, Simone. 'X-Strahlen, Radiometer und Hauteinheitsdosis. Die Entwicklung der Messverfahren und Maßeinheiten für Röntgenstrahlung in der medizinischen Physik von den Anfängen bis zur internationalen Standardisierung'. PhD diss., Universität Hamburg, 2015. http://ediss.sub.uni-hamburg.de/volltexte/2015/7181/pdf/Dissertation.pdf.

Goltermann, Svenja. *Die Gesellschaft der Überlebenden. Deutsche Kriegsheimkehrer und ihre Gewalterfahrungen im Zweiten Weltkrieg*. Munich: DVA, 2009.

Göring, Matthias H., ed. *Deutsche Seelenheilkunde. Zehn Aufsätze zu den seelenärztlichen Aufgaben unserer Zeit*. Leipzig: S. Hirzel, 1934.

Groddeck, Georg. *Die psychische Bedingtheit und psychoanalytische Behandlung organischer Leiden*. Leipzig: S. Hirzel, 1917.

Groddeck, Georg. 'Psychic Conditioning and the Psychoanalytic Treatment of Organic Disorders'. In *The Meaning of Illness: Selected Psychoanalytic Writings*, translated by Gertrud Mander, 109–31. New York: International Universities Press, 1977.

Gruppe Krebs. *Sonder-Katalog der Gruppe Krebs der wissenschaftlichen Abteilung der Internationalen Hygiene-Ausstellung in Dresden 1911*. Dresden, 1911.

Häberlen, Joachim C. *The Emotional Politics of the Alternative Left: West Germany, 1968–1984*. Cambridge: Cambridge University Press, 2018.

Hahn, Susanne. 'Moulagen in der Gesundheitsaufklärung'. In *Wachs—Moulagen und Modelle*, edited by Susanne Hahn and Dimitrios Ambatielos, 39–46. Dresden: Verlag des Deutschen Hygiene-Museums, 1994.

Haller, Lea, Sabine Höhler, and Heiko Stoff. 'Stress—Konjunkturen eines Konzepts'. *Zeithistorische Forschungen/Studies in Contemporary History* 11, no. 3 (2014): 359–81.

Hansen, G., and H. Vetterlein. *Arzt und Recht in der Deutschen Demokratischen Republik*. Leipzig: Thieme, 1959.

Hansen, G., and H. Vetterlein. *Ärztliches Handeln—Rechtliche Pflichten in der Deutschen Demokratischen Republik*. Leipzig: Thieme Verlag, 1959.

Harrington, Anne. *Reenchanted Science: Holism in German Culture from Wilhelm II to Hitler*. Princeton, NJ: Princeton University Press, 1996.

Harrington, Anne. 2016. 'Mother Love and Mental Illness: An Emotional History'. *Osiris* 31, no. 1 (2016): 94–115. https://doi.org/10.1086/687559.

Hellmann-Mersch, Birgit. 'Institutionen zur Krebsforschung und Krebsbekämpfung in Deutschland. Historischer Überblick und Analyse'. PhD diss., RWTH Aachen, 1994.

Helvoort, Ton van. 'Scalpel or Rays? Radiotherapy and the Struggle for the Cancer Patient in Pre-Second World War Germany'. *Medical History* 45, no. 1 (2001): 33–60.

Hernández Brotons, Fanny. 'The Experience of Cancer Illness: Spain and Beyond during the Second Half of the Nineteenth Century'. PhD diss., Carlos III University Madrid, 2017. https://e-archivo.uc3m.es/bitstream/handle/10016/26034/brotons_illness_tesis_2017.pdf?sequence=1&isAllowed=y.

Hess, Volker, Laura Hottenrott, and Peter Steinkamp. *Testen im Osten. DDR-Arzneimittelstudien im Auftrag westlicher Pharmaindustrie, 1964–1990*. Berlin: Be.bra Wissenschaft, 2016.

Hitzer, Bettina. 'Healing Emotions'. In *Emotional Lexicons: Continuity and Change in the Vocabulary of Feeling, 1700–2000*, edited by Ute Frevert, Monique Scheer, Anne Schmidt, Pascal Eitler, Bettina Hitzer, Nina Verheyen, Benno Gammerl, Christian Bailey, and Margrit Pernau, 118–50. Oxford: Oxford University Press, 2014.

Hitzer, Bettina. 'Oncomotions: Experiences and Debates in West Germany and the United States after 1945'. In *Science and Emotions after 1945: A Transatlantic Perspective*, edited by Frank Biess and Daniel M. Gross, 157–78. Chicago: University of Chicago Press, 2014.

Hitzer, Bettina. 'Krebs oder wie weit reicht die psychosomatische Medizin'. In *Auf der Suche nach einer anderen Medizin. Psychosomatik im 20. Jahrhundert*, edited by Bettina Hitzer and Alexa Geisthövel, 258–72. Frankfurt am Main: Suhrkamp, 2019.

Hitzer, Bettina. 'The Odor of Disgust. Contemplating the Dark Side of 20th-Century Cancer History'. *Emotion Review* 12 (2020): 156–67. https://doi.org/10.1177/1754073919897293.

Hitzer, Bettina. 'Körper zwischen Angst und Sicherheit. Krebs-Früherkennung im 20. Jahrhundert'. In *Entbehrung und Erfüllung: Praktiken von Arbeit, Körper und Konsum in der Geschichte moderner Gesellschaften*, edited by Gleb Albert, Daniel Siemens, and Frank Wolff, 273–88. Bonn: Dietz, 2021.

Hitzer, Bettina. 'Ein Gefühl von Gesundheit. Neue Perspektiven auf die moderne Medizin'. In *Was ist Gesundheit? Interdisziplinäre Perspektiven aus Medizin, Geschichte, Philosophie und Religion*, edited by Philip van der Eijk, Detlev Ganten, and Roman Marek, 312–21. Boston: DeGruyter, 2021. https://doi.org/10.1515/9783110713336-021.

Hitzer, Bettina, and Pilar León-Sanz. 'The Feeling Body and Its Diseases: How Cancer Went Psychosomatic in Twentieth-Century Germany'. *Osiris* 31, no. 1 (2016): 67–93. https://doi.org/10.1086/687591.

Hoeppner-Salazar, Evelyn. 'Krebsforschung und Krebsbekämpfung in Berlin bis zum Jahre 1945'. PhD diss., Freie Universität Berlin, 1986.

Hofer, Hans-Georg. 'Labor, Klinik und Gesellschaft. Stress und die westdeutsche Universitätsmedizin (1950–1980)'. *Zeithistorische Forschungen/Studies in Contemporary History* 11, no. 3 (2014): 382–405.

Holland, Jimmie C., and Julia H. Rowland, eds. *Handbook of Psycho-Oncology: Psychological Care of the Patient with Cancer*. New York: Oxford University Press, 1989.

Jackson, Mark. *The Age of Stress*. Oxford: Oxford University Press, 2013.

Jasen, Patricia. 'Malignant Histories: Psychosomatic Medicine and the Female Cancer Patient in the Postwar Era'. *Bulletin canadien d'histoire de la médicine = Canadian Bulletin of Medical History* 20, no. 2 (2003): 265–97.

Jensen, Uffa, and Daniel Morat, eds. *Rationalisierungen des Gefühls: Zum Verhältnis von Wissenschaft und Emotionen 1880–1930*. Munich: Wilhelm Fink, 2008.

Johach, Eva. *Krebszelle und Zellenstaat. Zur medizinischen und politischen Metaphorik in der Zellularpathologie Rudolf Virchows*. Freiburg: Rombach, 2008.

Jütte, Robert (with Wolfgang U. Eckart, Hans-Walter Schmuhl, and Winfried Süß). *Medizin und Nationalsozialismus. Bilanz und Perspektiven der Forschung*. 2nd edn. Göttingen: Wallstein, 2011.

Kaiser, Matthias. 'Zur Geschichte des Deutschen Zentralkomitees zur Erforschung und Bekämpfung der Krebskrankheit (1900–1933)'. PhD diss., University of Greifswald, 1988.

Kasper, August M. 'The Doctor and Death'. In *The Meaning of Death*, edited by Herman Feifel, 259–70. New York: Blakiston Division, McGraw-Hill, 1959.

Katz, Jay. *The Silent World of Doctor and Patient*. Baltimore: Free Press, 1984.

Kauz, Daniel. *Vom Tabu zum Thema? 100 Jahre Krebsbekämpfung in der Schweiz 1910–2010*. Basel: Schwabe, 2010.

Keating, Peter, and Alberto Cambrosio. *Cancer on Trial: Oncology as a New Style of Practice*. Chicago: University of Chicago Press, 2012.
Kleinman, Arthur. *The Illness Narratives: Suffering, Healing, and the Human Condition*. New York: Basic Books, 1988.
Klocke, Sonja E. *Inscription and Rebellion: Illness and the Symptomatic Body in East German Literature*. Rochester: Camden House, 2015.
Krecke, Albert. *Vom Arzt und seinen Kranken*. Munich: Lehmanns, 1932.
Kübler-Ross, Elisabeth. *On Death and Dying: What the Dying Have to Teach Doctors, Nurses, Clergy and Their Own Families*. New York: Routledge, 1969.
Kury, Patrick. 'Vom physiologischen Stress zum Prinzip "Lebensqualität": Lennart Levi und der Wandel des Stresskonzepts um 1970'. *Body Politics* 1, no. 1 (2013): 119–37.
Kutcher, Gerald. *Contested Medicine: Cancer Research and the Military*. Chicago: University of Chicago Press, 2009.
Kutcher, Gerald. 'A Case Study in Human Experimentation: The Patient as Subject, Object and Victim'. In *Cancer Patients, Cancer Pathways: Historical and Sociological Perspectives*, edited by Carsten Timmermann and Elizabeth Toon, 57–77. New York: Palgrave Macmillan, 2012.
Kütemeyer, Wilhelm. *Körpergeschehen und Psychose*. Stuttgart: Ferdinand Enke, 1953.
Kütemeyer, Wilhelm. 'Psychosocial Aspects of Cancer'. Paper presented at the Fourth International Conference on Psychosomatic Aspects of Neoplastic Disease 4.
Laukötter, Anja. '"Anarchie der Zellen". Geschichte und Medien der Krebsaufklärung in der ersten Hälfte des 20. Jahrhunderts'. *Zeithistorische Forschungen/Studies in Contemporary History* 7, no. 1 (2010): 55–74.
Lederer, Susan E. 'Dark Victory: Cancer and Popular Hollywood Film'. *Bulletin of the History of Medicine* 81, no. 1 (2007): 94–115. https://doi.org/10.1353/bhm.2007.0005.
Leopold, Ellen. *Breast Cancer, Women, and Their Doctors in the Twentieth Century*. Boston: Beacon Press, 1999.
Leopold, Ellen. *Under the Radar: Cancer and the Cold War*. New Brunswick, NJ: Rutgers University Press, 2009.
Lerner, Barron H. *The Breast Cancer Wars: Hope, Fear, and the Pursuit of a Cure in Twentieth-Century America*. Oxford: Oxford University Press, 2001.
Lerner, Barron H. 'Politician as Patient. John Foster Dulles Battles Cancer'. In *When Illness Goes Public. Celebrity Patients and How We Look at Medicine*, edited by Barron H. Lerner, 81–99. Baltimore: Johns Hopkins University Press, 2009.
LeShan, Lawrence. *You Can Fight for Your Life: Emotional Factors in the Treatment of Cancer*. Lanham, MD: Rowman and Littlefield, 1977.
LeShan, Lawrence. *Cancer as a Turning Point*. New York: Plume, 1990.
Liek, Erwin. *Der Kampf gegen den Krebs*. Munich: J. F. Lehmanns, 1924.
Liek, Erwin. 'Stand und Zukunft der Krebsbekämpfung'. *Praktische Karzinomblätter* 1 (1934): 1–7.
Lindner, Cornelia. 'Vinzenz Czerny (1842–1916). Leben und Wirken des Heidelberger Chirurgen und Krebsforschers im zeitgeschichtlichen Kontext'. PhD diss., Heidelberg University, 2007.
Lindner, Ulrike. *Gesundheitspolitik in der Nachkriegszeit. Großbritannien und die Bundesrepublik Deutschland im Vergleich*. Munich: Oldenbourg, 2004.
Linek, Jenny. *Gesundheitsvorsorge in der DDR zwischen Propaganda und Praxis*. Stuttgart: Franz Steiner, 2016.
Löwy, Ilana. 'La standardisation de l'inconnu: les protocoles thérapeutiques en cancérologie'. *Techniques & Culture* 25/6 (1996): 73–108. https://doi.org/10.4000/tc.507.

Löwy, Ilana. *Between Bench and Bedside: Science, Healing, and Interleukin-2 in a Cancer Ward*. Cambridge, MA: Harvard University Press, 1996.

Löwy, Ilana. 'Cancer: The Century of the Transformed Cell'. In *Science in the Twentieth Century*, edited by John Krige and Dominique Pestre, 461–77. Amsterdam: Routledge, 1997.

Löwy, Ilana. *Preventive Strikes: Women, Precancer, and Prophylactic Surgery*. Baltimore: Johns Hopkins University Press, 2010.

Löwy, Ilana. *A Woman's Disease: The History of Cervical Cancer*. Oxford: Oxford University Press, 2011.

Maehle, Andreas-Holger. 'Assault and Battery, or Legitimate Treatment? German Legal Debates on the Status of Medical Interventions without Consent, c. 1890–1914'. *Gesnerus* 57, nos. 3/4 (2000): 206–21.

Maehle, Andreas-Holger. '"God's Ethicist": Albert Moll and His Medical Ethics in Theory and Practice'. *Medical History* 56, no. 2 (2012): 217–36. https://doi.org/10.1017/mdh.2011.34.

Marks, David F. 'The Hans Eysenck Affair: Time to Correct the Scientific Record'. *Journal of Health Psychology* 24, no. 4 (2019): 409–20.

Mitscherlich, Alexander. 'Zur psychoanalytischen Auffassung psychosomatischer Krankheitsentstehung'. *Psyche* 7, no. 10 (1954): 561–78.

Mitscherlich, Alexander. 'Anmerkungen über die Chronifizierung psychosomatischen Geschehens'. *Psyche* 15, no. 1 (1962): 1–25.

Mitscherlich, Alexander, and Fred Mielke. *Doctors of Infamy: The Story of the Nazi Medical Crimes*. Translated by Heinz Norden. New York: Henry Schuman, 1949.

Mitscherlich, Alexander, and Fred Mielke. *Wissenschaft ohne Menschlichkeit. Medizinische und eugenische Irrwege unter Diktatur, Bürokratie und Krieg*. Heidelberg: Lambert Schneider, 1949.

Mitscherlich, Alexander, and Fred Mielke. *Medizin ohne Menschlichkeit. Dokumente des Nürnberger Ärzteprozesses*. Frankfurt am Main: Fischer, 1960.

Mitscherlich, Alexander, and Margarete Mitscherlich. *Die Unfähigkeit zu trauern. Grundlagen kollektiven Verhaltens*. Munich: Piper, 1967.

Mizrachi, Nissim. 'From Causation to Correlation: The Story of Psychosomatic Medicine 1939–1979'. *Culture, Medicine, and Psychiatry* 25, no. 3 (2001): 317–43. https://doi.org/10.1023/A:1011817010797.

Moamai, Marion. *Krebs schreiben. Deutschsprachige Literatur der siebziger und achtziger Jahre*. St. Ingbert: Röhrig Universitätsverlag, 1997.

Moll, Albert. *Ärztliche Ethik. Die Pflichten des Arztes in allen Beziehungen seiner Thätigkeit*. Stuttgart: Enke Verlag, 1902.

Moscoso, Javier. *Pain: A Cultural History*. Basingstoke: Palgrave Macmillan, 2012.

Moscoso, Javier. 'Exquisite and Lingering Pains: Facing Cancer in Early Modern Europe'. In *Pain and Emotion in Modern History*, edited by Rob Boddice, 16–35. London: Palgrave Macmillan, 2014.

Moscucci, Ornella. *Gender and Cancer in England, 1860–1948*. London: Palgrave Macmillan, 2016.

Moser, Gabriele. *Deutsche Forschungsgemeinschaft und Krebsforschung 1920–1970*. Stuttgart: Franz Steiner, 2011.

Müller, Frank Lorenz. *Der 99-Tage-Kaiser: Friedrich III. von Preußen—Prinz, Monarch, Mythos*. Munich: Siedler Verlag, 2013.

Mukherjee, Siddharta. *The Emperor of All Maladies: A Biography of Cancer*. New York: Scribner, 2010.

Noack, Thorsten. *Eingriffe in das Selbstbestimmungsrecht des Patienten. Juristische Entscheidungen, Politik und ärztliche Positionen 1890–1960*. Frankfurt am Main: Mabuse-Verlag, 2004.

Nolte, Karen. '"Telling the Painful Truth"—Nurses and Physicians in the Nineteenth Century'. *Nursing History Review* 16, no. 1 (2008): 115–34. https://doi.org/10.1891/1062-8061.16.115.

Nolte, Karen. *Todkrank. Sterbebegleitung im 19. Jahrhundert: Medizin, Krankenpflege und Religion*. Göttingen: Wallstein, 2016.

Parkinson, Anna M. *An Emotional State: The Politics of Emotion in Postwar West German Culture*. Ann Arbor: University of Michigan Press, 2015.

Patterson, James T. *The Dread Disease: Cancer and Modern American Culture*. Cambridge, MA: Harvard University Press, 1987.

Pelosi, Anthony J. 'Personality and Fatal Diseases: Revisiting a Scientific Scandal'. *Journal of Health Psychology* 24, no. 4 (2019): 421–39.

Perrin, George M., and Irene R. Pierce. 'Psychosomatic Aspects of Cancer'. *Psychosomatic Medicine* 21, no. 5 (1959): 397–412.

Pinell, Patrice. *The Fight Against Cancer: France 1890–1940*. Translated by David Madell. London: Routledge, 2002.

Plamper, Jan. *The History of Emotions: An Introduction*. Oxford: Oxford University Press, 2015.

Proctor, Robert N. *The Nazi War on Cancer*. Princeton: Princeton University Press, 2000.

Quitz, Andrea. *Staat, Macht, Moral. Die medizinische Ethik in der DDR*. Berlin: Metropol, 2015.

Reckwitz, Andreas. 'Affective Spaces: A Praxeological Outlook'. *Rethinking History* 16, no. 2 (2012): 241–58. https://doi.org/10.1080/13642529.2012.681193.

Reddy, William M. *The Navigation of Feeling*. New York: Cambridge University Press, 2001.

Reich, Wilhelm. *The Cancer Biopathy*. New York: Farrar, Straus and Giroux, 1974.

Rorschach, Hermann. *Psychodiagnostik. Methodik und Ergebnisse eines wahrnehmungsdiagnostischen Experiments (Deutenlassen von Zufallsformen)*. Bern, 1921.

Rosenberg, Charles. 'Holism in Twentieth-Century Medicine'. In *Greater than the Parts: Holism in Biomedicine, 1920–1950*, edited by Christopher Lawrence and George Weisz, 335–55. New York: Oxford University Press, 1998.

Rosenwein, Barbara. 'Worrying about Emotions in History'. *American Historical Review* 107, no. 3 (2002): 821–45.

Rosenwein, Barbara, and Riccardo Cristiani. *What Is the History of Emotions?* Cambridge: Cambridge University Press, 2018.

Scheer, Monique. 'Are Emotions a Kind of Practice (and Is That What Makes Them Have a History)? A Bourdieuan Approach to Understanding Emotion'. *History and Theory* 51, no. 2 (2012): 193–220.

Scheer, Monique. 'Topographies of Emotion'. In *Emotional Lexicons: Continuity and Change in the Vocabulary of Feeling 1700–2000*, edited by Ute Frevert, Monique Scheer, Anne Schmidt, Pascal Eitler, Bettina Hitzer, Nina Verheyen, Benno Gammerl, Christian Bailey, and Margrit Pernau, 32–61. Oxford: Oxford University Press, 2014.

Scheybal, Ulrike. 'Krebsforschung in der Zeit des Nationalsozialismus unter besonderer Berücksichtigung des Allgemeinen Instituts gegen die Geschwulstkrankheiten'. PhD diss., Leipzig University, 2000.

Schmaltz, Florian. *Kampfstoff-Forschung im Nationalsozialismus. Zur Kooperation von Kaiser-Wilhelm-Instituten, Militär und Industrie*. Göttingen: Wallstein Verlag, 2005.

Schnalke, Thomas. *Diseases in Wax—The History of the Medical Moulage*. Translated by Kathy Spatschek. Berlin: Quintessenz, 1995.

Schregel, Susanne. 'Konjunktur der Angst. "Politik der Subjektivität" und "neue Friedensbewegung", 1979–1983'. In *Angst im Kalten Krieg*, edited by Bernd Greiner, Christian Th. Müller, and Dierk Walter, 495–520. Hamburg: Hamburger Edition/HIS Verlag, 2009.

Schultz-Venrath, Ulrich, and Ludger M. Hermanns. 'Gleichschaltung zur Ganzheit. Gab es eine Psychosomatik im Nationalsozialismus?' In *Neues Denken in der Psychosomatik*, edited by Horst Eberhard Richter and Michael Wirsching, 83–103. Frankfurt am Main: Fischer, 1992.

Schwerin, Alexander von. 'Prekäre Stoffe. Radiumökonomie, Risikoepisteme und die Etablierung der Radioindikatortechnik in der Zeit des Nationalsozialismus'. *NTM: Zeitschrift für Geschichte der Wissenschaften, Technik und Medizin* 17, no. 1 (2009): 5–33. https://doi.org/10.1007/s00048-008-0324-z.

Schwerin, Alexander von. *Strahlenforschung: Bio- und Risikopolitik der DFG, 1920 bis 1970*. Stuttgart: Steiner, 2015.

Seyfarth, Carly. *Der 'Ärzte-Knigge'. Über den Umgang mit Kranken und über Pflichten, Kunst und Dienst der Krankenhausärzte*. Leipzig: Thieme Verlag, 1935.

Solomon, George Freeman. *From Psyche to Soma and Back: Tales of Biopsychosocial Medicine*. Bloomington, IN: Xlibris, 2000.

Sontag, Susan. *Illness as Metaphor*. New York: Farrar, Straus and Giroux, 1977.

Stearns, Peter N. *American Cool: Constructing a Twentieth-Century Emotional Style*. New York: New York University Press, 1994.

Stearns, Peter N. *American Fear: The Causes and Consequences of High Anxiety*. New York: Routledge, 2006.

Stierlin, Helm, and Ronald Grossarth-Maticek. *Krebsrisiken—Überlebenschancen. Wie Körper, Seele und soziale Umwelt zusammenwirken*. Heidelberg: Carl Auer, 1998.

Stiftung Deutsches Hygiene-Museum, ed. *'Rechtzeitig erkannt—heilbar'. Krebsaufklärung im 20. Jahrhundert*. Dresden: Sandstein, 2002.

Stolberg, Michael. *Die Geschichte der Palliativmedizin. Medizinische Sterbebegleitung von 1500 bis heute*. 2nd edn. Frankfurt am Main: Mabuse, 2013.

Süß, Sonja. *Politisch mißbraucht? Psychiatrie und Staatssicherheit in der DDR*. Berlin: Ch. Links, 1998.

Süß, Winfried. *Der 'Volkskörper' im Krieg. Gesundheitspolitik, Gesundheitsverhältnisse und Krankenmord im nationalsozialistischen Deutschland 1939–1945*. Munich: Oldenbourg Wissenschaftsverlag, 2003.

Tändler, Maik. *Das therapeutische Jahrzehnt. Der Psychoboom in den siebziger Jahren*. Göttingen: Wallstein, 2016.

Tarlau, Milton, and Irwin Smalheiser. 'Personality Patterns in Patients with Malignant Tumors of the Breast and Cervix: An Exploratory Study'. *Psychosomatic Medicine* 13, no. 2 (1951): 117–21.

Tausch, Anne-Marie. *Gespräche gegen die Angst. Krankheit als ein Weg zum Leben*. Reinbek: Rowohlt Verlag, 1981.

Timmermann, Carsten. 'Appropriating Risk Factors: The Reception of an American Approach to Chronic Disease in the Two German States, c. 1950–1990'. *Social History of Medicine* 25, no. 1 (2012): 157–74. https://doi.org/10.1093/shm/hkr051.

Timmermann, Carsten. '"Just Give Me the Best Quality of Life Questionnaire": The Karnofsky Scale and the History of Quality of Life Measurements in Cancer Trials'. In *Chronic Illness* 9, no. 3 (2013): 179–90. https://doi.org/10.1177/1742395312466903.

Timmermann, Carsten. *A History of Lung Cancer: The Recalcitrant Disease*. Basingstoke: Palgrave Macmillan, 2014.

Timmermann, Carsten, and Elizabeth Toon, eds. *Cancer Patients, Cancer Pathways: Historical and Sociological Perspectives*. New York: Palgrave Macmillan, 2012.

Toon, Elizabeth. '"Cancer as the General Population Knows It": Knowledge, Fear, and Lay Education in 1950s Britain'. *Bulletin of the History of Medicine* 81, no. 1 (2006): 116–38. https://doi.org/10.1353/bhm.2007.0013.

Virchow, Rudolf. *Die Cellularpathologie in ihrer Begründung auf physiologische und pathologische Gewebelehre*. 4th edn. Berlin, 1871.

Voswinckel, Peter. *50 Jahre Deutsche Gesellschaft für Hämatologie und Onkologie*. Würzburg: Murken-Altrogge, 1987.

Voswinckel, Peter. *Erinnerungsort Krebsbaracke. Klarstellungen um das erste interdisziplinäre Krebsforschungsinstitut in Deutschland (Berlin, Charité)*. Stuttgart: Georg Thieme Verlag, 2014.

Wagner, Gustav, and Andrea Mauerberger. *Krebsforschung in Deutschland. Vorgeschichte und Geschichte des Deutschen Krebsforschungszentrums*. Berlin: Springer, 1989.

Weiss, Burghard. 'Von der Hochvolt- zur Megavolttherapie. Strahlentherapie und Großtechnologie in Deutschland und den USA, 1925–1955'. In *100 Years of Organized Cancer Research. 100 Jahre organisierte Krebsforschung*, edited by Wolfgang U. Eckart, 137–41. Stuttgart: Georg Thieme, 2000.

Weizsäcker, Viktor von. 'Klinische Vorstellungen I–VI'. *Psyche* 1, no. 2 (1947): 258–93.

Weizsäcker, Viktor von. 'Körpergeschehen und Neurose. Analytische Studie über somatische Symptombildungen'. *Gesammelte Schriften*, Vol. 6: *Körpergeschehen und Neurose, Psychosomatische Medizin*, edited by Peter Achilles, 119–238. Frankfurt am Main: Suhrkamp, 1986.

Wheeler, John I., and Bettye McDonald Caldwell. 'Psychological Evaluation of Women with Cancer of the Breast and of the Cervix'. *Psychosomatic Medicine* 17, no. 4 (1955): 256–68.

Will, Herbert. *Die Geburt der Psychosomatik. Georg Groddeck, der Mensch und Wissenschaftler*. Munich: Urban & Schwarzenberg, 1988.

Witte, Wilfried. *Unerhörte Leiden: Die Geschichte der Schmerztherapie in Deutschland im 20. Jahrhundert*. Frankfurt am Main: Campus, 2017.

Wood, James M., M. Teresa Nezworski, Scott O. Lilienfeld, and Howard N. Garb. *What's Wrong with the Rorschach? Science Confronts the Controversial Inkblot Test*. San Francisco: Jossey-Bass, 2003.

Index

Note: Figures are indicated by an italic '*f*' respectively, following the page number.

For the benefit of digital users, table entries that span two pages (e.g., 52–53) may, on occasion, appear on only one of those pages.

Persons